Scotland's Health
and Health
Services

Scotland's Health and Health Services

Editors

Professor Kevin Woods
and
Sir David Carter

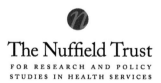

The Nuffield Trust
FOR RESEARCH AND POLICY
STUDIES IN HEALTH SERVICES

London: TSO

Published by TSO (The Stationery Office) and available from:

Online
www.tso.co.uk/bookshop

Mail, Telephone, Fax & E-mail
TSO
PO Box 29, Norwich, NR3 1GN
Telephone orders/General enquiries: 0870 600 5522
Fax orders: 0870 600 5533
E-mail: book.orders@tso.co.uk
Textphone 0870 240 3701

TSO Shops
123 Kingsway, London, WC2B 6PQ
020 7242 6393 Fax 020 7242 6394
68-69 Bull Street, Birmingham B4 6AD
0121 236 9696 Fax 0121 236 9699
9-21 Princess Street, Manchester M60 8AS
0161 834 7201 Fax 0161 833 0634
16 Arthur Street, Belfast BT1 4GD
028 9023 8451 Fax 028 9023 5401
18-19 High Street, Cardiff CF10 1PT
029 2039 5548 Fax 029 2038 4347
71 Lothian Road, Edinburgh EH3 9AZ
0870 606 5566 Fax 0870 606 5588

TSO Accredited Agents
(see Yellow Pages)

and through good booksellers

First published 2003

ISBN 0 11 703241 7

Printed in the United Kingdom for The Stationery Office

Contents

EDITORS' NOTE

The idea for this book came shortly after the turn of the millennium while one of us was browsing among the shelves of the Scottish Health Services Centre's library in Edinburgh in search of historical perspectives on Scotland's rural health services. An obvious starting place for such an endeavour was Gordon McLachlan's volume on the changes in Scotland's health and its health services since 1900. As the then Secretary of the Nuffield Provincial Hospitals Trust, McLachlan had played a vital role in turning Sir John Brotherston's idea for such a volume into published reality.[*] Could the story be brought up to date, the years between having witnessed so much change, and was it worth trying to peer in to the future as a new century unfolded? With a restored Scottish Parliament providing an unrivalled focus for debate about health in Scotland we decided it was. We approached the Nuffield Trust with our idea, and received in response not only encouragement but also financial help for our editorial task. We are indebted to John Wyn Owen, the current Secretary of the Nuffield Trust, for his interest and support.

We decided at the outset that this should be a book written by people in the thick of the action, people involved in the design and implementation of the changes that they narrate. We asked them to write an essay that could stand alone as an informed discussion of the issue in question, and also be a part of a larger story. We asked our authors to look back, and to look forward. We decided to apply a light editorial pen from the outset, knowing that the contributors we had chosen had undoubted expertise in the field in question. We knew that this would have some consequences for the final text but we judged them a price worth paying. Inevitably, there is on occasion, some overlap between the essays but we have not attempted to remove this altogether lest it undermine the coherence of the individual chapters. It might be said that the proximity of our contributors to the

---

[*] McLachlan G. (Ed.) Improving the Common Weal. Aspects of Scottish Health Services 1900–1984. A collation in honour of the late Sir John Brotherston. Edinburgh: Edinburgh University Press for the Nuffield Provincial Hospitals Trust, 1987.

events they discuss distorts their perspective on them, and that others viewing events from a different standpoint might offer a different account. Another of the challenges for us has been to keep pace with the continuing stream of changes affecting Scotland's health services. We have tried to include as much up to date material as possible but have had to draw a line under events occurring after the beginning of May 2003 and some of the chapters were completed in 2002. More time will be needed before mature judgements of the most recent changes and developments can be formed. So be it. At the least we hope we have provided an accessible and authoritative account on which others can build.

Many people have helped with this volume. Each contributor has cause to thank numerous people who have helped locate forgotten facts, obscure reports or jogged their memories. We cannot list them all, but we do wish to acknowledge their contribution. There are though a small number of people whose contribution has been so significant we must break silence. Susie Stewart took on the challenging role of working with us as Editorial Assistant and not only converted our various initial drafts in to the chapters that follow, but cheerfully kept us on our toes and to our timetable. In the course of our working lives in Scotland we have had cause to thank the many talented colleagues within the National Health Service with whom we have worked. Both of us have had the privilege of working during times of great change as senior members of the Scottish Office and its successor, the Scottish Executive Department of Health. There are many people we could mention but we wish, in particular, to acknowledge the contribution of Geoff Scaife, Head of the Health Department and Chief Executive of the NHS in Scotland during our time in St Andrew's House. Finally, we would like to pay tribute to Sam Galbraith, a remarkable man with whom we both worked. Having decided to forego a career as a leading neurosurgeon to become a politician and attempt to right the wrongs of the health service as he saw them, he was Scotland's Minister of Health in Donald Dewar's ministerial team during the passage of the Scotland Act 1998. As such he played an important part in enabling people in Scotland to decide what kind of health service they want in the future. It was a time of optimism and opportunity, and we are glad to have been part of it.

Kevin Woods and David Carter
May 2003

FOREWORD
John Wyn Owen

In 1982 Sir John Brotherston asked the Trustees of the Nuffield Provincial Hospitals Trust whether they would be interested in financing a history of the Scottish Health Service since 1900. The Trust agreed and published *Improving the Common Weal. Aspects of Scottish Health Services 1900–1984.* The then Secretary of the Trust and Editor of the volume, Gordon McLachlan, explained in the prologue that the Trust had acceded to the request because of 'the belief that time future is contained in time past and because Scotland has an identifiable persona separate from England and its regions … the Trustees approved the study in the hope of having, for comparative purposes, an analysis and review of developments and improvements in health services in a unique area of the United Kingdom.' It is, therefore appropriate that Professor Kevin Woods and Sir David Carter approached the Trust for support for a sequel, *Scotland's Health and Health Services*, which brings the story up to the beginning of May 2003. We are grateful to them and to their contributors for undertaking this task.

In its *Policy Futures 2000* report, the Trust recognised that we would see increasing diversity of health policy within the UK; this challenge, for those interested in policy analysis was carried in a headline in the *Financial Times* on 4th March 2003 – 'England and Scotland are taking different approaches to change. Old style health services aim to outdo the internal market.' The present volume sets a benchmark against which those with an interest can address the issues raised by Jennifer Dixon, Head of Health Policy at the Kings Fund, when she wrote recently that we have a huge natural laboratory in the UK for studying the outcome of different approaches to reform, but nobody seems to be using it.

In updating the history in Scotland, this volume will complement other forthcoming Nuffield Trust publications which record contemporary history and deal with issues relevant to future policy formulation: *History of the Post of the Chief Medical Officer* (Sheard and Donaldson), Brian Edwards' study of *The Executive Years of the NHS* and *Medicine and the Troubles – Enduring Values in Medicine and Health Care: the case of Northern Ireland* by James McKenna.

The editors acknowledge that more time will be needed before mature judgements of the most recent changes and developments can be formed but believe they have provided an accessible and authoritative account upon which others can build. I share their view.

John Wyn Owen CB
Secretary
Nuffield Trust
July 2003

ABOUT THE AUTHORS

DAVID BREWSTER MB ChB, MSc, FFPHM, MRCGP, DCH, DRCOG was appointed in 1995 as Director of Cancer Registration in Scotland and Consultant in Public Health Medicine at the Information and Statistics Division of the Common Services Agency of the National Health Service in Scotland. He graduated in medicine from Bristol University in 1981 and after nine years of clinical practice, began his public health medicine training in Edinburgh in 1990. He has been closely associated with the Scottish Cancer Therapy Network and is a member of the Scottish Cancer Group, which advises Ministers on the implementation of Cancer in Scotland: Action for Change. He is an Honorary Clinical Senior Lecturer in the Department of Community Health Sciences at Edinburgh University and his principal research interests are data quality, the epidemiology of cancer and cancer care, and socio-economic variations in risk and outcome.

GRAHAM BUCKLEY BSc, MB ChB, MD, FRCS (Ed), FRCP (Ed), FRCPS (Glasg), FRCGP is Chief Executive of NHS Education for Scotland. He was for seven years Chief Executive of the Scottish Council for Postgraduate Medical and Dental Education in Scotland. He began his career in General Practice and Geriatric Medicine in West Lothian and he has been Editor of the Journal of the Royal College of General Practitioners/ British Journal of General Practice and Medical Education. He is an External Examiner in Medical Education in the Universities of Dundee and Wales. He is also an External Examiner for the Graduate Entry Programme at St George's Hospital Medical School, London.

DAVID CARTER MD, FRCS (Ed), FRSE is immediate past Vice-Principal of Edinburgh University and Chairman of the Scientific Advisory Committee of the Cancer Research Campaign. He was Chief Medical Officer in Scotland from 1996–2000. He was previously Regius Professor of Clinical Surgery in Edinburgh (1988–1996) and St Mungo Professor of Surgery in Glasgow (1979–1988). He is a Fellow of the Royal Colleges of Surgeons of Edinburgh and England, the Royal College of Physicians of Edinburgh, the Royal College of Physicians and Surgeons of Glasgow, and the Faculty of Public Health Medicine. He is Vice-President of the Royal Society of Edinburgh, an Associate of the Institute of Medicine of the USA and a Founding Fellow of the Academy of Medical Sciences in the the UK. He is Chairman of the Health Foundation and Past President of the BMA. His surgical interests centred on hepatobiliary and pancreatic disease, he has published numerous surgical articles and texts and was co-editor of the British Journal of Surgery from 1986–1991. He was created Knight Bachelor in 1996 for services to medicine.

ANNA GREGOR FRCP (Ed) FRCR is Consultant in the Edinburgh Cancer Centre, Lead Clinician for Cancer in Scotland and Clinical Director of South East Scotland Cancer Network (SCAN). She is also Macmillan Lead Cancer Clinician for Lothian and Treasurer of the International Association for Study of Lung Cancer. She graduated from Charles University in Prague and the Royal Free Hospital School of Medicine in London with postgraduate studies at the Royal Free, Brighton General, Royal Northern, Brompton and Royal Marsden and the Western General in Edinburgh. From 1983–1987 she held a consultant appointment in the Beatson Oncology Centre in Glasgow and from 1987–1997 was Senior Lecturer in Clinical Oncology in the University of Edinburgh. She was Chair of the SIGN lung cancer guidelines development group. Her clinical interests include lung cancer management, neuro-oncology, quality improvements, health service management and patient involvement in health care planning.

PHIL HANLON BSc, MD, MRCGP, FRCP, FFPHM, DRCOG is Professor of Public Health at Glasgow University and advisor in Public Health strategies to the Scottish Executive. He was educated in the West of Scotland and graduated in medicine from Glasgow University in 1978. Following a period in which he gained clinical experience in adult medicine and general practice, he took up a research post with the Medical Research Council in the Gambia, West Africa. On returning to the UK, he completed a period of training in public health after which he was appointed to the post of Director of Health Promotion with the Greater Glasgow Health Board, leading a number of campaigns and initiatives. In 1994 Dr Hanlon moved to become a Senior Lecturer in Public Health at the University of Glasgow and was promoted to Professor in 1999.

ROSS LORIMER PRCPSGLASG, MD, D UNIV, F MED SCI, FRCP is currently President of the Royal College of Physicians and Surgeons of Glasgow. He graduated MB ChB from University of Glasgow in 1960 and subsequently MD with Honours in 1974. He was Consultant Physician and Cardiologist in the Royal Infirmary from 1992 to 2000. He was elected Honorary Professor in Medicine and Medical Cardiology by the University of Glasgow in 1991. Research interests have been in artherosclerosis and coronary heart disease. Recently he was the Chairman of the Task Force in Coronary Heart Disease/Stroke of the Scottish Health Executive.

ANGUS MACKAY OBE, MA, BSc, PhD, MB ChB, FRCP(Ed), FRCPSYCH trained in medicine and pharmacology at Edinburgh University, subsequently qualifying with a doctorate in neuropharmacology at the University of Cambridge, where he taught pharmacology at Trinity College. Responding to the pull from clinical medicine, he trained in psychiatry in Edinburgh and returned to Cambridge as Director of Clinical Research for the MRC Neurochemical Pharmacology Unit. He came back to Scotland in 1980 to be Physician Superintendent at the Argyll and Bute Hospital in Lochgilphead, a post he still occupies and the last such one in the United Kingdom. A fervent believer in eclectisism and the visible profile of practising clinicians in health service management, he has maintained an active interest in biological psychiatry, medicines regulation in the UK and Europe, mental health service development in Scotland, and a scientific approach to achieving value for money in health service provision. Previously Chairman of the Working Group on Mental Health Services in Scotland, recently psychiatric representative to the Committee on Safety of Medicines and Chairman of the Health Technology Board for Scotland, he is currently Honorary Professor in Psychological Medicine at the University of Glasgow, Honorary Fellow in Neuroscience at the University of Edinburgh and Director of Mental Health Services for Lomond and Argyll.

ALISON PETCH BA, MA, PhD has been Director of the Nuffield Centre for Community Care Studies at the University of Glasgow since 1993. She was previously responsible for the community care research theme at the ESRC/Scottish Office funded Social Work Research Centre at the University of Stirling. Her earlier career saw involvement in research on a range of health, housing and social care issues. She has acted as adviser to a number of Parliamentary Inquiries by the Scottish Affairs Committee at Westminster into the Closure of Psychiatric Hospitals (1995) and into the Implementation of Community Care (1997), and by the Health and Community Care Committee of the Scottish Parliament into Community Care (2000). She was a member of the Ministerial Care Development Group in Scotland, established to bring forward recommendations on the implementation of free personal care.

LEWIS RITCHIE OBE, BSc, MSC, MD, FRCP (Ed), FRCGP, FFPHM is James Mackenzie Professor of General Practice and Head of the Department of General Practice and Primary Care at the University of Aberdeen, appointed in 1992. He is a graduate in chemistry and medicine (University of Aberdeen) and public health (University of Edinburgh) and holds additional qualifications in computing science. He practises clinical medicine as a general practitioner at Peterhead where he became a principal in 1984. He was a consultant in public health medicine with Grampian Health Board (1987–1992) and continues in an honorary capacity. His R&D interests include: cardiovascular prevention, information technology, medicines assessment, oncology and intermediate care. He serves on a number of national advisory committees and currently chairs the Biomedical and Therapeutics Research Committee of the Chief Scientist Office, the Electronic Clinical Communications Implementation Advisory Board, and the National Pneumococcal Immunisation Programme.

DAVID STEEL MA DPhil is Chief Executive of NHS Quality Improvement Scotland. After 12 years as a Lecturer in Public Administration at the University of Exeter, during which time he served for five years as a member of the local health authority, he moved into NHS management in 1984 as Assistant Director of the National Association of Health Authorities. In 1986 he was appointed Secretary to the Health Board Chairmen's and General Managers' Groups and to the Scottish Health Management Efficiency Group (SCOTMEG). He joined the NHS Management Executive in the Scottish Office at its inception in 1990 as Director of Corporate Affairs, moving to the post of Head of Health Gain in 1995. He was Chief Executive of the Clinical Standards Board for Scotland from its establishment in April 1999 until its incorporation into NHS Quality Improvement Scotland in January 2003.

ANDREW TANNAHILL MB, ChB, MSc, FFPHM, FRCP (Edin, Glasg) is a Consultant in Public Health Medicine with NHS Argyll and Clyde and an Honorary Clinical Senior Lecturer in Public Health at the University of Glasgow. He studied Medicine at the University of Glasgow and Community Medicine at the University of Edinburgh. Trained in public health with Lothian Health Board, he worked as a Specialist in Community Medicine with East Anglian Regional Health Authority, leading the development of health promotion and becoming an Associate Lecturer at the University of Cambridge. Following a time as a Senior Lecturer in Public Health Medicine at the University of Glasgow and Honorary Consultant with Greater Glasgow Health Board, he spent 10 years as Chief Executive of the Health Education Board for Scotland (HEBS), a World Health Organisation Collaborating Centre. He has been a visiting professor to the University of Glasgow, and has held honorary appointments with the Universities of Dundee and Edinburgh.

NICOLA WALKER MB ChB, BSc, MRCP is currently a British Heart Foundation Clinical PhD Research Fellow in the Department of Medical Cardiology at the University of Glasgow. She is studying for a PhD and working at Glasgow Royal Infirmary. She graduated from the University of Glasgow with a first class honours BSc in Molecular Biology in 1993 and MB ChB with commendation in 1996. She completed her MRCP in 1999. Research interests include ventricular arrhythmias associated with acute myocardial ischaemia.

DAVID WALSH MA MSc is a Public Health Information Manager with NHS Health Scotland (formerly the Public Health Institute of Scotland). He is currently on secondment from the Information and Statistics Division (ISD) of NHSScotland, which he joined from Grampian Health Board in 1994. He has worked in a variety of information and statistics related roles during that time, including a wide range of projects within the area of medical record linkage, as well as seconded posts within both Argyll and Clyde (1996–1998) and Greater Glasgow (1998–2000) health boards. Within NHS Health Scotland he jointly leads the organisation's work on integrating data and information sources relevant to public health, developing and applying these data to support a range of analyses based on the socio-ecological model of health.

BRUCE WHYTE BSc, MSc is a Public Health Information Manager with NHS Health Scotland (formerly the Public Health Institute of Scotland). Previously, he has worked in various information analysis roles with Argyll and Clyde Health Board (1995–2001), the Information and Statistics Division of NHSScotland (1991–1995) and Grampian Health Board (1990–1991). During this time he has been involved in a wide variety of work, including medical record linkage, needs assessment, simulation modelling, and has carried out research at the Department of Public Health, University of Glasgow on the feasibility of compiling a new health-related database for Scotland. Within NHS Health Scotland he jointly leads the organisation's work on integrating data and information sources relevant to public health, developing and applying these data to support a range of analyses based on the socio-ecological model of health.

KEVIN WOODS BSc, PhD, MIHM, HON MFPHM was appointed to the newly endowed Lindsay Chair of Health Policy and Economic Evaluation, University of Glasgow in August 2000. He established and chairs The Scottish Health Services Policy Forum which promotes debate about health services policy in post-devolution Scotland. Previously he was Director of Strategy and Performance Management for the NHS in Scotland working in the Scottish Office (now Scottish Executive) Department of Health. He has held a number of general management positions in the NHS in England including that of General Manager of the Trent Regional Health Authority. He has published on the subjects of resource allocation, social deprivation and health care planning and his current research interests include health policy and political devolution, health system integration and health care rationing. He was elected Chair of the Scottish Association of Mental Health (SAMH), Scotland's largest mental health charity in November 2000.

1. Scotland's Changing Health System

Kevin Woods

Introduction

In the years since publication of the Nuffield Trust's book on the evolution of Scotland's health services,[1] published in honour of Sir John Brotherston, one of Scotland's most distinguished Chief Medical Officers, many changes have contributed to undeniable improvements in the lives and the health of Scotland's people. At the same time, however, a glance at the health service literature of the 1980s indicates that many of the problems that faced Sir John and his contemporaries are also present day problems. A time traveller, isolated from events in the intervening years, might be forgiven for thinking little had changed. The health of Scots was and remains relatively poor compared with people in other parts of the United Kingdom and Europe. Social inequalities in health status have worsened rather than improved. In the health service, concerns about resources, waiting times, staffing levels, organisation, and proposals for reform have continued to dominate professional, political and public discussion. New diseases have emerged; older health threats, thought to be contained or overcome, have returned in more challenging forms; scientific advance has created new treatment possibilities; and organisational health service structures have been changed and changed again. The enduring dilemma of how to meet these challenges links the concerns of 20 years ago with those of today.

There is, however, one striking change that has affected virtually every aspect of life in Scotland, and altered the context in which these concerns are debated – namely the devolution in 1999 of political power from the UK Parliament to Scotland. The establishment of the Scottish Parliament and the Scottish Executive has created a new focus for policy-making in many areas of government, and health and health care are central to their work.

The purpose of this chapter is to tell the story of the challenges and changes that have shaped Scotland's health services and faced its large and diverse workforce since the middle of the 1980s, to bring that story up to date and peer into the twenty-first century. It has not been a smooth progression. There has been constant policy change and organisational upheaval as policy-makers have sought new ways of improving health and addressing the complexities of a national health care system. Two underlying issues pervade the organisation of health care in Scotland, however, and it is important to consider these in setting the particular Scottish context. The first issue – common to the health debate in all parts of the United Kingdom but with a particular Scottish dimension – is the question of *health care funding* and how to meet growing demands within limited resources. The second issue is the impact of *distance*. Other parts of the United Kingdom include remote and rural areas, but in Scotland this is the norm outside the central belt of urban development between Edinburgh and Glasgow and the cities of Aberdeen and Dundee.

Funding

In common with other health care systems and with the NHS elsewhere in the UK, the National Health Service in Scotland has struggled to reconcile the demands made upon it with available resources. There are three main factors behind this problem: the changing demography of the population, in particular the growth in the proportion of the very elderly; the expansion of medical knowledge and the benefits of scientific and technological innovation which create new, and often costly, treatment possibilities; and the rising public expectations of the services provided.[2] This potent cocktail poses a stiff challenge to the NHS as a tax funded system aiming to be universal in its coverage, comprehensive in the range of services it provides, and largely free to the patient at the time of use.

In many other countries, one or more of these characteristics is often valued less than the others. Thus, co-payments by patients may play a larger role in the funding of care, some people may be excluded from obtaining certain services, or there may be less concern with the control of health care costs because these are borne directly by citizens, employers and private insurers. Looked at in this way, the ability of NHS to achieve a workable balance between the interests of taxpayers, patients, and professions may help to explain why it is has been successful in retaining widespread support.

Health Spending and the Barnett Formula

Claims about the inadequacy of health care services in Scotland are constant. Patients waiting for admission, doctors and nurses working unreasonable hours, inadequate or out-of-date equipment and so on provide a steady stream of stories to fill the newspapers and provide ammunition for opposition politicians to fault the government of the day. Accusations are often made that NHSScotland is 'underfunded' – a somewhat vague notion that suggests it has less than it needs by reference to some unstated yardstick. Increasingly, the European average level of health spending is used as a benchmark. The Organisation for Economic Co-operation and Development (OECD), for example, publishes data enabling such comparisons, and its latest data show that in 2000, the UK spent 7.3% of its Gross Domestic Product on health in contrast to an EU average of 8.0%, and the G7 group of industrialised countries of 9.3%.[3]

The overall figure for the UK disguises a more complex picture. In July 2000 the Scottish Health Minister told Parliament that health spending in Scotland had exceeded the EU average in 1997.[4] The Wanless Report[2] commissioned by the UK Treasury, and perhaps the most complete analysis of the health services' funding requirements yet undertaken, showed that per capita spending on health in 1999/2000 was £1271 in Scotland in comparison with a UK average of £1071 and a figure for England of £1041.

The higher spending in Scotland reflects the decisions of successive Scottish Office (and now Scottish Executive) ministers to give priority to health spending from within the resources transferred to them by means of the Barnett Formula*. This is the arrangement that determines Scotland's share of UK government spending programmes that fall within the competence of Scottish Ministers. It consists of two elements; the 'block', which is the accumulated spending level; and the 'formula', which adjusts the block annually by transferring to Scotland an amount proportionate to its population of increased UK public spending. When this arrangement was introduced in the mid 1970s Scotland's initial 'block' was larger than other parts of the UK. Over time the application of the formula

---

* The Barnett Formula is named after its inventor, Joel Barnett, Chief Secretary to the Treasury in the 1970s. It is discussed fully by Heald.[5]

was intended to result in a progressive convergence of public spending across the UK, a feature of the formula's operation that has come to be known as the Barnett 'Squeeze.'[5] It arises from the result of adding the same per capita increase in funds in England to Scotland's higher historic spending (the block) which arithmetically becomes a lower percentage spending increase in Scotland than in England. Convergence occurs faster when spending grows most rapidly. For many years public spending growth rates were low and the debate about convergence was primarily of academic interest, a situation now changing as public spending on health in the UK is increasing rapidly (see below).

The additional resources that Scottish ministers have chosen to allocate to health from the 'block' should of course be seen alongside Scotland's unenviable health record (chapter 2) that is often used to justify the need for them. The result is that on virtually every measure of resource input, whether it is the availability of hospital beds, the number of doctors and nurses in hospitals and the community, or the prescribing of medicines, Scotland's health care system is better resourced than any other part of the UK. The only exception to this general pattern is that Scotland has a much smaller independent sector of private and voluntary providers, and fewer people are privately insured for health care costs. This situation has not obviously altered the way the media, politicians, and pressure groups portray the health service in Scotland, nor has it eased the clamour for ever greater spending. The reality is that whatever is spent on health, it is unlikely to be enough and the search for better value, greater efficiency and effectiveness in health care spending will be as prominent in the future as it has been in the past.

Efficiency Savings

Pay is the largest element in the health service budget, a simple consequence of its labour intensive nature. Small changes in the real pay of NHS staff have large implications for the overall costs to the taxpayer. In order to avoid damaging industrial relations, the determination of pay levels for doctors and nurses is considered annually by Independent Pay Review Bodies whose recommendations are usually accepted by governments. Governments, however, have not always provided additional resources to the NHS to meet the entire cost of any increase and have argued that greater efficiency should release money to fill the gap. This drive for efficiency has taken different forms over the past decades.

During the Thatcher years, detailed analyses of particular activities were undertaken by one of her advisers, Sir Derek Rayner, to identify and where possible eliminate waste. During this time there was also an emphasis on the generation of additional income from the sale of some NHS services – for example, occupational health care – by developing private wings attached to NHS hospitals, and by letting space to retailers in hospital foyers. Perhaps the most controversial of these strategies was the compulsory competitive tendering of certain support activities that led to the 'contracting out' of domestic, laundry and catering services.

Annual 'efficiency targets' were set throughout the 1990s – subsequently called Cash Releasing Efficiency Savings (CRES) and Cost Improvement Programmes (CIPs) – ranging in value between 1% and 3% of budgets. These schemes were integral to the funding of the health service; without them the books of individual NHS Trusts did not balance and various accounting manoeuvres became commonplace in order to meet demanding financial targets. Unsurprisingly, these were unpopular measures, and whatever the reality of their objectives, they were widely regarded as euphemisms for 'cuts' in the NHS.

Private Finance Initiative

In the middle of the 1990s a new approach to the supplementation of tax funding emerged in the form of the Private Finance Initiative (PFI). Aimed at expanding the resources available for capital spending, the PFI was designed to enable the NHS to pay, over lengthy periods, typically 25 years, the costs of private bank loans used to fund the construction and facilities management of new hospitals. In this way the NHS obtained new buildings without the capital cost appearing on the public spending balance sheet, an important goal of government macro-economic policy. Before a scheme could be approved for funding under the PFI, it was necessary to demonstrate that it was better value for money over the lifetime of the contract than was a 'public sector comparator'. These highly technical financial analyses required a calculation of the risks transferred to the private sector by these deals – for example, the cost of long-term maintenance. The basis of such calculations has been contested and PFI schemes have been dogged inevitably by political and academic controversy.[6]

Begun under the Conservative governments of the 1990s, PFI – re-branded as Public Private Partnerships (PPP) – has become a central plank of the Labour – Liberal Democrat Scottish Executive's policies to renew public services infrastructure, opposed only by the Scottish National Party. A number of new NHS hospitals have been built and are now open, including two district general hospitals in Lanarkshire and the new Royal Infirmary of Edinburgh, at Little France on the south side of the city where a new university medical school has also been built. Expanding the role of the private and independent sectors in the delivery of publicly funded health services has become a central tenet of Labour NHS policy in England[7] but has not been replicated in Scotland. This is a prominent example of policy divergence[8] that was underlined by the Scottish Executive's acquisition in June 2002 of Scotland's largest former private hospital, HCI at Clydebank, to act as a national centre to reduce waiting times.[9]

Priorities and New Approaches to Funding

In comparison with efforts to manage the supply side of the health care funding equation, little has been done to influence the demand side. User charges – for example, payments for GP appointments or bed and breakfast charges for hospital stays – have found little support, although prescription charges for most people have been increased annually in line with inflation. The costs of dental and ophthalmic services are increasingly paid for in whole or part by individuals with appropriate age and income exemptions as governments adjust entitlement to public services. There has, however, been no politically sponsored debate as yet about the limits to a publicly funded health care system or the relative priorities within it, as became popular in Sweden, New Zealand, and the Netherlands in the 1990s. Instead the NHS in Scotland has tended to leave local health boards to make difficult decisions within a national framework. This has resulted in accusations that a post-code lottery of care has been created with some treatments – such as, for example, interferon drugs for multiple sclerosis – available in some parts of Scotland but not others.[10]

The nearest Scotland came to a different approach was the work undertaken in the 1980s by the SHAPE and SHARPEN initiatives[11, 12] (see below). More recently, the creation in 2000 of the Health Technology Board for Scotland (HTBS) represented a modest attempt to guide the use of resources on new technologies scientifically in the light of the evidence of their clinical and cost effectiveness.

In contrast to this rather *ad hoc* approach to determining the relative priority of particular patient groups, the geographical distribution of the NHS budget has spawned a small industry of analysts to calculate the share of the national cake that each of Scotland's 15 health boards should receive. It is an enquiry with a relatively long tradition, beginning with the work of the SHARE committee in the 1970s.[13] This committee aimed to measure need for health care in each health board by taking account of demography and mortality. The result was a differentiation between boards with more than their fair share (above target funding) and those with less. Over time the plan was to level up the allocations by distributing more of annual NHS growth money to those boards below target than those above. It took until the end of the 1990s before parity was achieved. The decline in the size of Glasgow's population meant that it was the big loser throughout the period despite its massive health and deprivation problems.

In practical terms, redistribution was slow because the overall real growth rates in the NHS budget averaged only 2.2% in the 1980s and 2.5% in the 1990s, much of which was absorbed by pay and price costs that were rising by about 1–2% more than the GDP deflator throughout this period.[14]

In 1997 Sam Galbraith, then Minister for Health, decide to review the SHARE formula. It had been criticised for three reasons: it did not measure adequately the effects of social deprivation on health care need; it did not address the additional costs of delivering services in rural Scotland; and new data and new analytical techniques had become available to measure relative needs more accurately.

The Arbuthnott Review and Real Growth

Sir John Arbuthnott, at that time Principal of Strathclyde University, was appointed to lead the review. His report,[15, 16] published shortly before the new Parliament became established in July 1999, had the distinction of being one of the first topics to be the subject of an inquiry by the newly established Health and Community Care Committee. The report's proposals, which were accepted by Ministers were designed to guide growth in the NHS budget towards health board areas like Greater Glasgow with its high levels of social deprivation and Highland which experiences the effects of rurality and distance discussed below. The rate of convergence among the board areas under the Arbuthnott Formula is likely to be quicker than it was with SHARE because the variance between the boards is smaller, and the rate of growth in the overall budget for health care is now expanding much faster than at any time in the recent past.

On occasion over the past 15 years governments have departed from the long-term trends in spending growth referred to earlier with substantial injections of resources, usually in response to a particularly acute 'crisis' when the political temperature has risen to an uncomfortable degree, or because of an impending election, or to ease the wheels of organisational reform. The Treasury has usually taken the view, however, that health care spending is a cost to be minimised because it is one of the largest components of overall public spending. The most recent budgets of the present Chancellor of the Exchequer suggest that this view may have changed, at least for the time being. Having commissioned the Wanless Report to take a 20-year perspective on the funding needs of the NHS as currently conceived, and having accepted its view that health care is an investment rather than a cost, the 2002 Budget has promised annual real growth in NHS spending of over 7.5% for the next five years.[17]

In accordance with the Barnett Formula Scotland received its proportionate share of this growth and Scottish Ministers have chosen to allocate it to health even though they have discretion to spend it on other services if they wish. As public spending on health is increasingly rapidly so is the rate of convergence and Scotland's ruling politicians may, at some point, come to the same conclusion as some of their counterparts in Wales and Northern Ireland that a new formula for public spending is in their interest. The Scottish National Party has already reached this view, campaigning for greater 'fiscal autonomy' with the power to raise and spend tax revenues. How this issue unfolds is bound to have important implications for NHS funding; indeed so substantial is the NHS as a component of Scottish public spending that those implications are likely to play a part in the debate about the merits of the different options. Even though Scotland's health budget is planned to grow by 50% over the next five years,[18] it looks as though the dilemma of how to pay for health care in Scotland is here to stay.

Impact of distance[†]

Although rural life brings with it some specific health hazards,[19, 20] the main causes of illness and death are the same in rural Scotland as elsewhere – namely, coronary heart disease, stroke, cancer, and mental illness. Statistics of life expectancy indicate that on average rural dwellers live longer than people in urban areas. This supports the idea of an idyllic rural life, but, in reality, rural communities contain within them a very diverse mix of people. Some earn a good living in urban areas, returning each evening to their rural lives – a group described by the sociologist Ray Pahl as 'urbs in rure.'[21] Others struggle to exist on low incomes associated with fishing, farming, and seasonal employment.[22] Some again, who may have moved to rural areas in search of peace and tranquillity, depend on social benefits or modest retirement incomes only to experience growing isolation as age erodes their mobility.

The lower levels of illness reported in rural areas are in part a consequence of difficulty in attending services in the first place and it is, therefore, vital to look beyond the headline statistics in this context. This is the problem of 'distance decay' or 'friction of distance'[23, 24] where the further people live from a service the less likely they are to use it. Numerous studies have shown how this affects the use of health services, including accident and emergency departments, outpatients and screening services. Unsurprisingly, the more specialist the service the more willing are patients to travel. The unresolved question in many of these studies, however, is the impact of distance on the outcome of the patient's condition. A recent study of cancer survival in Scotland, for example, has found that patients who lived further away from a cancer centre were less likely to have their cancer diagnosed (and treated) before death in the cases of stomach, breast and colorectal cancer, and showed poorer survival in the case of prostate and lung cancer.[25] There was no evidence that living in a small community was a factor in affecting outcome, but the distance of such communities from a cancer centre was significant. Despite the many arrangements made to meet the needs of rural populations in Scotland, the tyranny of distance continues to exert its influence.[26, 27]

[†]This section of the chapter draws on an article first published in the British Journal of Health Care Management [27] and is used with the permission of its editor.

Successive reports have considered ways of mitigating the problem of rural access.[18–32] These have usually focused on improving transport and communications, on better integration of services and on enhancing the conditions of service and remuneration of family doctors. New surgeries and health centres have been built in many places, the air ambulance service has been extended and improved to enable speedy transfer of patients, and financial assistance has been provided to ease the cost burden of travel for the less affluent. The Associate GP scheme introduced in 1990 has supplemented the GP Retainer arrangements and Inducement Practice Scheme, established to encourage doctors to take on practices in the most remote parts of Scotland. These have eased but not eliminated the burden of out-of-hours on-call duty.[33, 34]

With regard to the provision of hospital services, decisions about where to treat are not clear cut, and this ambiguity about what can and should be done in smaller hospitals bedevils the development of hospitals in rural areas.[35] A number of factors, including quality, convenience, cost, and outcome have to be balanced. The understandable fear of rural communities is that moves to centralise services in the name of quality or efficiency involve real costs to them.

The Acute Services Review published in 1998,[36] led by Scotland's Chief Medical Officer (see chapter 9), considered these matters in some detail, finding the evidence on hospital size, clinical outcomes, and cost efficiency to be ambiguous, but also observing that as medicine becomes increasingly specialised it is essential to maintain specialist skills through regular practice. This requirement is not easily satisfied by the kind of cases presenting in sparsely populated areas, where breadth of skill and experience are arguably more important than depth of specialist knowledge. In the past, for example, surgical services in remote parts of Scotland developed by using GPs as anaesthetists and single-handed surgeons who performed a range of surgical procedures, some of which would be the province of their specialist colleagues in urban areas. As well as placing a considerable burden on those who practice in these circumstances because of the on-call requirements and professional isolation, such arrangements are increasingly being challenged on the grounds of safety and quality. A further complication is that the Royal Medical Colleges are no longer prepared to approve the training of junior doctors in these situations and this calls into question the feasibility of delivering such services at all unless additional consultant cover is available.[37]

In weighing these factors, health planners in Scotland face difficulties in striking a balance between considerations of safety, quality, convenience, and cost. Safety is clearly paramount but there is a trade-off to be made among the other three concerns. Most argument about rural hospitals reflects differences of view about the preferred trade-off and has often resulted in an uneasy relationship between the health authorities and the people they serve.

The Acute Services Review offered proposals intended to help reconcile these concerns – for example, the use of modern digital communications to support telemedicine – and these are discussed further in chapter 9. The Review's most important recommendation, specifically for rural health care, was for the creation of a Remote and Rural Areas Resource Initiative (RARARI).[38] This was established in 1999 and provides a valuable focus for rural practice. Although its work has only just begun, the centre has the potential to provide the help, support, and fellowship so vital to the maintenance of skills and morale among the professionals that serve Scotland's rural communities.

Meeting the Challenges: Organisational change in the NHS

It is sometimes said that the NHS needs a rest from organisational change, a period of calm when the functions (and names) of organisations within it are given time to become established before they are changed once more. If the past is a guide, those who hope for such organisational peace and quiet are likely to be disappointed. This is mainly because political leaders who are temporarily entrusted with Scotland's health service have only a short time in which to make their mark. The pressures on them are intense; the complexity of the service, the pressing nature of its problems, and their own political commitments force a search for organisational panaceas.

In a review of the experience in OECD countries Naylor and colleagues[39] concluded 'that improvements in health care are not contingent on the drafting of grand blueprints or the ability of politicians and public servants to pull big policy levers. Health care improvement starts from the ground up. It requires tenacious work to understand what does and does not work in real life and the engagement of countless providers and patients, institutions and communities. Similarly, most policy movement seems to be incremental, driven by experience and evidence, rather than theory or ideology.'

Nonetheless, it seems unlikely that politicians will ever be able to resist the temptations of the quick organisational fix that has been the experience in Scotland since 1985, a period in which three distinct organisational eras have been identified.[40] The first, lasting until 1989, can be described as the end of *hierarchy*, when the traditional 'command and control' model on which the NHS was founded, was swept away by a Conservative government's enthusiasm for *markets* and competition. This second era lasted until 1997 when Tony Blair's New Labour government rejected these ideas and sought a 'third way' based on 'partnership'. During this current era, *networks* have emerged as a preferred organisational model. In reality this may be too neat a classification; there is seldom a clear-cut point of change, but there are without doubt very different political philosophies guiding policy development in each period and it provides a helpful route through the changes that have taken place.

Hierarchy: 1985–1990

For most of its existence the health service in Scotland has been organised and reorganised much in common with other parts of the UK. Undoubtedly, the NHS in Scotland has retained a distinct identity – a service within a service,[41] and it is possible to point to a number of differences in its organisation at various times. For the most part, however, these have amounted to structural nuances in arrangements determined principally by UK governments, and implemented in Scotland by its Secretaries of State and their health ministers. Consequently, between 1948 and 1974, the NHS in Scotland had the same tripartite structure as England. Health management responsibilities were divided among 55 local authorities, responsible for community health and environmental health services; 55 Executive Councils administering contracts with independent providers of family practitioner services; and five Regional Hospital Boards and 65 Hospital Management Committees responsible for hospital services.[42]

By the start of the 1970s, concerns about a lack of integrated health management led to consideration of the reform of this structure and in 1974 the Scottish Office adopted a model that unified the administration of health care in 15 new geographically defined Health Boards, some of which were divided for operational management purposes into districts. The combination within Health Boards of responsibilities for primary care as well as hospital and community health services differed from the arrangements in England, as did the absence of a regional administrative level. Appointed by and accountable to the Secretary of State for Scotland, the Health Boards (whose boundaries have survived, if not their form nor function, to the present day) became the focus for the administration of Scotland's health service, operating in a hierarchical organisational model reaching from the Scottish Home and Health Department in St Andrew's House in Edinburgh to the most distant island communities. Consensus management – the making and taking of decisions by teams – was the managerial fashion of the day, and in an era of ever tightening financial constraint, the search for greater efficiency in public spending and the delivery of health care became the dominant theme in the Scottish health service.

One of the novelties of the 1974 reorganisation in Scotland was the creation of the Scottish Health Service Planning Council to advise the Secretary of State for Scotland on the discharge of his (health service) functions 'at his request or its own initiative.'[43] With membership drawn from the 15 Health Boards, university, and other interests, the Planning Council was responsible for two reports that have had a lasting influence on the planning of the NHS in Scotland. Following on from the 1976 SHARE report that had addressed the geographical distribution of health care resources among the health boards, SHAPE[11] and SHARPEN[12] sought to give greater priority to the needs of the elderly, the mentally ill, and the learning disabled at the relative expense of acute hospital care where improved efficiency was to yield resources for reinvestment. In many ways these remain unfulfilled ambitions: in 1985/6 the share of hospital and community health revenue spending on general and acute hospital services was 41%[44] and in 1999/00 it was approximately 46%.[15]

The search for greater efficiency informs much of the health service policy pursued in Scotland since the middle of the 1980s. Sir Kenneth Stowe (Permanent Secretary of the Department of Health in England) has published a fascinating account of political thinking in this era.[45] Its relevance to Scotland derives from the process of 'administrative devolution' whereby ideas developed in Whitehall were 'tartanised' or adjusted for Scottish circumstances and implemented by Scottish Ministers.

An example of organisational tartanisation was the announcement of the abolition in November 1983 of the districts set up under the Health Boards in 1974 and their replacement with 'Units of Management'. This was a significant change in the light of events in England. In the previous month the Secretary of State for Health, Norman Fowler, received and accepted the recommendations of an NHS Management Inquiry under the Chairmanship of Roy Griffiths – then Managing Director of the supermarket group, Sainsbury's – with far-reaching and longstanding consequences for the NHS.[46] Malcolm Rifkind, the Secretary of State for Scotland, soon announced that he intended to adopt the recommendations of the inquiry, prominent among which was the idea that the NHS needed a general management function. Consensus management was out of fashion, condemned for creating confusion and delay, and hindering the effective leadership of local health services. Instead all local health bodies were to appoint a general manager with clear executive authority. Hunter[43] has noted that a similar recommendation had been made 20 years previously in Scotland, but not acted upon. The Farquharson-Lang Report[47] had been concerned with the administrative practices of hospital boards and had come to the conclusion that a chief executive appointed on merit should lead them.

Although the general management function is now well established in the health service, in the middle of the 1980s there were doubts and uncertainties about its likely effects. If the appointment of general managers caught the headlines, Griffiths' recommendation for clinicians to have an enhanced role in management was an equally important proposal of long-term influence. At a national level, the report led to a series of changes in the internal organisation of the Scottish Home and Health Department. A Supervisory Board for the NHS (The Health Services Policy Board) was set up under the Chairmanship of the Minister for Health and Social Work, and a new senior civil service position – the Under-Secretary for NHS Management, Finance and Operational Planning – was created as a focal point for NHS management. In time, these changes led to the establishment of the NHS Management Executive, which continued in existence until 2000, and the appointment of the first Chief Executive of the NHS in Scotland in Don Cruickshank, recruited from the Virgin Group.

In retrospect, these changes can be seen as another instalment in the long running search for improved organisational effectiveness in the NHS. Charged with the provision of a universal, (almost) comprehensive health service, from within strictly limited exchequer funding, the NHS organised as a bureaucratic hierarchy appeared to some to be increasingly unsuited to the reconciliation of these competing demands. Over the years, increases in spending, structural change, and the adoption of various management fads and fashions were reasonably successful in enabling governments to continue to run the service along the lines on which it had been set up in 1948. At the end of the 1980s, however, the possibility of an entirely new approach to the resolution of these problems began to emerge.

Markets: 1991–1997

Prompted by growing public concern over financial problems in many parts of the NHS, and a particularly disturbing case in November 1988 of a small baby in Birmingham, whose heart surgery had to be cancelled five times because of staff shortages, the Prime Minister, Margaret Thatcher, announced on the television programme, Panorama, that she would be conducting a review of the NHS[48, 49]. The review was conducted under great secrecy and speculation grew on what it might prescribe.

When the review was published in the document *Working for Patients*,[50] it revealed a set of ideas completely different from anything previously tried in publicly funded health systems anywhere. At its heart was the development of an internal market within the NHS, by creating new organisations – NHS Trusts – that would compete with each other to win service contracts from health authorities transformed into purchasers of health care. By enabling money to follow patients, competition would reward those Trusts that provided better quality, value for money services. It was argued that Adam Smith's invisible hand could achieve the reconciliation of need, demand and supply that had eluded governments administering the NHS by centralised command and control. A particularly novel innovation was the creation of GP Fundholding where an individual general practice could acquire part of a health authority's budget and purchase a designated set of services at its own hand without reference to the health board (chapter 8).

Based on the concept of managed competition, developed by the American economist Alain Enthoven,[51, 52] the internal market represented the most radical departure in health care policy in the UK since the NHS was founded. Here were untested ideas to be implemented wholesale in the largest public service in the land.

Reflecting on the changes that had swept across the NHS, Rudolf Klein[53] suggested that they had shifted the goals of long established health policy. Instead of conceiving of the NHS as a 'church' it should be more appropriately regarded as a series of 'garages'. Klein quoted Barbara Castle, Secretary of State for Health in the 1970s: 'the NHS is a church. It is the nearest thing to the embodiment of the Good Samaritan that we have in any aspect of our public policy.' In the new system, Klein detected a secularisation of policy, whereby patients became consumers, and the NHS a satisfier of individual wants, a repairer of people, rather than a promoter and contributor to broader social goals. NHS Trusts were the new garages, and consumers (patients) were advised that they had new representatives when in need of repair in the form of fundholding GPs and Health Boards responsible for the negotiation of service contracts with the garage owners. The publication of the Citizen's Charter, and its NHS derivative, the Patient's Charter, gave added impetus to these ideas, leading the Chief Executive of the NHS in Scotland to attempt a wholesale process of change described in the Scottish Office's *Framework for Action*.[54]

Detailed guidance to the NHS on how to set up Trusts[55] and to GPs on how to become fundholders[56] was issued from Edinburgh, and succeeded in attracting some support in the face of doubts among many about the wisdom of the reforms and their suitability to Scottish circumstances. In a country that had led the opposition to Mrs Thatcher's poll tax, and where Conservative MPs represented a small minority of Scotland's Westminster constituencies, there remained a strong preference for the NHS as a church, rather than a garage. Writing about the NHS in Scotland just before these particular reforms emerged, T Drummond Hunter,[41] (p220), appears to have seen straws blowing in the wind, and urged the Scottish people, 'to turn society the right way up, first by subordinating the state to the aspirations of its citizens for self determination and, secondly, by organising society on a genuinely collective and interdependent basis so that it is at last able to meet the needs of its members both for basic wellbeing and for fullness of life'.

From an initial band of enthusiasts, the number of NHS Trusts in Scotland grew until all the former directly managed units of the mainland Health Boards became NHS Trusts, as did the Scottish Ambulance Service. By the end of 1996 there were 47 NHS Trusts in Scotland. The exceptions were the Island Health Boards where, for reasons of scale, it was impractical to create separate NHS

Trusts. Instead these Boards attempted to distinguish between their purchasing and providing functions by restructuring their internal management arrangements. Fundholding also grew in significance as the initial scheme designed primarily for larger practices was amended in scope to enable the participation of smaller practices. Although an early evaluation[57] of six 'shadow' fundholding groups (including 50 GPs) suggested that the scheme had delivered some benefits for patients and the expansion of primary care services, the scheme never achieved the uptake observed in England .[58] At the end of 1996 43% of Scotland's population was registered with a GP fundholding practice[59] the highest level of coverage being in Grampian. As increasing proportions of health board budgets were devolved to fundholding practices, and NHS Trusts cut their links with their previous masters, the role of health boards came under scrutiny. A new word entered the NHS vocabulary – commissioning. No longer responsible for providing services, and progressively handing over some of their newly acquired responsibilities as health care purchasers to GP fundholders, health boards were encouraged to exercise oversight of local health systems, 'holding the ring' in emergent health care markets through their strategic planning responsibilities.

The Shields Report[60] gave greater definition to the commissioning role, placing emphasis on the concept of health gain. This imprecise term envisaged health boards systematically assessing population health status, evaluating the effectiveness of services, and determining the relative priority of competing claims on resources. As a concept, it brought back into focus the need to address the determinants of health, many of which lie outside the direct control of the health service. Health alliances between the NHS and others, notably local authorities, able to contribute to improved population health were encouraged. This evolution of roles was certainly unstated and perhaps unforeseen by the architects of *Working for Patients* and provided some comfort for those who preferred the NHS as a church rather than a garage. It also provided a link with a separate strand of policy that had been gathering impetus from the beginning of the 1990s – how to address Scotland's reputation as the sick man of Europe? The scale of the problems had been described in *Scotland's Health: A Challenge to Us All*[61]. On the eve of the 1997 general election Scotland's Secretary of State, Michael Forsyth, published a White Paper that attempted to strengthen the connections between these strands by weaving a tartan of policy initiatives aimed at health improvement.[59] With an eye on the gathering momentum for political devolution the separate identity of the NHS in Scotland was acknowledged in the paper's title, *The Scottish Health Service*. Its subtitle, *Ready for the Future*, attempted to capture the paper's other theme, that the necessary restructuring to establish the internal market was complete and a period of organisational calm would follow when the fruits of unprecedented change would be gathered. It was not to be.

Networks: 1997 onwards

In May 1997 Donald Dewar became Secretary of State for Scotland in Tony Blair's New Labour Government. His key priority was to deliver devolved government for Scotland, and most other policy issues came some way behind. But the Scottish Labour manifesto had made some important promises about the NHS, including early action to abolish the internal market. The proposals were not long in coming in the shape of a White Paper, *Designed to Care: Renewing the NHS in Scotland* [62] that was published in December 1997. This promised an NHS 'for the people of Scotland that offers them the treatment they need, where they want it, and when.'

As in the past, there were many common features with health policy elsewhere in the UK. Six themes can be identified: (i) a new emphasis on public health; (ii) the promotion of partnership working; (iii) the pursuit of service integration; (iv) a concern with the quality of clinical practice; (v) a search for improvements in access to care through reductions in waiting lists and times; (vi) a determination to tackle inequalities in both health status and health care[63]. With the prospect of political devolution increasingly likely, however, *Designed to Care* offered a distinctively different organisational model that reflected important policy differences between Scottish Office Ministers and their Whitehall colleagues over the role of GPs in the management of budgets for secondary health care[64, 65].

The Scottish model retained separate roles for Health Boards and NHS Trusts. The former were to focus on public health and strategic planning. The latter, hitherto competitors, were amalgamated in Acute Hospital Trusts (AHTs) and Primary Care Trusts (PCTs). Fundholding became yesterday's fad, condemned for its bureaucracy and injustices, its statutory basis being undone, among other things, in new legislation enacted by the Westminster Parliament in the form of the Health Act, 1999. Single AHTs served individual health boards other than in Glasgow where size dictated that two were created. Similarly, single PCTs served whole health board populations (apart from Argyll and Clyde because of geographical and other practical reasons) and, for the first time, brought together primary care, community health services and specialist services for the mentally ill, elderly and learning disabled. The only exceptions to this pattern were the Island Boards because of their size and the retention of a combined acute and primary care trust serving West Lothian.

In an attempt to achieve greater integration of care and develop a community focus, Local Health Care Co-Operatives (LHCCs) were encouraged, voluntary combinations of GPs operating within and accountable to the PCT. Joint Investment Funds (JIFs) were invented as a successor to fundholding with the aim of encouraging the integration of primary and secondary care, though the label was something of a misnomer as no new fund was actually created. Instead the emphasis was on the redesign of existing services and the reallocation of their associated resources. Although the JIFs did not catch on, the idea of 'local health systems' of Board and Trusts, working to common objectives described in the Health Improvement Programmes they were required to produce, did. As partnerships within the NHS began to strengthen, government policy also encouraged joint working between the NHS, local government and others who could contribute to the process of health improvement and especially to the dismantling of barriers between health and social care.

In rejecting the ideas of the market and resisting a return to hierarchy with its reliance on top-down management, the Labour Government was attempting to give expression in the NHS to the Prime Minister's belief in the political idea of the 'Third Way.'[66] The emphasis on partnership acknowledged that solutions to enduring problems depended on the combined efforts of many individuals and organisations. Patients were seen to value continuity of care on their journey through the services of numerous providers associated with the complexity and increasing specialisation of modern medicine. The increased need for patient referral can stretch lines of communication to breaking point and leave everyone involved frustrated by unnecessary delay, and duplicated or neglected administrative and clinical processes. The emergence of 'partnership' as the new guiding concept of health care organisation at this time signalled an explicit attempt to manage these complications of service networks. In the words of

Designed to Care the aim was to develop, 'a partnership between different parts of
the NHS in Scotland to promote the integration of care and provide patients
with a seamless service'[62] (p8). These ideas were developed further in the Acute
Services Review (see chapter 9) in which the concept of Managed Clinical
Networks was articulated with the aim of building managerial support for
important clinical relationships.

Political Devolution

If these policies were far-reaching in their implications for Scotland's health
services, wider political and constitutional changes, unfolding concurrently, had
the undeniable potential to be of far greater long-term significance. The
establishment of the Scottish Parliament in Edinburgh in July 1999 devolved
political control from the UK Parliament at Westminster to 129 newly elected
members (MSPs) and to the Scottish Executive, the political administration
responsible for the government of Scotland.

The Scotland Act of 1998 granted primary legislative powers and full executive
power to these institutions for those policy areas within their competence. The
Act was designed to devolve competence unless it was specifically reserved to
Westminster, and thus most health and NHS policy became the concern of
Scotland's new politicians at Holyrood. Only a small number of policy topics in
health[§] were reserved including, for example, the regulation of the health
professions and abortion, the rationale of UK ministers who made these
decisions being that it would be undesirable to have the possibility of different
legislation guiding policy and practice in these areas either side of the border.[67]

Health and the NHS have been prominent features of the Parliament's activities.
The first legislation enacted in September 1999 was the Mental Health (Public
Safety and Appeals) (Scotland) Act 1999, provoked by the need to close a legal

---

[§] Detailed information explaining the Parliament's powers and procedures can be found
elsewhere (www.scottish.parliament.uk) and the early years of its activities and those of the
Scottish Executive (www.scotland.gov.uk) have been closely studied through the work of the
Constitution Unit's (www.ucl.ac.uk/constituion-unit) devolution monitoring projects[68, 69] that
have co-ordinated the observations and analyses of a network of scholars throughout the UK. As
far as health and the NHS is concerned detailed accounts of events in Scotland can be found at
www.dph.gla.ac.uk/shspf and a UK analysis in Woods.[64]

loophole that allowed the release from the State Hospital at Carstairs[#] of a patient, Mr Noel Ruddle, because he no longer suffered from a mental illness amenable to treatment. These events illustrated a number of novel features and intriguing consequences of the new political institutions. The speed at which legislation was brought forward to deal with a particularly Scottish problem exceeded the previous possibilities at Westminster. The Liberal Democrat Minister for Justice (Mr Jim Wallace) introduced the legislation to Parliament on behalf of the Coalition Executive, which had been formed by Labour and the Liberal Democrats as an almost inevitable consequence of the new electoral system partly based on proportional representation.

The new Minister for Health and Community Care was Susan Deacon, the first woman to hold the post in Scotland and appointed as one of 11 members of First Minister Donald Dewar's Cabinet or Executive. To her fell the job of implementing the commitments made in the health section of the coalition's *Programme for Government*[69] with formidable challenges to be met while the newly created machinery of government and Parliament became established.

Hazell and Jervis[70] attempted to capture the views of senior figures in Scotland's health services in 1997/98. In common with the popular mood that had given overwhelming support to devolution, expectations were high. Those interviewed saw the opportunities for Scotland to develop distinctive policies – 'Scottish solutions for Scottish problems' – and to build a new political consensus that would help tackle Scotland's poor health record and the enduring problems of the NHS; and to find innovative policies free from the controlling influence of Whitehall.

It was not long before events intruded on the air of optimism. The winter of 1999/2000 brought some familiar NHS problems to the top of the political agenda. The inevitable increase in influenza type illness put health services and the government under increased pressure, as numerous media reports highlighted the difficulties faced by some patients requiring admission to hospital. These difficulties had been particularly serious a year earlier, but a new factor, the fear that the 'millennium bug' would cause computer systems to fail as

---

[#] For high security mentally disordered offenders.

the clocks chimed midnight on New Year's Eve 1999 added a new dimension to the usual cocktail of health service problems. In the event, only isolated, minor hitches occurred. The problems of winter however, precipitated a change in UK government policy with profound implications for health services throughout the whole country.

In February 2000 the Prime Minister, in a move reminiscent of Margaret Thatcher, surprisingly announced on national television that he planned to increase health spending to the 'European average' a direct response to accusations laid by leaders of the medical profession that the winter crisis had its origins in the relatively low level of UK health spending compared to other European countries, notably France and Germany. Despite the uncertainty over what this commitment might actually mean in reality, it undoubtedly offered the prospect of significant additional resources finding their way to the NHS in Scotland as a consequence of the operation of the Barnett Formula.

Within a few weeks the Chancellor of the Exchequer announced details of the new resources. Although the Scottish Executive could have chosen to allocate the 'health consequential' (as these monies are referred to in the jargon of government accounting), to other services, they decided not to and the NHS in Scotland, therefore, benefited. Accompanying the spending announcements was the news that the UK government intended to produce a plan for the 'modernisation' of the NHS in England, subsequently published in July 2000. [71] Scottish Ministers had a choice. Post devolution they had no need to follow suit; they could have produced something completely different or, as in the era of administrative devolution, they could have produced a Scottish version of the English proposals. They chose an approach closer to the last of these possibilities than the others, and towards the end of 2000 *Our National Health: A plan for action, a plan for change* was published. [72]

Compared with its English equivalent, the Scottish plan laid greater emphasis on public health, and announced a 'rewiring' of NHSScotland, itself a new brand name for the health service. Health Boards and NHS Trusts were retained but brought together in 'unified boards of governance'. The membership of these NHS Boards, as they have come to be designated, included people appointed to them by Ministers from among the elected members of local authorities and NHS staff representatives. The aim was to 'to simplify, improve and rationalise the current local decision-making arrangements' without embarking on another restructuring of the NHS[72] (p28). Nonetheless, the Plan also announced a 'high-level review of the management and decision-making in the NHS', followed in May 2002 by the First Minister, Jack McConnell, announcing that the Executive would be publishing a White Paper which duly appeared at the end of February 2003.[73]

The integration of services and the devolution of decision-making within a national system of organisational performance management were at its heart. Since patients want improved access, fewer bottlenecks, and continuity of care, the logic of the paper was that joining up services is a desirable objective: joining up services required joining up organisations within NHS Scotland under the umbrella of NHS Boards. To avoid these becoming old-fashioned command and control posts of the pre-Thatcher NHS hierarchy, however, they were told to design effective arrangements for the devolution of operational management to the front line. Supported by a 'massive' redesign effort and a £29 million Change and Innovation Fund the intention was to put the patient at the heart of the NHS. Just in case those at the front line strayed from their new responsibilities a strengthened regime of monitoring and inspection was introduced to send early warning signals to the Executive, which, like a good shepherd, would guide the wayward flock in the desired direction.

Abolishing NHS Trusts (a bit of Scottish Labour's unfinished business in ridding the NHS of the hated internal market) was the headline catching proposal that paved the way for greater integration. The paper did not actually say how NHS Boards were to structure themselves, but left them to come up with their own ideas on how to 'strengthen corporate working [that does not] result in greater central control over operational matters'.

Within this general framework two ideas were given prominence. First was the accelerated development of Managed Clinical Networks. NHS Boards were to work together in regional groupings to progress their introduction. Second was the idea of Community Health Partnerships (CHPs), operating divisions of NHS Boards charged with the management and development of an expanding range of integrated primary care, community health, and social care services. CHPs were to evolve from the network of Local Health Care Co-Operatives (LHCCs), which were judged to have been making good progress as 'responsive and inclusive organisations'. That these ideas were of little interest to the media at the time of publication should not detract from their importance as vehicles for the integration of care. The paper left unspecified the detailed means by which this was to be achieved, however, requiring NHS Boards to come up with a development path for LHCCs. Some people might have expected more central guidance on this (and on the structuring of other operating divisions) but the discretion given to Boards offered the advantage of enabling them to come up with arrangements that suit the varied circumstances found throughout Scotland.

At the time of writing it is unclear if the most recent White Paper will lead as intended to the effective management of complex service networks or lead back to a reliance on hierarchy and top down management as Ministers seek to achieve the delivery of important political commitments. The present Minister for Health and Community Care, Mr. Malcolm Chisholm, favours the former[74] but this may prove difficult given the intensification of parliamentary and public scrutiny since 1999 that has placed the Executive's health policies under an intense spotlight.

The scrutiny of public policy and public bodies is fundamental to the work of the Parliament, and health and the NHS have been prominent in this aspect of its work. The size of the health budget, about 30% of the total expenditure of the Executive, and its insatiable appetite for additional spending is part of the explanation. So too, is the nature of health care. It provides personal services that everyone will need at some point in their lives and is provided by the largest workforce in Scotland (chapter 11). Interest is heightened by the fact that the NHS is the single largest public service under the direct management control of the Executive. Unlike education there are limited roles for elected representatives in local government, and unlike agriculture, fisheries, or industrial policy, responsibility is not shared with political institutions in Westminster, Brussels and Strasbourg.

The Minister of Health and Community Care sits at the apex of Scotland's largest nationalised service, and every event within it, good or bad, is rapidly politicised. While this has been true since 1948, the creation of the Scottish Parliament has intensified this dynamic. According to the Health Plan there were 50 debates on health and community care matters in the first 18 months of its existence compared with only one short adjournment debate at Westminster in the period immediately preceding devolution. There has also been an upsurge

in the number of parliamentary questions asked by MSPs, and the Health
Minister regularly answers oral questions in the parliamentary chamber. The
novel creation of a 'Petitions Committee' has given people the opportunity to
bring their local concerns to national prominence, and has been used to good
effect by them.[75] A standing Health and Community Care Committee has the
power of pre-legislative scrutiny, and indeed can initiate legislation at its own
hand, while the Parliament's Audit Committee takes a close interest in the health
budget and the financial stewardship of NHS bodies. Last, but by no means
least, the proceedings of all of these components of the post-devolution health
policy-making process are closely monitored and reported by Scotland's large
and active media.

Conclusion

There is a danger that the formal account of the policies, events, and changes
that have been described in this chapter does not do justice to the people involved
in them. Change is seldom easy for those it affects, and it is important to bear in
mind that the NHS in Scotland is not an anonymous organisational construct.
At times those involved may have felt like soldiers in the army of the Grand Old
Duke of York. That this large and talented workforce has been able, by and large,
to accommodate and adapt to unfolding events, grand designs, and new
possibilities is a testament to its commitment to the idea of a national health
service. In the labour intensive service that is the NHS people and personalities
shape and influence the grand designs of policy architects, incorporating them
in to established practice. At times there have been vigorous disputes between
politicians directing the service and the staff delivering it, to such an extent that
occasionally staff and their representatives have expressed outright opposition
to the politicians' ideas. Tales of notable characters, tragedies, scandals,
successes, and failings abound in the folklore of the service. Thousands of lay
people have contributed their time, knowledge, and skills to the management
challenges of Scotland's largest public service. Politicians and others have come
and gone as judgments have formed on their suitability for the job in hand. Some
are remembered, but many have been quickly forgotten as others took on the
fascinating dilemmas that characterise health care administration. Most of
those who have contributed to the progress of the NHS often joined it with a
sense of vocation they were able to fulfill, for it remains a service for and about
people, and a reflection of the society it serves.

REFERENCES

1. McLachlan G. (Ed.) *Improving the Common Weal. Aspects of Scottish Health Services 1900–1984.* A collation in honour of the late Sir John Brotherston. Edinburgh:Edinburgh University Press for the Nuffield Provincial Hospitals Trust, 1987.

2. Wanless D. *Securing Our Future Health: taking the long-term view.* London: The Stationery Office, 2002.

3. OECD. *Health Data 2002: a comparative analysis of 30 countries.* CD-ROM. Paris: OECD,2002.

4. The Scottish Parliament. Official Report. 24 July 2000.

5. Heald D, McLeod A. *Beyond Barnett? Financing Devolution.* In: Devolution in Practice. Adams J, Robinson P (eds).London: Institute for Public Policy Research, 2002.

6. Institute for Public Policy Research. *Building Better Partnerships.* Final Report of the Commission on Public Private Partnerships. London: IPPR, 2000.

7. Department of Health. *For the Benefit of Patients: A Concordat with the Private and Voluntary Healthcare Provider Sectors.* London: Department of Health, 2000.

8. Keating M. Devolution and Public Policy in the UK: Divergence or Convergence? In: *Devolution in Practice.* Adams J, Robinson P (eds). London: IPPR, 2002.

9. Scottish Executive. News Release, SEHD, 126/2002 28 June 2002.

10. The Scottish Parliament, Official Report, Written Answers, S1W-11380.

11. The Scottish Office. *Scottish Health Authorities Priorities for the Eighties.* Edinburgh: HMSO, 1980.

12. The Scottish Office. *Scottish Health Authorities Priorities for the Eighties and Nineties.* Edinburgh: HMSO, 1988.

13. The Scottish Office. Scottish Health Authorities Resource Equalisation: The Report of the Working Party on Revenue Resource Allocation. Edinburgh: HMSO, 1977.

14. Personal communication, Scottish Executive Health Department, 2002

15. The Scottish Executive. *Fair Shares for All: The National Review of Resource Allocation for the NHS in Scotland.* (Chairman: Sir John Arbuthnott) Edinburgh: The Stationery Office, 1999.

16. The Scottish Executive. *Fair Shares for All: Final Report.* Edinburgh: The Stationery Office, 2000.

17. H M Treasury. The 2002 Budget, April 17, www.hm-treasury.gov.uk/budget.

18. The Scottish Parliament. Official Report, 19 April 2002.

19. McKie L, MacPherson I. Health Issues in Remote and Rural Areas. *Health Bulletin* 1997, 55 (5).

20. Mungall I. Rural Disease. In: *Rural Health Care.* Cox J, Mungall I (eds).Oxford: Radcliffe Medical Press, 1999.

21. Pahl RE. *Urbs in Rure: The Metropolitan Fringe in Hertfordshire*. London: London School of Economics, 1965 .

22. Clark GM. Health and Poverty in Rural Scotland. *Health Bulletin* 1997, 55 (5).

23. Bentham CG. Proximity to Hospital and Mortality from Motor Vehicle Accidents. *Social Science and Medicine* 1986,23: 1021–1026.

24. Stark C, Reay L, Shiroy C. The Effect of Access Factors on Breast Screening Attendance on Two Scottish Islands. *Health Bulletin* 1997, 55 (5).

25. Campbell NC, Ritchie L, Sharp L, Cassidy J, Little J. Rural Factors and Survival from Cancer: An Analysis of Scottish Cancer Registration. *British Journal of Cancer* 2000, 82 (11): 1863–1866.

26. Blainey G.1966, *The Tyranny of Distance*. Melbourne: Sun Books, 1966.

27. Woods KJ. The Overthrow of a Tyrant: Prospects for Rural Health in Scotland. *British Journal of Health Care Management* 2001, 7 (8): 316–321.

28. The Report of the Highlands and Islands Medical Committee. (Chairman: Sir John Dewar) House of Commons, Cmnd Paper 6559. London: HMSO, 1912

29. The Report of the Committee on Scottish Health Services. House of Commons, Cmnd Paper 5204. London: HMSO,1936.

30. General Medical Services in the Highlands and Islands. Report of a committee appointed by the Secretary of State for Scotland. (Chairman: The Lord Birsay) House of Commons, Cmnd Paper 3257. London: HMSO,1967.

31. Health Care Services in Remote and Island Areas in Scotland. The Scottish Health Services Advisory Council. Edinburgh: HMSO,1995.

32. Barnes l, Gould J. Strategies for Success in Rural Care: Creating Effective and Accessible Health and Social Care Services in Rural Areas: A Practical Guide. London: National Council for Voluntary Organisations, 1997.

33. Steiner E, Mathieson D. What is an Associate GP? *Scottish Medicine* 1994, 14 (4): 12–13.

34. Marshall L. Inducement Practitioners, Associates and the Doctors' Retainer Scheme. In: *Rural Health Care*. Cox J, Mungall I (eds).Oxford: Radcliffe Medical Press, 1999.

35. Ritchie LD. *Community Hospitals in Scotland: Promoting Progress*. Aberdeen: Department of General Practice and Primary Care, University of Aberdeen, 1996.

36. The Scottish Office Department of Health. *The Review of Acute Hospital Services*. Edinburgh: The Stationery Office, 1998.

37. The Royal College of Surgeons of Edinburgh. *Surgery in Hospitals Serving Isolated Communities*. Edinburgh: RCS,1995.

38. The Scottish Executive.The Remote and Rural Areas Resource Initiative. Tweedale Buildings, High Street, Fort William, PH33 6EU. 2002. www.rarari.org.uk.

39. Naylor D, Karey I, Handa K. Measuring Health System Performance: Problems and Opportunities in an Era of Assessment and Accountability. Paper in *Measuring up: Improving Health Systems Performance in OECD Countries*. OECD Conference, Ottawa, 5 November 2001.

40. Harrison A. *Making the right Connections: the design and management of health care delivery*. London: King's Fund, 2001.

41. Hunter TD. 1989, A Service within a Service: The National Health Service in Scotland. In: *Success and Crisis in National Health Systems: A Comparative Approach*. Field MG (ed). London: Routledge, 1989.

42. Levitt R. *The Reorganised National Health Service*. London: Croom Helm, 1976.

43. Hunter DJ. *Managing the NHSiS: Review and Assessment of Research Needs*. Scottish Health Service Studies, 45. Edinburgh: Scottish Office, 1986.

44. The Scottish Office. *Scottish Health Authorities Priorities for the Eighties and Nineties*. Table A–2, p1, HMSO, Edinburgh: HMSO, 1988.

45. Stowe K. *On Caring for the National Health*. London: Nuffield Provincial Hospitals Trust, 1988.

46. Griffiths R. 1983, NHS Management Inquiry, Department of Health, London.

47. The Scottish Office. *Administrative Practice of Hospital Boards in Scotland*. Chairman: Farquharson-Lang. Edinburgh: Scottish Office, 1966.

48. Edwards B. *The NHS: a Manager's Tale*. London: Nuffield Provincial Hospitals Trust, 1993.

49. Rivett G. *From Cradle to Grave: Fifty Years of the NHS*. London: King's Fund, 1998.

50. Department of Health. *Working for Patients*. London: HMSO, 1989.

51. Enthoven AC. *Reflections on the Management of the NHS: An American looks at Incentives to Efficiency in Health Services Management in the UK*. Occasional Paper 5. London: Nuffield Provincial Hospitals Trust, 1985.

52. Enthoven AC. *In pursuit of an improving National Health Service*. London: Nuffield Trust, 1999.

53. Klein R. The Goals of Health Care: Church or Garage? In: *Health Care UK* 1992/93. Harrison A (ed).London: King's Fund, 1993.

54. Scottish Office. *Framework for Action*. NHS Management Executive. Edinburgh: HMSO, 1991.

55. Scottish Office. *NHS Trusts: A working guide*. Edinburgh: NHS Management Executive,1990.

56. Scottish Office. *Funding General Practice*. Edinburgh: NHS Management Executive.1990.

57. Howie, JGR, Heaney DJ, Maxwell M. *General Practice Fund-Holding: Shadow Project – an Evaluation*. University of Edinburgh Department of General Practice, 1995.

58. Audit Commission. *What the Doctor Ordered: A Study of GP Fundholders in England and Wales*. London: HMSO, 1996.

59. Scottish Office. *The Scottish Health Service. Ready for the Future*. Edinburgh: HMSO, 1997.

60. Scottish Office. *Commissioning Better Health*. Report of a Working Group. (Chairman: Professor Sir Robert Shields) NHS Management Executive, Edinburgh: NHS Management Executive, 1997.

61. Scottish Office. S*cotland's Health: A Challenge to Us All*. Edinburgh: HMSO, 1992.

62. Scottish Office. *Designed to Care: Renewing the NHS in Scotland*. Edinburgh: HMSO,1997.

63. Woods KJ. Health policy and the NHS in the UK 1997–2002. In: *Devolution in Practice*. Adams J, Robinson P (eds). London: IPPR, 2002.

64. Woods KJ. The Development of Integrated Health Care Models in Scotland. *International Journal of Integrated Care* 2001, 1: 3. www.ijic.org.

65. Hudson B, Hardy B. Localization Partnership in the 'New NHS': England and Scotland Compared. *Public Administration* 2001, 79 (2): 315–335.

66. Giddens A. *The Third Way*. Oxford: Polity, 1998.

67. Hazell R (ed). *The State and the Nations 2000*. Exeter: Imprint Academic, 2000.

68. Trench A (ed). *The State of the Nations 2001*. Exeter: Imprint Academic, 2001.

69. The Scottish Executive. *Programme for Government*. Edinburgh: The Stationery Office, 1999.

70. Hazell R, Jervis P. *Devolution and Health*. London: The Nuffield Trust, 1998.

71. Department of Health. *The NHS Plan. A Plan for Investment. A Plan for Reform*. London: The Stationery Office, 2000.

72. The Scottish Executive. *Our National Health: A Plan for Action, A Plan for Change*. Edinburgh: The Stationery Office, 2000.

73. The Scottish Parliament. Official Report 2002, May 22. www.scottish.parliament.uk . *Partnership for Care: Scotland's Health White Paper*, The Scottish Executive Department of Health, February 2003. Edinburgh: The Stationery Office,

74. Chisholm M. Report of the Scottish Health Services Policy Forum, 13 May 2002. www.dph.gla.ac.uk/shspf

75. The Scottish Parliament. Health and Community Care Committee.Report on Strathcathro Petition PE13, 9th Report, 1999. www.scottish.parliament.uk.

2. The Health of Scotland

Phil Hanlon, David Walsh and Bruce Whyte

Introduction

Health is complex. It is a multidimensional construct, comprising physical, mental, social and even spiritual dimensions, each with positive (wellbeing, good function) and negative (disease, loss of function) components.

The mechanisms by which health is improved are equally complex. The health status of the population of Scotland, for example, emerges from a highly complex hierarchy of interacting systems of causation. These include genetic inheritance, biological factors, the physical circumstances in which people grow up – for example, housing, air quality, working environment – the social environment – for example, levels of support and trust – personal behaviour – for example, smoking, diet, exercise – and, crucially, access to resources that give control over life. It is now well understood that these determinants operate over the whole life course.[1]

Given this level of complexity, it is impossible even to conceptualise a situation where a few pieces of summary data could be used to describe adequately the health of a whole nation. The work on which this chapter is based is part of an ongoing project being conducted by the Public Health Institute of Scotland (PHIS) (now NHS Health Scotland) that recognises this complexity and seeks to address it by collecting as wide a range of data as possible, with such data assigned to appropriate 'domains'. For this chapter, only a few selected indicators from each domain have been included, analysed in three simple ways: (i) comparisons of Scotland with other European countries; (ii) examination of trends over time; and (iii) analysis of differences (inequalities) within Scotland itself. Two additional sections examining the more specific areas of children's health and communicable disease in Scotland alone are also included. This briefer presentation does not give a comprehensive picture of the health of Scotland but it does provide enough information to highlight many of the health challenges that emerge from a larger analysis.

Life expectancy

Figure 2.1a shows life expectancy at birth for males in 1998 for Scotland compared to a wide range of European countries. Although not shown here, the picture for female life expectancy, in terms of Scotland's position relative to these other European nations, is almost identical. What emerges is that Scotland's life expectancy lags behind almost all other Western and Northern European nations. Only the poorer Eastern European countries fare worse.

Figure 2.1a   Life expectancy at birth, males, 1998

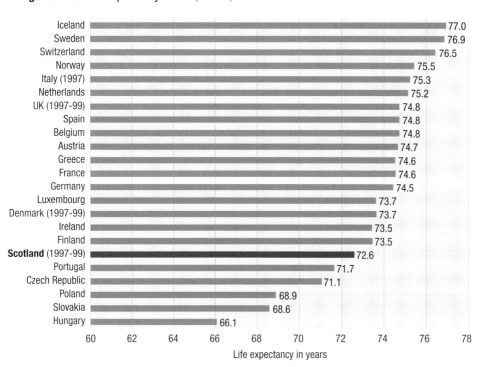

Some have expressed the view that this is not a surprise given Scotland's legacy of heavy industry and relative poverty. The past two decades, however, have witnessed profound changes in Scottish society, so although our current 'league position' is poor, it would be interesting to know if we are beginning to catch up. Figure 2.1b shows that life expectancy for males in Scotland has risen over the past decade (1990 to 2000), from 71.4 to 72.8 years. Previous analysis[2] has

Figure 2.1b Life expectancy at birth, males, Scotland 1990–2000

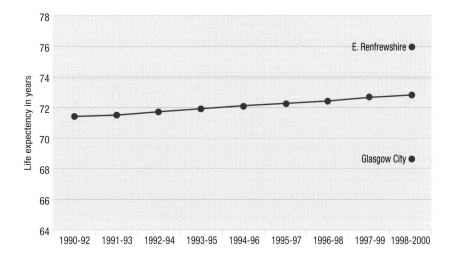

shown, however, that the rate of improvement is currently not rapid enough for Scotland's relative position in this league table to improve.

These figures also demonstrate a feature that will be a recurring theme: inequalities in health within Scotland. For the years 1998–2000, male life expectancy in the 'best' local authority area (East Renfrewshire) was seven years higher than that in the 'worst' (Glasgow City) even though these two areas lie only a few miles apart.

Infant mortality and low birthweight

Although Scotland's overall life expectancy is low compared to much of Europe, death rates in infancy are, comparatively, much better than age-specific death rates in adult life. Figures 2.2a and 2.2b show rates of infant mortality for Scotland compared to Europe in 1999 (figure 2.2a), and as a trend over a 20-year period (figure 2.2b). The first of these figures shows that Scotland, with an infant mortality rate of 5 per 1000 live births in 1999, compares favourably with a large number of European countries. This position has been maintained over a 20-year period as a result of rates more than halving since 1980.

Figure 2.2a Infant mortality: rate per 1000 live births, 1999

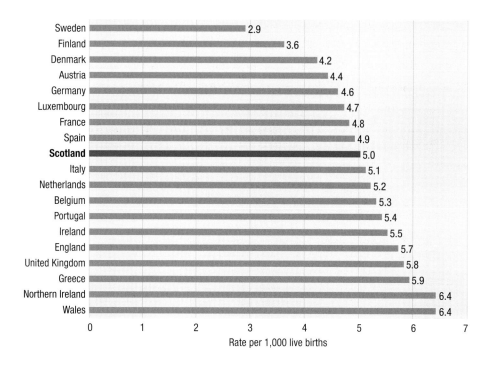

Rate per 1,000 live births

Figure 2.2b Infant mortality: rate per 1000 live births, 3 year rolling averages, 1980–2000

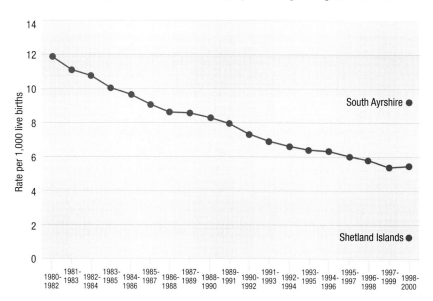

Despite this good news, two issues of concern set this finding in context. First, inequalities in infant mortality persist. The average rate for 1998–2000 for South Ayrshire (9.3 per 1000 live births), for example, is 40% higher than the national figure, and seven times higher than the area with lowest rate, Shetland (1.3 per 1000 live births) – although, given the small number of such events at a local authority level, this measure is liable to considerable fluctuations over short periods. Secondly, although Scotland has been successful in reducing infant deaths, other indices of health in infancy are less favourable. Figure 2.3a shows for 1998 the percentage of all live births which were categorised as being of low birthweight (< 2500 grams). Scotland's position compared to most other

Figure 2.3a Low birthweight births as percentage of all live births, 1998

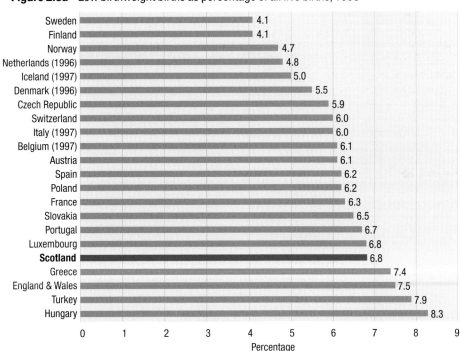

European countries is again poor and the trend (figure 2.3b) appears to suggest a worsening of the situation. This chart also demonstrates the variation in low birthweight births across Scotland. At the end of the period, the proportion of low birthweight births in Glasgow was more than twice that in Shetland: 8.7% compared to 4.1%.

Figure 2.3b   Low birthweight births as percentage of all live births, 3 year rolling averages, Scotland 1980–1998

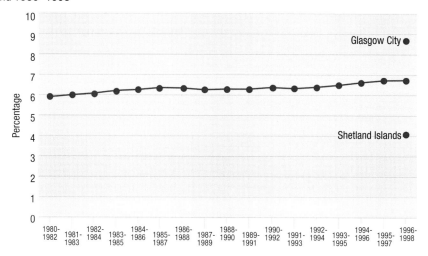

Illness and disease

Figure 2.4a shows age-standardised mortality rates for *cancer* (all malignant neoplasms) for Scotland and a range of European nations in 1997. Of the 22 countries listed, Scotland has the third highest rate for this cause of death. In terms of trends (figure 2.4b), there is evidence of the beginning of a decline in the cancer mortality rate during the last decade. This figure also shows that, at the end of period, Glasgow City again had the highest rates of cancer mortality among Scottish local authority areas.

Figure 2.4a Malignant neoplasms: age-standardised mortality rates per 100,000 population, 1997

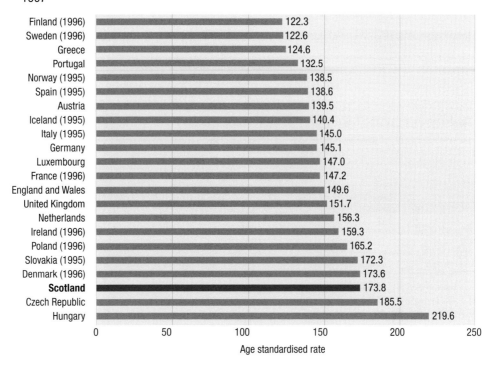

Figure 2.4b Malignant neoplasms: age-standardised mortality rates per 100,000 population, 3 year average, Scotland 1974–2000

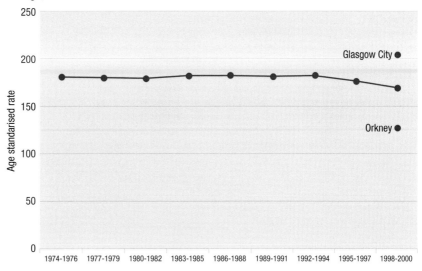

Figures 2.5a and 2.5b show similar data for deaths from *ischaemic heart disease*.
Once more, Scotland fares very badly in comparison with the other European
countries (figure 2.5a). Unlike cancer, however, there has been a marked
improvement over the past 25 years (figure 2.5b), with rates almost halving
between 1974 and 2000. This downward trend has also been observed for deaths
from *strokes* (cerebrovascular disease). The decline in these two causes of death –
given their prevalence over the past 25 years – would account for much of
Scotland's improved life expectancy during this period. Although this is good
news, the rate of decline in heart disease and stroke in most highly industrialised
nations has been as or more rapid: thus, Scotland's relatively poor league table
position remains.[2]

Figure 2.5a Ischaemic heart disease: age-standardised mortality rates per 100,000
population, 1997

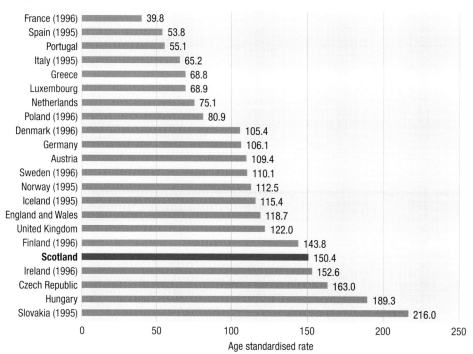

Figure 2.5b Ischaemic heart disease: age-standardised mortality rates per 100,000 population, 3 year averages, Scotland 1974–2000

300
250
200
150
100
50
0
Age standardised rate
Inverclyde
Borders
1974-1976
1977-1979
1980-1982
1983-1985
1986-1988
1989-1991
1992-1994
1995-1997
1998-2000

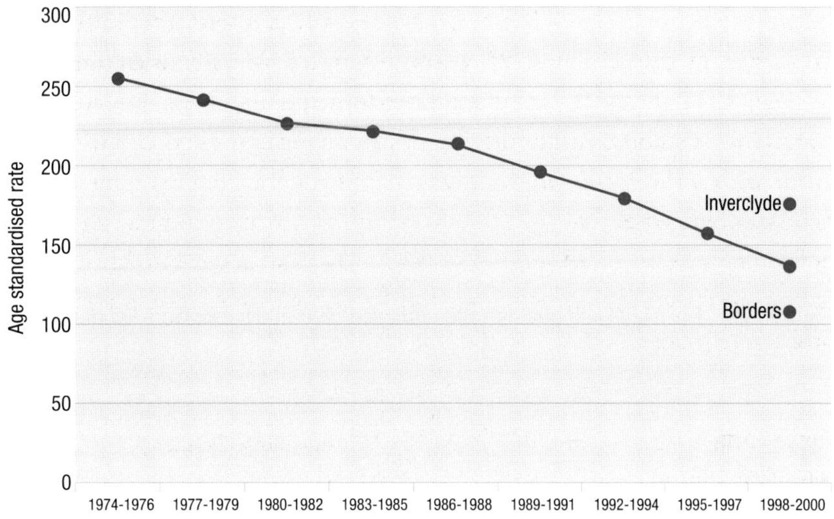

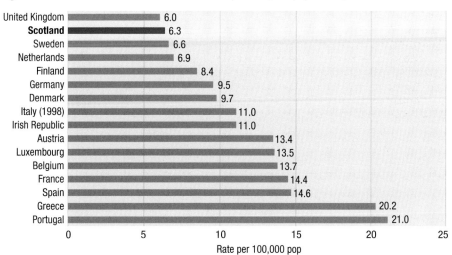

Road accident mortality

By way of contrast, road accident mortality is an area where Scotland compares very favourably with other European nations. As can be seen from figure 2.6a, in 1999 the United Kingdom as a whole had the lowest rates of road accident mortality in the European Union – 6.0 per 100 000 population – and the figure

Figure 2.6a Road accident deaths: crude rates per 100,000 population, 1999

United Kingdom 6.0
Scotland 6.3
Sweden 6.6
Netherlands 6.9
Finland 8.4
Germany 9.5
Denmark 9.7
Italy (1998) 11.0
Irish Republic 11.0
Austria 13.4
Luxembourg 13.5
Belgium 13.7
France 14.4
Spain 14.6
Greece 20.2
Portugal 21.0
0
5
10
15
20
25
Rate per 100,000 pop

for Scotland that year (6.3 per 100 000) is only marginally higher. The trend over a 12-year period (figure 2.6b) has been generally downward, particularly between 1989 and 1994, when rates fell from 11.1 to 7.0, a reduction of almost 40%. Rates vary considerably across the country, however, with rural areas such as Borders, Highland, Orkney, and Dumfries and Galloway showing the highest rates. Indeed, the average rate for Borders between 1996–2000 was, at 15.2, twice the national rate and five times the rate of the area with the lowest figure, East Dunbartonshire.

Figure 2.6b   Road accident deaths: crude rates per 100,000 population, Scotland 1989–2000

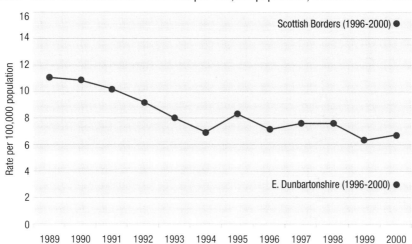

Mental health

This is a domain for which there are currently relatively few indicators that can be used to describe Scotland's position adequately. Figure 2.7a shows age-standardised death rates per 100 000 population for *suicide and deliberate self-harm* in 1997. Although death rates from this type of cause in Scotland are far from the highest in Europe, two points should be noted. First, suicide is the leading cause of death among men aged 15–34 years in Scotland. Secondly, as is illustrated in figure 2.7b, the trend is upwards, with a 50% rise between 1974 and 2000. In addition, between 1998 and 2000, Dundee City had the highest suicide rate, with a figure seven times that of the area with the lowest rate, the Western Isles (Eilean Siar) – although, as with infant mortality, the relatively small number of such events at a local authority level should be borne in mind.

Figure 2.7a Suicide/self-inflicted injury: age-standardised death rates per 100,000 population, 1997

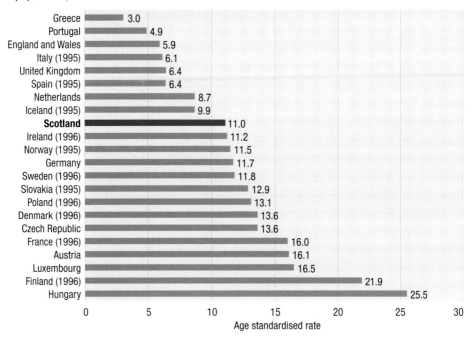

Figure 2.7b Suicide/self-inflicted injury: age-standardised mortality rates per 100,000 population, 3 year averages, Scotland, 1974–2000

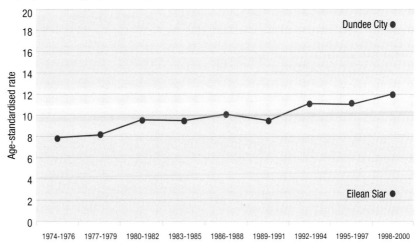

Life circumstances

The fact that life circumstances influence health has been recognised in recent policy documents.[3] Again, only a few of a large number of indicators are presented here, but those shown reflect the general pattern. The first of these is the proportion of all households that are *lone parent households*. Unfortunately, comparative European data are not easily obtainable for this particular indicator. However, in 2001 the figure for Scotland was 6.6%, slightly higher than the figure for both England (6.0%) and Wales (6.0%), and projections (figure 2.8) show that this figure is likely to rise to about 8% in 10 years' time. These projections also show the large difference between the 'highest' and 'lowest' local authority areas: predicted figures of 13% of households in Glasgow compared to 3% in Orkney.

Figure 2.8 Lone parent households as percentage of all households: projections for Scotland 1998–2012

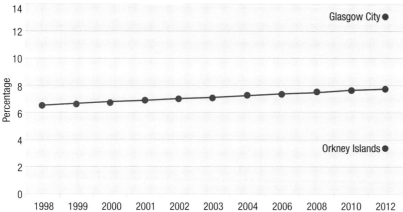

Figure 2.9a shows, for a more limited set of European countries, the estimated percentage of the population who were a victim of one (or more) of a number of crimes* in 1999. The figures range from 15% (Portugal, Northern Ireland) to 26% (England & Wales), with Scotland set in the lower half of the table with 23%. In terms of all reported crimes, figure 2.9b shows the rate per 10 000 population in

* Car theft, burglary, robbery, motorcycle theft, assault, sexual offences, personal theft, attempted burglary, bicycle theft, theft from a vehicle, car vandalism.

Figure 2.9a Victimisation Risk: percentage of people victimised once or more in the previous year by any of 11 crimes, 1999

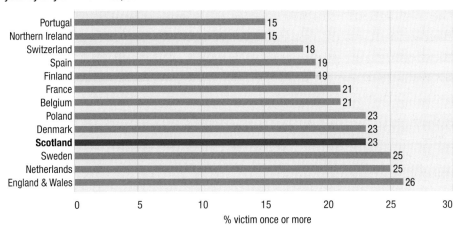

% victim once or more

Figure 2.9b Number of Crimes Recorded by the Police by 100,000 population, 1992–2001

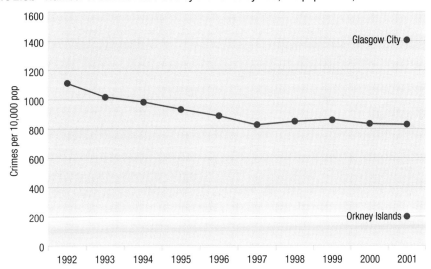

Scotland between 1992 and 2001. The trend has generally been downward although there is evidence of stabilisation in the rate from 1997 onwards. The figure also illustrates, yet again, the large differences between local authority areas: in 2001 the crime rate of Glasgow City was seven times higher than that of Orkney.

Figure 2.10a shows, again for a slightly more limited number of European countries, the proportion of the total population that is deemed to be living in 'low income' households.[†] With 20% of the Scottish population falling into this category in 1996–1997, Scotland again compares badly with the other nations for which data are available. Two further points are worth noting. First, although not shown here, this figure has remained fairly constant over the past seven or

Figure 2.10a Low income: percentage of population living in low income households, 1996

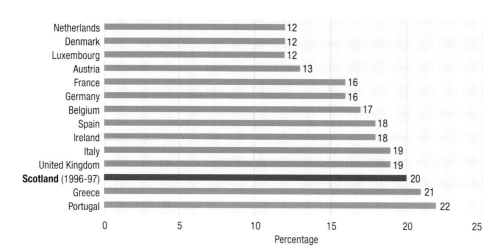

eight years. Secondly, although data are not available at a local authority level, this measure *can* be broken down for different sections of the population (figure 2.10b). In 2000–01, one in four children (25%) and one in five (20%) pensioners were living in a low income household.

Figure 2.11a shows the International Labour Organisation (ILO) estimate of *unemployment* for a range of countries in 1999. For reasons of comparability, this is expressed as a percentage of the total population of each country which, although not an ideal way in which to analyse such data, does at least give an indication of Scotland's position compared to the other nations. Again, Scotland is in the lower half of the league table. An alternative measure of unemployment, the number of actual claimants expressed as a proportion of the

---

[†] Definition: Percentage of population living in households with an income (before housing costs) of less than 60% of the country's median income in that year.

Figure 2.10b Low income: percentage of population living in low income households, Scotland 1994–2001

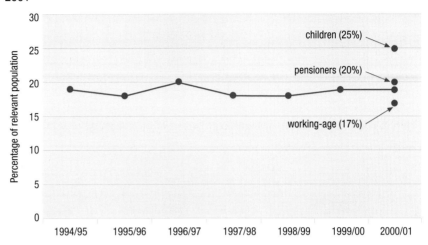

Figure 2.11a Unemployment: ILO estimate expressed as percentage of total population, 1999

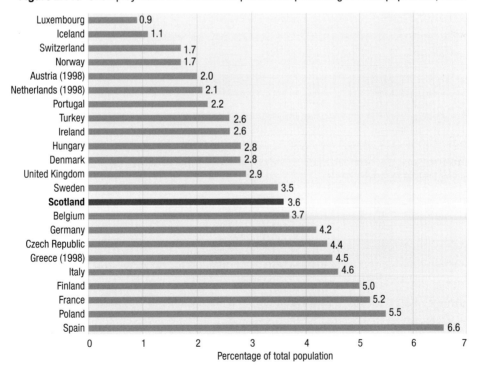

working age population, is shown for Scotland in figure 2.11b for a six-year period between 1996–2001. What is apparent from this is that, although claimant unemployment has fallen considerably over this period, inequalities are again evident within the country: the local authority area with the highest rate of unemployment, Dundee City, has almost five times the rate of the area with the lowest rate, Aberdeenshire.

Figure 2.11b Unemployment: claimant count expressed as percentage of working-age population, Scotland 1996–2001

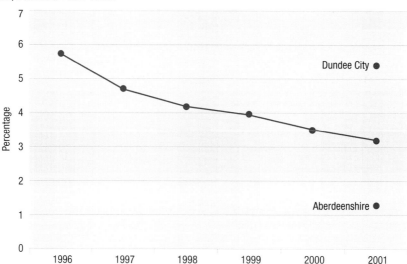

Self-perceived health

Much of the evidence presented in this chapter depicts a rather gloomy picture of Scotland's health. Interestingly, however, it would appear that most Scots perceive their own health to be good. Figure 2.12 shows the percentage of the population who, in surveys, reported their health as being 'good' or better. At 77%, the figure for Scotland is higher than many countries which have superior health records for a range of indicators – for example, Spain, Germany, Italy, Finland. Although not shown here, analysis within Scotland (based on a slightly different question on self-assessed health from the Scottish Household Survey) suggests that this is true throughout the country. The area with the highest percentage of adults rating their health as 'good' or 'fairly good' is the Shetland Islands (94%); however, the figure for the 'lowest' area – Glasgow City – is also very high: 79%.

Figure 2.12   Self-perceived Health Status of Adults: percentage of population aged 15 years or over reporting their health to be 'good' or better

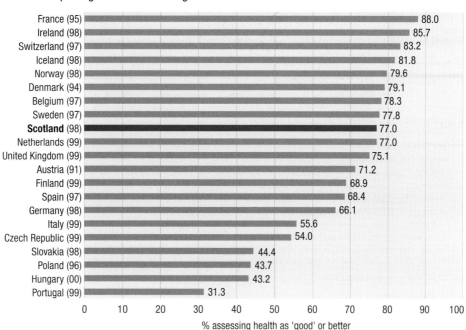

% assessing health as 'good' or better

Behaviour

Figure 2.13a shows the percentage of the female population (aged 15+ years) who are daily smokers. As these results are derived from different surveys (involving different methodologies, questions, sample sizes and structures), one must obviously exercise great caution in making direct comparisons between countries. Nonetheless, it is apparent that Scotland has a high proportion of smokers compared to other European countries. That said, the general trend for smoking – at least until the mid 1990s – has been downwards (figure 2.13b). But with 30% of all adults still smoking in 1999–2000 (the same as in 1994), and with some evidence that the downward trend in smoking prevalence has halted, there are clearly no grounds for complacency.

Figure 2.13a Percentage of Female population aged 15 years and over who are Daily Smokers

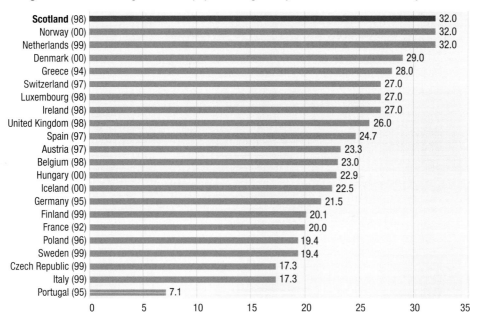

Figure 2.13b Percentage of Adults (16+) Smoking in Scotland, 1978–2000

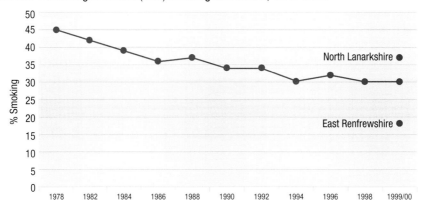

Figure 2.14 shows the percentage of the female population (aged 15 years or over) categorised as 'obese'.[§] Again, different survey methodologies – together with the different years of data which are available for different countries – make direct comparisons problematic, but the underlying picture is apparent:

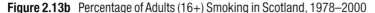

[§] Obesity defined as having body mass index (BMI) of 30 or greater.

Figure 2.14   Percentage of Female Population (15+) that are Obese (BMI > 30)

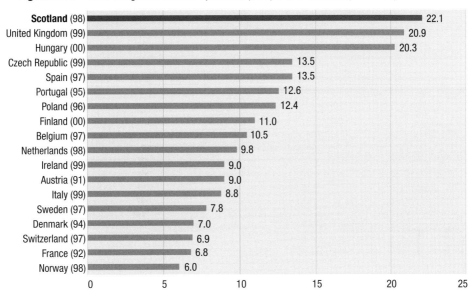

Scotland has a very high rate of obesity, and this has obvious implications for health. Accurate trend data for Scotland are not readily available, but the indications are that the problem is worsening. Data from two years of the Scottish Health Survey (1995 and 1998) have shown a rise in adult obesity in both males and females: from 16.1% to 18.8% for males, and from 17.4% to 20.9% for females.

Health of children

Much of what has already been discussed in this chapter gives a picture of children's health in Scotland: for example, infant mortality, low birthweight, road accidents, life circumstances. A range of other indicators could be used to illustrate further the health of children in Scotland, but just two have been chosen as they highlight important issues: dental health and immunisation.

Figure 2.15 shows the percentage of 5-year-old children free from dental caries in Scotland between 1987 and 2000. There has not been much variation over the period, although there has at least been some improvement in the last five to six years – from 38% in1993–1994 to 45% in 1999–2000. This, however, is still well short of the national target of 60% by the year 2010.

Figure 2.15   Percentage of 5 year-olds free from dental caries, Scotland, 1987–2000

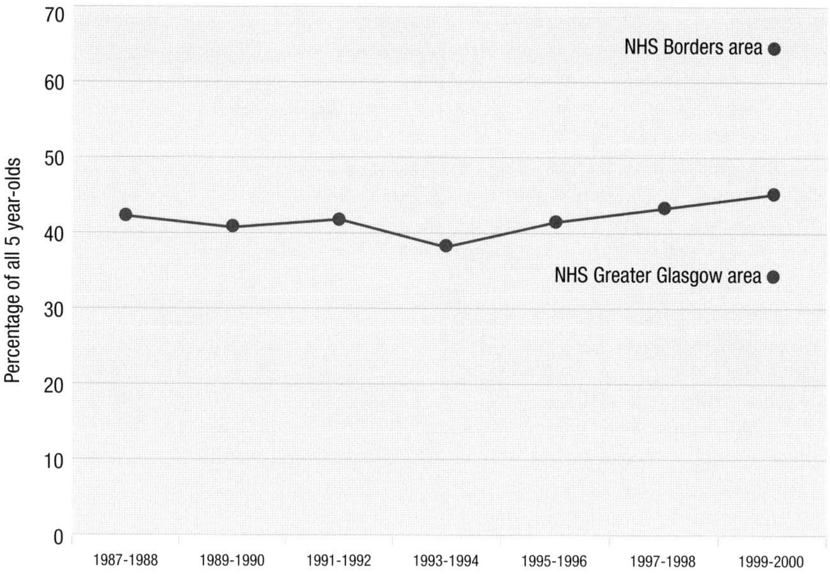

Within Scotland, currently only one NHS board area – Borders – has already achieved this target (65% in 1999–2000), although others – for example, Shetland and Grampian (not graphed) – are very close. At the other end of the scale, NHS Greater Glasgow area has the lowest proportion: just 34% of 5-year-olds were dental caries free in the last year for which data are available. Thus, there is a 30% difference between the 'best' and 'worst' areas of the country with regard to this health indicator, and as such it is a further graphic illustration of Scotland's inequalities in health.

Immunisation rates make an interesting contrast. Generally, the uptake rate for most childhood vaccinations in Scotland has, since the mid 1990s, consistently stood at around 97% at 2 years of age. As such, it illustrates how, with effort, the health service can overcome the gradient normally associated with deprivation. Figure 2.16, however, shows the uptake rate for the mumps, measles and rubella (MMR) vaccine. It shows that the average annual rate in Scotland of approximately 93% uptake dropped sharply in 2002 to 86%. The on-going public debate regarding the safety of this vaccine is clearly behind this decrease, and it is reflected in all NHS board areas of the country. Within Scotland, the NHS board area with the lowest uptake in 2002 was Highland (79.5%), while Dumfries and Galloway achieved the highest uptake: 93%.

Figure 2.16   Immunisation uptake rate for MMR at 2 years old, Scotland 1993–2002

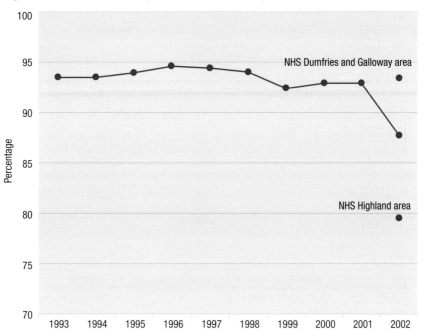

Communicable Disease

Historically, communicable and infectious diseases have been associated in Scotland, as elsewhere, with threats to the health of the population on a large scale: the outbreaks of typhoid and cholera in the middle of the 19th century are an obvious example. In more recent times, however, improved living standards, medical advances and effective public health preventative measures have meant that the proportion of the Scottish population affected by this category of disease has diminished to relatively small levels. Over this period there has been a change in emphasis towards major chronic diseases such as heart disease, cancer and stroke. This general decrease in risk to the population from infection can be viewed as a public health success story. An interesting, more recent example is measles. As recently as 1970 the total number of measles notifications was almost 25 000. In 2001, the figure was little over 300.

The fact that such a relatively small proportion of today's population is affected by communicable diseases is perhaps sometimes lost amid the widespread coverage given to some of these conditions in the media. With that in mind, it is worthwhile considering a small number of these conditions which have been placed firmly in the media spotlight in recent years: two longstanding conditions – *E. coli* and salmonella – and two newer diseases, new variant Creutzfeldt-Jakob disease (vCJD) and HIV/AIDS.

E. Coli 0157

The *E. coli* outbreak in Lanarkshire in 1996 has been well documented, with subsequent, smaller outbreaks the focus for further media attention. Recent figures, however, show that the number of confirmed *E. coli* cases in Scotland is still relatively small. As can be seen from Figure 2.17, between 1992 and 2000 the number rose from 115 cases at the beginning of the period to just over 500 in 1996 (around half of which were attributable to the Lanarkshire outbreak), before falling again in recent years to less than 200 in the year 2000 – a figure equating to less than four cases per 100 000 total population.

Figure 2.17   Laboratory-confirmed cases of E. Coli 0157, Scotland, 1992–2000

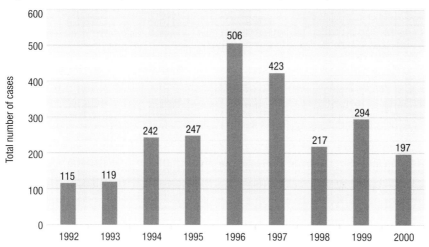

Salmonella

The confirmed number of salmonella infections in Scotland over a similar time period has been considerably larger, peaking in 1997 at almost 3500 (Figure 2.18). Since then, however, the numbers have dropped sharply, down to less than 1800 in the year 2000, with provisional, unconfirmed data for 2001 (not graphed) suggesting that the number of infections has decreased further to approximately 1500 (or less than 30 per 100 000 population) – a reduction of more than one-third from the 1991 level.

Figure 2.18   Laboratory-confirmed cases of Salmonella, Scotland, 1991–2000

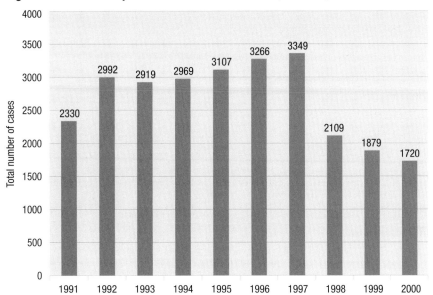

vCJD

The current level of confirmed vCJD cases is extremely small. Although specific Scottish figures are not available, the total for the United Kingdom has not surpassed 30 cases per year since it was first recorded in 1995. In the most recent year for which data are available – 2001 – the number of confirmed cases was 20. This, however, is not to underestimate possible future increases in the incidence of this condition, given the potentially lengthy, although much debated, incubation period of the disease.

HIV/AIDS

Figure 2.19 shows the numbers of new HIV infections, AIDS registrations and HIV/AIDS related deaths between 1990 and 2001.

As a result of HIV infected individuals surviving longer, the chart shows that while the number of new HIV infections has risen since 1991 (a 22% increase from 140 in that year to 171 in 2001), both the number of people diagnosed with AIDS and the number of HIV/AIDS related deaths have fallen sharply over the period: a 27% drop in the former (from 63 to 46), and a 53% decrease in deaths (from 74 to 35).

Figure 2.19 New HIV infections, AIDs registrations and HIV/AIDs deaths in Scotland, 1990–2001

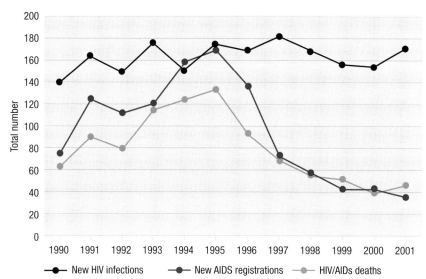

Despite this, however, public health challenges remain in relation to this condition. Figure 2.20, for example, shows that of new HIV infected individuals, an increasingly large proportion are heterosexuals (as opposed to injecting drug users and homosexual/bisexual men). This may suggest increasing apathy towards the 'safe sex' message in this largest at risk group.

This selected review of infection has shown that, in general, a relatively small proportion of the population is affected by communicable diseases in this country, especially when compared to the major chronic conditions such as heart disease. That is not, however, a reason for complacency. New challenges will present themselves – for example, the issue of hospital acquired infections – while particular subgroups of the population will always be at greater risk and, therefore, require specific targeting of effort and resources – for example, the elderly, drug users, young sexually active.

There is a clear need, therefore, for the maintenance and development of the prevention programmes and surveillance systems which are currently in place to ensure continued success in this field.

Figure 2.20   HIV infections by exposure category and year, Scotland 1990–2001

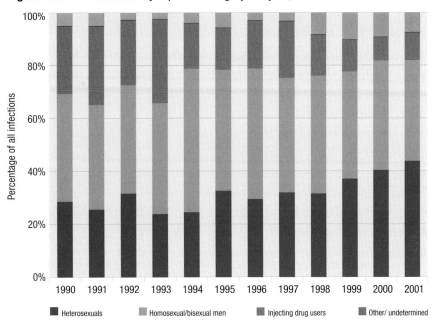

Discussion

The data presented show quite clearly that, despite improvements in recent decades, Scotland's health status and key determinants of health lag behind comparable countries in Northern and Western Europe. In addition, it is recognised that Scotland has the worst health in the United Kingdom, worse even than comparable regions like the industrial North-East of England.[4] Unfortunately, projected trends suggest that Scotland is unlikely to change its relative position.

It is likely that the reasons for Scotland's poor health arise from a large number of effects operating across the whole life course. Three examples illustrate this. First, factors that adversely affect birthweight create influences that manifest themselves years later as chronic disease in middle age.[5] Secondly, behaviours, habits and skills acquired during childhood and early adolescence have a profound influence on educational outcomes, job prospects and levels of disease later in life.[6] Thirdly, lifestyles in middle life have an effect on rates of chronic diseases, such as heart disease, cancer and diabetes, in older age.

The importance of the distribution of wealth as a determinant of health has emerged in recent years.[7] The mechanism that explains these observations is the subject of debate but the observation is not questioned. The gradient of health inequalities within Scotland is sharper than elsewhere in Great Britain.[2] Today we see cities like Edinburgh, which are fully integrated into the international economic system, groan under the benefits of tourism, investment and inward migration, while the formerly industrial centres struggle to keep their population and services at a viable level.

The situation is complex, however, and Scotland's health problems cannot be fully explained by economics alone. Although the former Strathclyde region has the worst health in Scotland, for example, the health divide between Scotland and England affects nearly all the Scottish regions.[2] It is also true that the proportion of the health gap between the two countries that can be explained by 'deprivation' (or at least the census variables that act as proxies for deprivation) has decreased in recent decades.[2] We need to understand these 'non economic' or cultural factors. Scottish culture and society has been changing rapidly. The structures which formerly played a key role in integrating individuals into larger social processes (unions, churches, professions, political parties) have all suffered loss such that in half a lifetime they have all but vanished (the maximum level of employment in manufacturing was reached in 1969, the maximum membership of the Church of Scotland in 1957). Because self-confidence and individual identity are social products, they suffer when group and community features such as family solidarity, educational stability and social integration are eroded. Many people in Scotland lack confidence in their ability to control their own lives and destiny. This expresses itself in many ways including a variety of behaviours, such as smoking, drinking, work patterns, eating patterns, relationships, that are damaging to health.

Disruptions, analogous to the social changes we have seen in Scotland in the past 50 years, have occurred before. At the beginning of the industrial revolution, alcohol consumption, crime and illegitimacy – to quote just three indices – were substantially higher in most UK cities than they are today.[8] What emerged in that period was a reaction to the social disorder that accompanied the upheavals brought about by the industrial revolution. Victorian society deliberately sought to create institutions and instil values that would create order. Thus, in time, emerged co-operative societies, modern police forces, health visitors, universal education, orphanages and much else. These were supported by grass roots efforts to create and sustain a whole series of informal norms and behaviours that in their time were important for social cohesion. The fact that these eventually became outmoded and now often seem illiberal to our modern eyes does not mean that they were not important in their time.

From this logic it is clear that the health of the people of Scotland will improve as new societal structures develop to meet the needs of the emerging future. The paradox, however, is that this process cannot be *managed* into existence. The role of leadership is to capture the emerging vision of Scotland and facilitate its creation. Public health advocates have a clear interest in the success of this project.

Summary of the argument

- Scotland has poor health by UK and EU standards

- Poverty and inequalities in wealth and power are crucial features of the problem

- There are also cultural influences on health that have to be confronted

- Health improvement requires societal change

- The lesson of history is that societies can adapt to meet new threats and challenges

From this the diagnosis of Scotland's health problems at the beginning of the 21st century is clear. There is also convincing evidence that the spectrum of interventions is proving successful in our attempts to combat many of these issues. Our rate of progress in improving health in Scotland, however, is not sufficient to improve our position relative to our UK and European counterparts. As a consequence, the Scottish Executive in 2003 is launching an integrated action plan for health improvement which pulls together the efforts of the whole programme for government as well as several health improvement programmes in an attempt to achieve the required step change in Scotland's health.

REFERENCES

1. Kuh D, Ben-Shlomo Y. (eds.) *A Life Course approach to Chronic Disease Epidemiology*. Oxford:Oxford Medical Publications, 1997.

2. Hanlon P *et al. Chasing The Scottish Effect – Why Scotland needs a step-change in health if it is to catch up with the rest of Europe*. Glasgow: Public Health Institute Of Scotland, 2001.

3. The Scottish Office Department of Health. *Towards a Healthier Scotland*. Edinburgh: The Stationery Office, 1998.

4. Fitzpatrick J, Griffiths C, Kelleher M, *Geographic Inequalities in Mortality in the United Kingdom during the 1990s*. London: ONS Health Statistics Quarterly 07, Autumn 2000.

5. Barker DJP. (ed). *Fetal and infant origins of adult disease*. London: BMJ Publications Group, 1992.

6. Goleman D. *Emotional Intelligence*. London: Bloomsbury,1995.

7. Wilkinson RG. *Unhealthy Societies*. London: Routledge, 1996.

8. Fukuyama F. *The Great Disruption*. New York: Touchstone. 1999.

Data descriptions and sources

Figures	Description	Sources
2.1a, 2.1b	Male life expectancy at birth	OECD Health Data 2001; General Register Office for Scotland (GRO(S)); Office for National Statistics (ONS)
2.2a, 2.2b	Infant mortality: deaths of children under the age of 1 year expressed as a rate per 1000 live births in the same year	ONS; GRO(S)
2.3a, 2.3b	Low birthweight births: live births with a weight of less than 2500g expressed as proportion of all live births in the same year	OECD Health Data 2001; Information & Statistics Division (ISD) SMR2/SMR02 data
2.4a, 2.4b	Age-standardised mortality rates (standardised directly to WHO world population) for malignant neoplasms	World Health Organisation (WHO); GRO(S)

Figures	Description	Sources
2.5a, 2.5b	Age-standardised mortality rates (standardised directly to WHO world population) for ischaemic heart disease	WHO; GRO(S)
2.6a, 2.6b	Road accident deaths expressed as crude rates per 100 000 population	ONS; GRO(S)
2.7a, 2.7b	Age-standardised mortality rates (standardised directly to WHO world population) for suicide/deliberate self-harm	WHO; GRO(S)
2.8	Lone parent households expressed as percentage of all households	Scottish Executive
2.9a	Crime: victimisation risk – percentage of those surveyed who had been victimised once or more in the previous year by any of the 11 crimes covered by the survey – that is, car theft, burglary, robbery, motorcycle theft, assault, sexual offences, personal theft, attempted burglary, bicycle theft, theft from a vehicle, car vandalism.	International Crime Victims Survey 2000
2.9b	Crime: number of crimes recorded by the police per 10 000 population	Scottish Executive
2.10a, 2.10b	Percentage of population living in households with an income (beforehousing costs) less than 60% of the country's median income	Eurostat; Department of Work & Pensions' (DWP) Households Below Average Income (HBAI) data set; Scottish Executive (SE)

Figures	Description	Sources
2.11a	International Labour Organisation (ILO) estimate of number of unemployed expressed as percentage of total population;	OECD Health Data 2001; SE Scottish Economic Statistics 2002;
2.11b	Unemployment claimant count expressed as percentage of working age (15–64 years) population	NOMIS
2.12	Self-perceived Health Status of Adults: % of population aged 15 years or over reporting their health to be 'good' or better	OECD Health Data 2001; Scottish Health Survey; (SHS);
2.13a	Smoking: % of female population aged 15 years and over who are daily smokers;	OECD Health Data 2001; Scottish Health Survey; General Household Survey;
2.13b	Smoking: % adults smoking in Scotland aged 16 years and over	Scottish Health Survey; Scottish Household Survey
2.14	Obesity: % of female population that are obese (BMI over 30, aged 15 years+)	OECD Health Data 2001; Scottish Health Survey
2.15	Percentage of 5-year-olds free from dental caries	ISD (SKIPPER)
2.16	Immunisation uptake rate for MMR at 2 years old	ISD (SKIPPER)
2.17	Laboratory-confirmed cases of *E. coli* 0157	Scottish Centre for Infection and Environmental Health (SCIEH)

3. Promoting Health in Scotland

Andrew Tannahill

Introduction

This chapter traces the development of national policy, strategy and priorities for the promotion of health in Scotland, and discusses the roles and contributions of various players at national, local and international levels. The work of the Health Education Board for Scotland is considered in some depth, and the chapter concludes by identifying issues and challenges for evaluation and delivery in the times ahead.

National policy, strategy and priorities

The first national policy statement dedicated to the promotion of health in Scotland was *Health Education in Scotland*,[1] published in March 1991 by The Scottish Office. The most immediate tangible outcome of the policy statement was the creation of a special health board – the Health Education Board for Scotland (HEBS) – to replace the Scottish Health Education Group (SHEG) as the national agency for health education. *Health Education in Scotland* recognised the promotion of good health as a focus for the whole spectrum of Scottish Office responsibilities, and set out roles of The Scottish Office Home and Health Department, HEBS, health boards, local authorities, voluntary organisations, employers, the mass media, and the public. Its declared intention was 'to stimulate a wide-ranging and concerted effort to create a healthy Scotland'. Another policy statement, *Scotland's Health: A Challenge to Us All*, followed in 1992,[2] and referred to a new priority within the NHS – improving health in addition to health care. At the same time, it emphasised the contributions to be made across government functions and departments, and placed a more explicit emphasis on environmental influences on health. 'Variations' in health relating to socioeconomic status and wealth were acknowledged. A number of initiatives were presented, including:

- creation of an interdepartmental group on health strategy, chaired by the Chief Medical Officer, to co-ordinate health-related activities across the range of Scottish Office responsibilities

- commissioning of a group of experts to make dietary recommendations and detail the dietary changes that were needed, leading to the setting of Scottish dietary targets[3]

- drawing up of a national dental strategy for Scotland (subsequently produced as an oral health strategy[4])

- establishment of a Scottish health survey, to measure and report on the health of the population, examine lifestyle, and monitor changes over time

Scotland's Health: A Challenge to Us All became an umbrella heading for a succession of initiatives and documents, the first example of a uniting slogan for various strands of central government strategy and action for better health in Scotland.

The change in UK government in 1997 prompted a review of health improvement policy and strategy. In February 1998, a consultation document entitled *Working Together for a Healthier Scotland*[5] was issued. This received a favourable response and was taken forward through the subsequent White Paper, *Towards a Healthier Scotland*,[6] published in February 1999. Key features included:

- identification of tackling inequalities in health as the overarching aim and priority

- co-ordinated three-level approach, with action on life circumstances, lifestyles and health topics

- new set of national priorities (see Table 3.1).

TABLE 3.1 National priorities for Scotland's health, 1999

Overarching priority: tackling inequalities

Priorities by action level

Improved life circumstances*	_Lifestyles_	_Health topics_
	• Less smoking, drug misuse and alcohol misuse	• Child health
		• Dental and oral health
	• A healthier diet	• Sexual health, including teenage pregnancies and sexually transmitted diseases
	• More physical activity	
		• Coronary heart disease (and stroke)
		• Cancer
		• Mental health
		• Accidents and safety

*Life circumstances include, for example, the general environment, unemployment, poverty, poor housing

The metaphor of a jigsaw was used to convey the multiple interlocking pieces of effort needed to achieve a healthier Scotland. As well as setting out an array of new developments, the White Paper drew together a host of existing initiatives across many aspects of Scottish life. A sustained programme of associated social and economic change was seen as central to improving health, with social inclusion as an important banner for strategy and action. Education, not just health education, was acknowledged as contributing to health prospects, while the creation of new community schools would 'offer children and their families integrated education, social work, family support, and health education and promotion services'.

The list of lifestyle priorities in the Health White Paper (Table 3.1) was very similar to that in *Scotland's Health: A Challenge to Us All*, but there were some significant differences. A major new focus for action was child health. The attention in this regard was not only on health in earlier life but also on investment in health in the longer term, acknowledging the evidence that childhood experiences, exposures and learned behaviours affect health in adulthood. The addition of mental health and stroke reflected their inclusion in the list of NHS clinical priorities. The replacement of HIV and AIDS by sexual health was prompted by concerns over incidence rates of sexually transmitted infections more widely, and teenage pregnancy. The broadening out of accidents to accidents and safety marked both a widening of concern to include non-accidental injury and the incorporation of the 'positive health' dimension of actively cultivating safe environments and behaviours. The previous priority of exercise became physical activity, in the light of accumulated evidence that even moderate physical activity is good for health in a number of important ways.

New targets for health and health-related behaviour were presented. In the spirit of 'putting the jigsaw together' and giving momentum to delivery of the White Paper's vision, action relating to a range of agencies and community settings was set out. Four flagship health demonstration projects were announced, concerned respectively with: early childhood (*Starting Well*); sexual health among young people (*Healthy Respect*); prevention of heart disease (*The Heart of Scotland* – which subsequently took shape as *Have a Heart Paisley*); and colorectal cancer (*Cancer Challenge*).

In autumn 1998, the Minister for Health commissioned from the Chief Medical Officer a review of the public health function in Scotland. The remit was 'to re-assess the role, relationships and locus of public health medicine and public health dentistry to ensure the optimal use of all available resources in the drive to safeguard and improve Scotland's health'. The review report[7] was published in December 1999. From the perspective of promoting health, significant outcomes of the review included the establishment of the Public Health Institute of Scotland (PHIS), and the attention given to the development of health boards as public health organisations. The latter area was taken further through Scottish Executive Health Department guidance on the role of NHS boards in improving health (January 2002), and through the Scottish Directors of Public Health Group and PHIS joint report on NHS boards as public health organisations (April 2002).[8]

The Chief Medical Officer's review stressed the multidisciplinary and multiagency nature of public health. Another important outcome was the creation of a full-time public health post within the Convention of Scottish Local Authorities (COSLA). This has provided a national focal point for developing the public health role and capacity of councils. COSLA has produced reports on local authorities as public health organisations and, with the Scottish Executive, has provided guidance for community planning partnerships on preparing joint health improvement plans.

The review of the public health function was complemented by a review led by the Chief Nursing Officer, the report of which (*Nursing for Health* [9]) appeared in March 2001, with 77 recommendations. Among these were the introduction of public health practitioners based in local health care co-operatives (LHCCs), and the establishment of public health nursing (bringing together health visiting and school nursing) with fresh thinking being given to how best it can contribute to health improvement.

Months before the CMO's review report was published, the Scottish Parliament came into being. One of its early debates, in September 1999, resulted in endorsement of the White Paper as the foundation for action to improve the health of the people of Scotland, thus providing valuable continuity of momentum. Early in its existence, the Scottish Executive committed itself to build a 'Health Promotion Fund'. Details of this were announced in March 2000, in the context of a programme to 'wage war on ill health' using a £26m Scottish share of one year's hypothecated UK tobacco tax. On implementation it was renamed the Health Improvement Fund. *Working Together for Scotland: A Programme for Government* [10] indicated that the Health Improvement Fund would invest more than £100m over four years, and gave commitments to: encourage every school to become a health promoting school; provide fresh fruit in nursery schools; provide free toothbrushes and toothpaste for 100 000 children in Scotland; and develop a strategy to tackle alcohol misuse.

In December 2000, the Scottish Executive captured its strategy for health in post-devolution Scotland in *Our National Health: A Plan for Action, a Plan for Change.* [11] This plan presented itself as 'a shift from the development of policy to the delivery of change'. It reinforced the established vision of a concerted national effort to improve health and reduce health inequalities. The NHS was seen as having an important part to play in this, working in partnership with other agencies, with communities, with patients and with the public at large. A commitment was given to making the NHS truly a national *health* rather than a national *illness* service. Emphasis was placed on linking local health plans to community planning processes co-ordinated by local authorities, who would be helped to become public health organisations.

Our National Health described a number of specific developments for health improvement, some already in train, others new. These included:

- deployment of the Health Improvement Fund

- establishment of a national health promoting schools unit

- investment in the *Scotland's Health at Work* health promoting workplace award scheme

- appointment of a national co-ordinator to give a new drive to putting the Scottish diet action plan[12] into practice

- launch of the Physical Activity Task Force[13]

- implementation of the action plan for dental services in Scotland,[14] including free toothbrushes and toothpaste for young children

- rollout of best practice in the provision of smoking cessation services

- development of a plan of action on alcohol misuse (subsequently produced as *The Plan for Action on Alcohol Problems*[15])

- a new package of expenditure on drugs misuse

- increased resources for tackling sexually transmitted and blood-borne infections.

The focus of attention in the evolving national policy has progressively broadened out. In summary, there has been a widening of the vision of:

- health – to encompass wellbeing, fitness and quality of life, not just ill-health; and paying more attention to social and mental dimensions alongside the physical

- determinants of health – including life circumstances as well as lifestyles, with an increased emphasis on tackling inequalities

- action to improve or promote health – including policies relating to specific health or behavioural issues, such as tobacco fiscal policy; and, more fundamentally, action to promote social inclusion[16] and social justice[17,18]

- people and agencies seen as having parts to play, in partnership – within the NHS, health care as well as health promotion; beyond the NHS, organisations in all sectors; and with the public and communities actively involved.

These trends have been accompanied by a changing vocabulary. 'Health education' was largely superseded by 'health promotion' in the early 1990s. Other terms have waxed and waned since then. 'Health gain' received some currency in the middle years of the decade and is still used to an extent, mainly with regard to quantifying improvements in health through particular interventions. More recently, 'health development' has emerged – for example, in the name and role of the Health Development Agency in England (which replaced the Health Education Authority) and within the World Health Organisation (WHO) HEALTH21 strategy.[19] That term chimes with the notion of developing capacity, in and across all sectors of society, for the promotion of health, and with the drawing of a parallel between health promotion and organisational development. Also there has been a resurgence of the term 'public health', in association with 'health improvement'. These two terms, used singly or together, have begun to eclipse 'health promotion', and some confusion has arisen. Health improvement is *not* a synonym for health promotion: rather, it is the *goal* of health promotion – and should be the goal of health care services. Health promotion can be viewed as a function within the public health function, with public health additionally having parts to play in improving the health outcomes of health care. Amid the linguistic imprecision, the term health promotion has shown some signs of falling into disuse but it still usefully delineates a particular realm of activity and set of competencies within the wider health improvement and public health drive.

At the time of writing, a new 'Health Improvement Challenge' publication from the Scottish Executive is anticipated. This is expected to set health improvement efforts in the context of four themes: early years, teenage transition, workplace and community.

Health Education Board for Scotland

The Health Education Board for Scotland (HEBS) came into being on 1 April 1991, replacing the Scottish Health Education Group (SHEG) which had been formed in 1980 through merger of the Scottish Council for Health Education (founded in 1943) and the Scottish Health Education Unit (established in 1968). SHEG had built up a reputation as an innovator in social marketing, working hand in hand with advertising agencies and social marketing researchers to produce memorable health education advertising on television, in the cinema, and using other mass media and sponsorship of sporting competitions and events. It developed an overarching campaign theme *Be All You Can Be* which covered advertisements on specific topics such as smoking and alcohol. The *Be All You Can Be* slogan became very well known in Scotland, and continued to be cited by the public in health education market research long after it had ceased to be used. SHEG was also known for pioneering work in a number of other areas, including the international development of the health promoting school concept, and training for health professionals and others.

An important early task for HEBS was to decide how it could best use its resources to play its part in addressing the national priorities and targets set out in *Health Education in Scotland*. An important driver was the need to enhance collaboration with other partners, a consideration which informed the development of its strategic plans.[20, 21]

Arena-centred approach to programmes

A distinctive aspect of the strategy HEBS adopted was to centre programmes on 'arenas' for health education/promotion. This involved combining a co-ordinated and strategic general public programme, using high-profile mass media, with strategic programmes that supported the development and delivery of health promotion in a range of settings and sectors: health service, schools, the voluntary sector, the workplace and other informal and formal community settings (through the community programme).

The rationale for this approach was presented in detail in a joint HEBS/WHO publication.[22] In summary, an arena-based approach facilitates:

- co-ordination of effort, reducing the risk of wasteful and potentially counterproductive duplication and competition

- broadening out of the view of health and its determinants, beyond a focus on individual health/ill-health and lifestyle behavioural topics

- promotion of a general health promotion ethos and commitment in settings and sectors combined with use of mass media

- development of comprehensive and sustainable strategies in each setting/sector

- building of health promotion capacity (including competencies) of relevance across a range of health and behavioural topics

- blending of 'top-down' views of needs and priorities with a 'bottom-up' perspective

- tailoring of methodologies to particular settings/sectors

- coverage of the right topics in the right ways at the right times in a given setting or sector

The arenas on which HEBS chose to centre its programmes are shown in Table 3.2. The approach had the added benefit of keeping the number of programmes to a manageable level.

TABLE 3.2 HEBS arena-centred programmes

● General public	● Community	● Health service
● Schools	● Voluntary sector	● Workplace

Setting- and sector-centred programmes

Reference was made above to the notion of building health promotion into settings and sectors. This 'building in' concept is qualitatively different from the more traditional alternatives of 'dropping in' action on discrete health and behavioural topics on top of existing activities or 'bolting on' a block of health promotion activity alongside existing day-to-day business. In essence, health promotion has much in common with organisational development. Health promotion programmes centred on arenas such as the workplace, health service and schools can help to incorporate health improvement as a goal for organisational development in these settings. Programmes centred on a sector, such as the voluntary sector, can help to instil a health focus in its development. Similarly, parallels can be drawn between organisational development and community development – the focus in the latter case is on a defined community rather than a single organisation or setting. Community development has been legitimised increasingly as a key approach to health promotion, and the HEBS community programme promoted and supported its use.

During the 1990s, the HEBS setting- and sector-based programmes and their underlying concepts grew in strategic focus and significance, building on their origins as largely producers of resources and training opportunities.

General public programme

To many people, the most visible face of HEBS was the general public programme. In its first four years, HEBS delivered high-profile mass media initiatives on each of the health/ill-health and lifestyle topic priorities set out in *Scotland's Health: A Challenge to Us All*. The flagship initiative during this period was the *Smokeline* advertising campaign, service and self-help guide.[23] Another campaign that captured the public's imagination involved a television and cinema advertisement featuring Gavin Hastings, former captain of the Scotland rugby team.[24, 25] Once all the major topics had been covered, and the HEBS 'brand' had firmly taken root, the decision was taken to adopt a new strategy for the general public programme.

The new approach initially involved two tracks – one for young people, the other for adults. Each track featured an overarching television advertisement under which there were separate advertisements on individual lifestyle topics. In 2001,

HEBS added a third track, for children and families. The young people's strategy, built around the slogan *Think About It*, featured advertisements and resources on smoking, alcohol, drugs and sexual health. The adult campaign centred on Scotland's 'Big 3' killers using the slogan *You Can Save a Life – Your Own*. It included numerous advertisements on smoking, healthy eating and physical activity, in the form of practical 'top tips' to 'beat the Big 3'.

HEBS advertisements became part of the fabric of Scottish life. The tone, content and flair of the young people's campaign were very highly rated by the media-literate 'target' audience. HEBS and its contracted advertising agencies ensured that the profile of health education rose well above the 'worthy but dull'. A striking example of the power of the young people's campaign is the story of *Stinx*. This fictitious girl band first appeared in a pop video-style TV advertisement in the HEBS *Think About It* series, singing a song that debunked the spuriously fashionable and glamorous image of smoking. News reached HEBS of pupils singing the song in school playgrounds, and of young people stopping smoking as a result of the advert. Young people from across Scotland emailed HEBS in enthusiastic praise of the advert and the influence it was having, and there were pleas to release the song as a CD. The resulting disc reached the Top 10 in the Scottish singles charts and the Top 50 in the UK chart (despite only having been released in Scotland). The song was also made available for downloading from the HEBS website. The related exchanges of emails between young people and HEBS press and PR team are likely to have added to HEBS's positive reputation as an 'in touch' organisation.

TV advertising work was supplemented or complemented by other forms of advertising, including posters (on sexual health or drugs) in the toilets of universities and clubs, outdoor posters, and cinema, press and radio advertisements. The advertising was supported by resources made available to the public directly (through record shops, pharmacies, travel agents and airports), and through telephone helplines (Smokeline, HEBS*line*, Fitline). The general public programme's strategic approach enabled HEBS to maintain a high profile for the young people's and adult campaigns, obtain the maximum longevity and value from the advertisements, and achieve continuity and progression of campaign themes by refreshing the advertising. It also meant that other HEBS programmes, specialist health promotion services and others had coherent and sustained backdrops for their efforts.

Special projects programme

Alongside its arena-centred programmes, HEBS created the special projects programme to enable the organisation and help others to respond to urgent threats to health and capitalise on new opportunities and to play its part in international and national special events such as World AIDS Day, No Smoking Day, and Mental Health Week. Developments in childhood immunisation provided a major focus for the work of the programme.

Lifecourse-centred programmes

National policy and strategy has come to place increasing emphasis on particular stages in the lifecourse as foci for health services and health improvement action. In keeping with this, HEBS introduced the three programmes shown in Table 3.3.

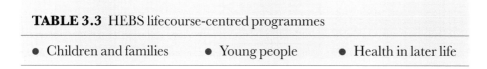

TABLE 3.3 HEBS lifecourse-centred programmes

● Children and families	● Young people	● Health in later life

These cross-cutting programmes were intended to work synergistically with other relevant programmes (for example, schools, community, voluntary sector) to ensure coherent approaches to promoting health at these lifestages. The approach adapted *Our National Health*'s notion of 'a lifetime of care' to 'a lifetime of health'.

Other functions and outputs

HEBS programmes were supported and complemented by a number of other functions and outputs.

Health information – HEBS was a pioneer in harnessing information technology for health promotion. The HEBSWEB website, for example, provided ready access to a huge range of information, resources and services, including full text HEBS publications and the Health Promotion Library Scotland.

Learning and development – HEBS played a key part in helping people in a range of roles and agencies to fulfil their potential as health promoters. *Promoting Health:*

A Short Course was an example of successful cascade training, whereby training was provided for trainers in health promotion units across Scotland and these trainers in turn ensured the delivery of training to health promoters working at local levels. Increasingly, learning and development resources were designed for HEBSWEB.

Research and evaluation – This function played lead roles in: informing the development of HEBS programmes and other outputs; evaluating the organisation's activities; presenting the evidence base for strategies and action on specific topics; and fostering research and evaluation skills beyond HEBS.

International role – HEBS was a WHO Collaborating Centre for health education programme development and evaluation, working within the context of the Ottawa Charter for Health Promotion[26] and the HEALTH21 strategy.[19] In this capacity, the organisation had inputs to a number of WHO policy and strategy developments, and delivered a number of specific pieces of work, including top level development workshops for countries of Central and Eastern Europe, and a health promoting school training resource. HEBS also played an international role through membership of the European Network of Health Promoting Agencies (ENHPA).

Public Health Institute of Scotland

The Public Health Institute of Scotland (PHIS) came into being in January 2001, as a direct result of the Chief Medical Officer's review of the public health function in Scotland. Its stated aims were to protect and improve the health of the people of Scotland by working with the relevant agencies and organisations to:

- increase understanding of the determinants of health and ill health

- help formulate public health policy

- increase the effectiveness of the public health endeavour.

These aims were translated into three work strands:[27, 28]

- developing the public health information base

- developing the public health evidence base

- developing the public health skills base

PHIS produced a number of publications of relevance to the promotion of health. These included health profiles of all Scottish parliamentary constituencies;[29] a joint paper with the Information and Statistics Division of the Common Services Agency on the *Scottish Effect* (a label given to the excess of deaths in Scotland not accounted for by deprivation);[30] and a report on health inequalities produced with the HEBS-funded Health Promotion Policy Unit of the University of Glasgow.[31]

NHS Health Scotland

Early in 2003, the Scottish Executive Health Improvement Strategy Division confirmed that, with effect from 1 April, HEBS and PHIS would come together under a single board of governance. The new organisation, to be known as NHS Health Scotland, is to deliver health improvement programmes at national level and employ knowledge about health and its determinants in a way that will influence policy and practice in Scotland.

Promoting Health at local levels

Mirroring the situation at national level, all local organisations, in all sectors, have parts to play in improving health. Specialist health promotion services within the NHS encourage and help the various players to fulfil their potential. The main locus for these services has been health boards (now known as NHS boards). The 1990s was a period of significant (albeit variable) expansion and increased prominence of such services. The purchaser-provider development in health care led to various attempts to split health promotion between the two sides of that divide, and in some areas the transferring of health promotion operations to NHS trusts. Option appraisals in a number of areas later on in the decade came out in favour of locating the services within health boards. The rising emphasis on health improvement and public health has led in some NHS boards to new approaches to the organisation, deployment and indeed naming of health promotion services and specialists.

Deployment of health promotion specialists has been influenced by a trend towards multiprofessional and multiagency health improvement activities centred on particular localities, within the contexts of community planning, local health planning, social inclusion partnerships (SIPs), development of the public health roles of local authorities and local health care co-operatives (LHCCs), and various other developments. The capacity to promote health at local levels has been enhanced by the establishment of public health practitioner posts in LHCCs and health improvement officer positions in local authorities (the latter jointly funded by the Scottish Executive, NHS boards and councils). There are suggestions that the focus of health promotion specialists should shift further towards localities. This would reinforce the more local health improvement efforts and teams, and enhance sensitivity to the needs and circumstances of different localities. On the other hand, it is important to ensure that locality-centred work has the benefit of coherent larger-scale strategies relating to specific health and lifestyle topics, particular arenas or settings, and different stages in the lifecourse. Furthermore, care is needed to avoid spreading the available health promotion specialist resource in any given NHS board area too thinly, losing or diffusing specific areas of expertise, and creating professional isolation. Whatever balance is struck between area-wide and more local remits, good working links between health promotion specialists and the other public health professionals referred to above offer exciting new scope for multi-disciplinary health improvement efforts in localities, and will facilitate NHS inputs to community planning.

Evaluation issues

One of the most commonly asked questions is 'Does health promotion work?' This is comparable to asking 'Does health care work?' and in both cases the question can be addressed at two levels. First, does health promotion, or health care, work *overall?* Just as no-one would deny that, taken as a whole, health care has had major effects on morbidity and mortality, no-one should doubt that health promotion as a whole (including policy measures, preventive services and communication for health) has had an important impact on health and disease. The second level of consideration concerns the effectiveness of *particular* interventions. There is a good deal of evidence of effective health promotion interventions.[32, 33] As with health care, however, not all interventions have been fully evaluated, some practice is based more on theory, experience or common sense than on evidence, and interventions in different hands, in different places or at different times can give different results. This last point is more relevant in health promotion than in health care, since the interventions often involve human efforts to motivate and persuade, and they take place in the context of other influences that might be crucial to success or failure. Other issues come more to the fore in health promotion than in health care. Outcomes can be difficult to assess with confidence – for example, there may be 'desire-to-please bias' in self-reporting of behaviour; the effects of health education may be delayed or decay over time; an intervention of interest can be difficult to isolate from other influences; and, in attempting to isolate an intervention through a randomised controlled trial (RCT) design, the control group may be influenced by the mere act of obtaining baseline data.

To elaborate on this last point, gathering study baseline data (for example, by asking people about aspects of their health-related behaviour) may be enough to trigger a change in behaviour, resulting in an appreciable amount of behavioural change in a total study population (intervention and control groups) that is eclipsed by a lack of significant differences in levels of change between intervention and control groups. A report published by WHO in 1998[34] advised policy-makers that 'the use of randomised controlled trials to evaluate health promotion initiatives is, in most cases, inappropriate, misleading and unnecessarily expensive'. This has implications for the usefulness of effectiveness reviews that place a high value on the use of the RCT methodology.

One of the problems of health promotion evaluation is the frequent difficulty of attributing desired outcomes to particular interventions. At a whole population level, for example, teasing out the extent to which various individual anti-tobacco interventions have contributed to the decline in smoking prevalence has been likened to 'unravelling gossamer with boxing gloves'.[35]

In a related vein, it is helpful to think of outcomes in terms of the degree of closeness to an intervention.[36] The closer a measurable change to the precise and realistic objectives of a given intervention, the greater the prospect of attributing the change to the intervention in question. With regard to an educational initiative on healthy eating, for example, changes in awareness, beliefs, attitudes and know-how may be observable and to a greater or lesser degree (depending on the robustness of the research design) attributable to the intervention. One is much less likely to be able to gauge the extent to which the initiative contributed to any reduction in diet-related morbidity or mortality – or, if no such reductions are observed or there are upward trends in relevant diseases, to judge the extent to which the intervention prevented or slowed deterioration against a tide of negative influences. Linking the initiative to trends in dietary behaviour presents an intermediate degree of difficulty.

This all makes perfectly good sense, and yet there remains a widespread tendency to place inappropriate expectations on what can be achieved by individual health promotion interventions, in terms of both the nature and extent of positive changes. A randomised controlled trial of a specially designed schools sex education programme in Scotland, for instance, has reported no evidence of reduction in sexual activity or sexual risk taking compared with conventional sex education.[37] This has been taken by some to indicate that sex education in schools does not work. A possible explanation for the findings is that conventional sex education is already fulfilling the potential for teacher-delivered class-based education to influence sexual behaviour. More fundamentally, the study can be looked upon as raising issues as to the prime purpose of schools sex education – to inform choice or to influence behaviour directly? The new programme was associated with increased knowledge among pupils, and there can surely be no doubt that informed choices are preferable to uninformed ones. Even if school-based sex education could be shown not to affect behaviour directly, it could still reasonably be viewed as a desirable component in an overall strategy.

The jigsaw analogy is widely used in describing health improvement action, but it tends not to be followed through logically to evaluation considerations. It is unrealistic to expect a single piece to yield the full picture, and there is a danger that key pieces viewed in isolation will be discarded – only to be missed later on. The situation is actually more complicated than that of a jigsaw in which interlocking pieces add together to make a whole: for example, influences on health can interact synergistically with each other. Reference has been made to the difficulty of isolating the effects of a particular intervention. The crucial point *here* is that it is artificial and potentially destructive to pursue such a line of enquiry to an excessive degree.

The foregoing discussion underlines the need to take a *systems* approach to health improvement efforts and their evaluation. Here, individual interventions of different types are seen as parts of a system in which the general policy, social and economic environment plays a crucial role. Underlying this is the application of available evidence and coherent theories that give cause to expect that the system overall will promote health. The 'theory of change' approach to designing and evaluating a comprehensive community initiative[38] takes this further by encouraging articulation of envisaged overall outcomes and of the contributions expected from each of its components, taking account of contextual factors in which the initiative is set; and evaluating processes and outcomes of relevance to that articulation. The thinking behind the theory of change can be applied beyond community-based initiatives (such as the health demonstration projects), to looking at the health improvement potential and performance of the 'whole system' at a local, regional, national or international level. In taking this forward, however, allowance has to be made for the fact that interventions at a given level may add up to more or less than their sum as a result of synergy, duplication or even inhibitory effects of one influence on another. The likely effects of influences from higher levels must also be taken into account – for example, local anti-smoking efforts take place within the context of national policy on tobacco taxation and advertising, nationwide mass media campaigns and so on.

Despite the complications and difficulties faced, each intervention in a given 'system' should be appraised to an appropriate degree, using suitable methods, against its specific and realistic objectives. There is a pressing need to step up such evaluation, and to develop evaluation capacity in terms of both skills among those who deliver health improvement action and the number of available researchers. Process evaluation can help understanding of how the components of the system interlink and interact, while the performance of a system as a whole can be assessed by monitoring trends in indicators of population health and lifestyle behaviours. Finally, there is a need for further development of valid and easily applied measures of individual and collective wellbeing.

Challenges for delivery

In looking to the future for promoting health in Scotland, three categories of challenge stand out – volume, co-ordination and capacity. One of the most remarkable features of the present day is the number and scale of developments that are recognised and introduced as contributing to population health improvement. For people who are committed to the promotion of health, this gives rise to an uneasy dichotomy of feelings. On the one hand, health and its determinants in the broadest sense are at the forefront of national and local agendas. At the same time, practical difficulties arise from the sheer volume, rate and complexity of new strategies, initiatives and imperatives that impact on workloads and workplans at all levels of the system. More initiatives mean more things to co-ordinate and to evaluate on the ground. The new developments often bear new specific labels, arise from different funding streams, and are channelled through different agencies and sectors. It is a real challenge to pull them together in ways that make good sense and good use of available human resources. The need to bid for specific funds, often in tight timescales, adds to the demands. Moreover, the pilot or short-term nature of many initiatives makes it difficult to embed positive developments as sustainable good practice.

A co-ordination challenge is posed by the trend towards locality-centred multiagency health improvement. It is important that those involved in individual localities do not have to spend their time on the wasteful and unreliable business of needlessly reinventing wheels. It does not make sense, for example, to have people in communities all over Scotland trying to find out for themselves the key features of a health promoting school or other setting, or the evidence base for action on specific health or lifestyle topics or stages of the lifecourse. A logical part of a specialist health promotion function is to feed into locality-centred teams the evidence- and theory-based strategies relating to settings, topics and lifestages. Health promotion specialist members of locality teams can provide a good bridge for two-way communication between specialists concerned with these strategies and local health improvement action.

The issues of volume and co-ordination are clearly relevant to the question of capacity to deliver. Considerable challenges face existing personnel, whether primarily engaged in public health or being encouraged to incorporate a health improvement dimension into their everyday work in any of a range of fields. Many people repeatedly meet the same set of individuals in the course of different initiatives or undertakings and networking and group working can feel as though they are becoming the main job at the expense of actually delivering change for the better. At the same time, for health services, healthcare professionals and others, redeployment of existing resources (human and other) to 'fire prevention' is inhibited by the fact that there is still 'fire-fighting' to be done – and by the fact that people and organisations may feel that they are trained, geared and motivated more to fight fires than to prevent them.

Against the above background, the continual addition of new jobs to the overall mix is more than welcome. It does, however, add to the challenge of joining up all the players and their activities. Moreover, new jobs tend to be filled by people from longer-established posts, which can in turn be difficult to fill in the face of limited overall capacity.

The notion of capacity involves numbers and competencies of people, and how they are deployed. If a step change in Scotland's health is to be achieved, there is a need to take a coherent overview of the necessary workforce and skills mix in the various sectors, building on the public health function and *Nursing for Health* reviews. A crucial aspect of this is to work out how best to deploy and join up a range of public health professionals to strengthen health improvement action at local levels, within the context of wider NHS redesign. This has to be combined with identifying and meeting the shared and distinctive learning and development needs of different players, existing and future. For all this to happen, investment in people and skills for health improvement must be firmly positioned as legitimate and mainstream.

REFERENCES

1. The Scottish Office Home and Health Department. *Health education in Scotland* – a national policy statement. Edinburgh: The Scottish Office, 1991.

2. The Scottish Office. *Scotland's health: a challenge to us all* – a policy statement. Edinburgh: HMSO, 1992.

3. The Scottish Office. *The Scottish diet* – report of a working party to the Chief Medical Officer for Scotland. Edinburgh: The Scottish Office Department of Health, 1993.

4. The Scottish Office. *The oral health strategy for Scotland*. Edinburgh: The Scottish Office Department of Health, 1995.

5. The Scottish Office Department of Health. *Working together for a healthier Scotland* – a consultation document. Edinburgh: The Scottish Office Department of Health, 1998.

6. The Scottish Office. *Towards a healthier Scotland* – a white paper on health. Edinburgh: The Stationery Office, 1999.

7. Scottish Executive. *Review of the public health function in Scotland*. Edinburgh: Scottish Executive, 1999.

8. Scottish Directors of Public Health Group, and Public Health Institute of Scotland. *Delivering better health: NHS boards as public health organisations*. Glasgow: Public Health Institute of Scotland, 2002.

9. Scottish Executive. *Nursing for health* – a review of the contribution of nurses, midwives and health visitors to improving the public's health. Edinburgh: Scottish Executive, 2001.

10. Scottish Executive. *Working together for Scotland: a programme for government*. Edinburgh: Scottish Executive, 2001.

11. Scottish Executive. *Our national health: a plan for action, a plan for change*. Edinburgh: Scottish Executive, 2000.

12. The Scottish Office. *Eating for Health* – a diet action plan for Scotland. Edinburgh: The Scottish Office Department of Health, 1996.

13. Physical Activity Task Force. *Let's make Scotland more active* – a strategy for physical activity: a consultation. Edinburgh: Scottish Executive, 2002.

14. Scottish Executive. *An action plan for dental services in Scotland*. Edinburgh: Scottish Executive, 2000.

15. Scottish Executive. *Plan for action on alcohol problems*. Edinburgh: Scottish Executive, 2002.

16. Scottish Executive. *Social inclusion – opening the door to a better Scotland* – strategy. Edinburgh: Scottish Executive, 1999.

17. Scottish Executive. *Social justice … a Scotland where everyone matters*. Edinburgh: Scottish Executive, 1999.

18. Scottish Executive. *Social justice … a Scotland where everyone matters* – milestone sources and definitions. Edinburgh: Scottish Executive, 1999.

19. World Health Organisation Regional Office for Europe. *HEALTH21: an introduction to the health for all policy framework for the WHO European Region*. Copenhagen: World Health Organisation, 1998.

20. Health Education Board for Scotland. *Strategic plan 1992 to 1997*. Edinburgh: Health Education Board for Scotland, 1993.

21. Health Education Board for Scotland. *Strategic plan 1997 to 2002*. Edinburgh: Health Education Board for Scotland, 1997.

22. Tannahill A. *Health education and health promotion: from priorities to programmes*. Edinburgh: Health Education Board for Scotland/World Health Organization, 1994.

23. Platt S, Tannahill A, Watson J, Fraser E. Effectiveness of antismoking telephone helpline: follow up survey. *British Medical Journal* 1997; 314: 1371–5.

24. Wimbush E, MacGregor A, Fraser E. The impacts of a national mass media campaign on walking. *Health Promotion International* 1998; 13: 45–53.

25. Tannahill A. Leader: 'You don't have to … ': walking to a healthier nation. *British Journal of Sports Medicine* 2000; 34: 79–80.

26. World Health Organisation. *Ottawa Charter for Health Promotion.* Geneva: World Health Organisation, 1996.

27. Public Health Institute of Scotland. *What is PHIS?* Glasgow: Public Health Institute of Scotland, 2001.

28. Public Health Institute of Scotland. *Work programme November 2001.* Glasgow: Public Health Institute of Scotland, 2001.

29. Public Health Institute of Scotland. Glasgow: *Profiles of the health of people in each of the Scottish parliamentary constituencies.* Glasgow: Public Health Institute of Scotland, 2001.

30. Hanlon P *et al. Chasing the 'Scottish Effect'.* Glasgow: Public Health Institute of Scotland, 2001.

31. Blamey A, Hanlon P, Judge K, Muirie J (eds). *Health inequalities in the new Scotland.* Glasgow: Public Health Institute of Scotland, 2002.

32. International Union for Health Promotion and Education. *The evidence of health promotion effectiveness: shaping public health in a new Europe* – a report for the European Commission. Part one – core document. Brussels/Luxembourg: European Commission/International Union for Health Promotion and Education, 1999.

33. International Union for Health Promotion and Education. *The evidence of health promotion effectiveness: shaping public health in a new Europe* – a report for the European Commission. Part two – evidence book. Brussels/Luxembourg: European Commission/International Union for Health Promotion and Education, 1999.

34. World Health Organisation Regional Office for Europe, Health Canada, Centers for Disease Control and Prevention. *Health promotion evaluation: recommendations to policy-makers* – report of the WHO European working group on health promotion evaluation. Copenhagen: World Health Organisation, 1998.

35. Chapman S. Unravelling gossamer with boxing gloves: problems in explaining the decline in smoking. *British Medical Journal* 1993; 307: 429–32.

36. Nutbeam D. Evaluating health promotion – progress, problems and solutions. *Health Promotion International* 1998; 13: 27–44.

37. Wight D, Raab G, Henderson M, Abraham C, Buston K, Hart G, Scott S. Limits of teacher delivered sex education: interim behavioural outcomes from randomised trial. *British Medical Journal* 2002; 324: 1434–3.

38. Connell JP, Kubisch AC. Applying a theory of change approach to the evaluation of comprehensive community initiatives: progress, prospects and problems. In: Fulbright-Anderson K, Kubisch AC, Connell JP (eds). *Approaches to evaluating community initiatives.* Volume 2 – theory, measurement and analysis. Washington DC: The Aspen Institute, 1998.

4. Coronary Heart Disease in Scotland

Nicola Walker and Ross Lorimer

Introduction

If our task had been to review changes in cardiological practice in Scotland over the past 50 rather than 15 years, the picture would have been very different. Fifty years ago the ravages of rheumatic heart disease were the dominant features. Even then, however, the prevalence of the different forms of heart disease was beginning to change. In 1956, in the classic Scottish textbook of medicine, Davidson[1] noted that coronary atheroma and hypertension had become the principal causes of heart disease in middle and old age. Rheumatic fever remained the most common cause of heart disease in childhood, adolescence and early adult life but its incidence was beginning to fall as housing and social conditions improved and penicillin became available as an effective means of preventing recurrent episodes of rheumatic fever. Nowadays acute rheumatic fever has disappeared and mitral stenosis is rare except in the immigrant population. Valvular disease of the heart, however, has not gone away. There is a residuum of longstanding mitral valve disease along with an increase in aortic valve disease, especially aortic stenosis, as a consequence of degenerative change and valvular calcification. The thrust of cardiological practice in the past 15 years has been directed towards Coronary Heart Disease (CHD). This will be looked at in two ways: firstly, by reviewing the epidemiology of CHD and secondly, by reviewing the changes in terms of prevention and management.

Epidemiology

Worldwide there have been very significant reductions in the death rate from acute myocardial infarction (AMI). Unfortunately, Scotland and Northern Ireland retain the highest incidence of myocardial infarction death but there are hopeful signs (see Tables 4. 1 and 4.2). An estimated half a million Scots have some form of CHD, of whom 180 000 require treatment for symptomatic disease. The disease remains much more common in men; at any age the absolute risk of a coronary event in women is about one-fifth that of men.

TABLE 4.1 Acute Myocardial Deaths in Scotland 1990 – 1999
(Number by age and sex)

	1990	*1991*	*1992*	*1993*	*1994*	*1995*	*1996*	*1997*	*1998*	*1999*
Male										
15–44	103	105	97	89	65	62	56	56	66	62
45–64	1659	1591	1589	1489	1256	1159	1059	1041	1018	933
65–74	2342	2324	2251	2210	2046	1892	1818	1527	1553	1455
75+	2692	2662	2569	2550	2265	2254	2232	2105	2056	2115
Female										
15–44	31	18	27	22	13	15	21	19	19	17
45–64	663	666	560	518	465	458	366	354	347	328
65–74	1505	1475	1457	1400	1227	1191	1035	966	919	834
75+	3715	3813	3665	3773	3245	3284	3024	2916	2831	2832

SOURCE: General Registrar's Office for Scotland

TABLE 4.2 Acute Myocardial Deaths in Scotland 1990 – 1999
(Crude rate per 100 000 by age and and sex)

	1990	*1991*	*1992*	*1993*	*1994*	*1995*	*1996*	*1997*	*1998*	*1999*	*% decline* *1999–* *2000*
Male											
15–44	9.0	9.2	8.6	7.9	5.8	5.5	5.0	5.0	6.0	5.6	37.6
45–64	308.6	295.2	289.2	267.2	223.0	204.1	185.5	181.5	175.8	159.5	48.3
65–74	1238.6	1210.9	1159.1	1121.7	1023.1	954.7	922.2	777.5	790.3	741.3	40.1
75+	2531.4	2485.2	2401.4	2418.9	2175.6	2074.5	1997.9	1833.1	1757.0	1774.9	29.9
Female											
15–44	2.8	1.6	2.4	2.0	1.2	1.4	1.9	1.7	1.7	1.6	43.3
45–64	114.5	115.1	95.3	87.2	77.7	76.2	60.6	58.4	56.8	53.2	53.5
65–74	606.6	592.0	580.7	552.2	479.4	473.3	416.1	391.4	374.6	342.2	43.6
75+	1689.1	1727.9	1669.5	1742.1	1519.0	1499.3	1363.0	1301.3	1256.6	1255.3	25.7

SOURCE: General Registrar's Office for Scotland

Death rates for AMI are indeed falling but not as rapidly as one would wish. In Scotland, over the past 15 years the mortality rate from CHD has fallen from 29% to 23% of all deaths.[2] Although age-adjusted mortality has declined by approximately 30% to 40% from its peak in the early 1970s, approximately 12 500 Scots die each year from CHD. Many of these deaths occur prematurely. The reduction in mortality has affected both sexes, all age groups and all Carstairs deprivation categories (DEPCAT). There remains a gap to be closed. The deprived continue to have a higher incidence of CHD than those who are affluent (Figures 4.1a–d).

Figure 4.1a Acute Myocardial Infarction standardised rates per 100,000 by DEPCAT Group in Scotland *(Males aged 15–64 years) People living in relative affluence are in groups 1 and 2 while those living in the greatest deprivation are in groups 5, 6 and 7.*

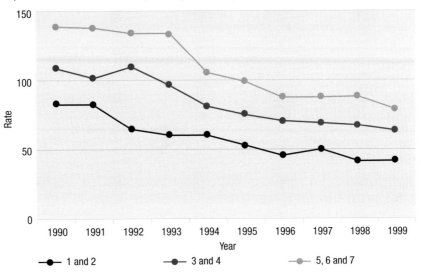

Figure 4.1b Acute Myocardial Infarction standardised rates per 100,000 by DEPCAT Group in Scotland *(Males aged 65 years and over).*

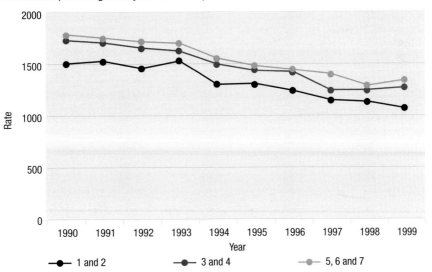

Figure 4.1c   Acute Myocardial Infarction standardised rates per 100,000 by DEPCAT Group in Scotland *(Females aged 15–64 years)*

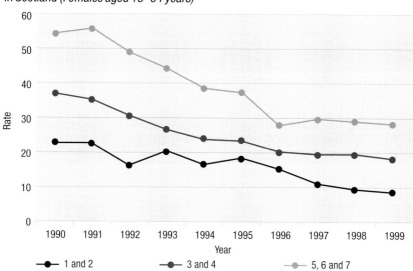

Figure 4.1d   Acute Myocardial Infarction standardised rates per 100,000 by DEPCAT Group in Scotland *(Females aged 65 years and over)*

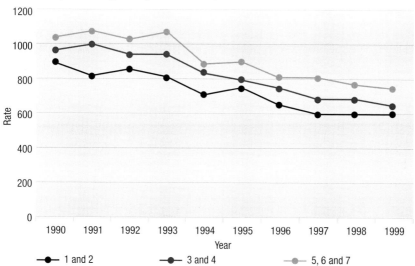

Although the mortality of CHD and number of admissions after AMI are falling, the disease continues to make an increasing impact on the population as illustrated by the number of patients treated for angina. In the 10 years to 1997 this number rose from 5522 to 11 352, a rise matched by the increasing load on cardiology and cardiothoracic surgery outpatient departments.

The practice of cardiology in dealing with CHD has changed very considerably in the past 30 years with the rate of change accelerating in the past 15. We now have a much better appreciation and understanding of risk factors and many effective pharmacological innovations have been developed. Interventional strategies and patterns of investigation and management have changed. We have also seen a growing realisation that the death rate from CHD is not immutable and can be influenced positively.

CHD task force

The report of the Scottish Office's Acute Services Review in June 1998 [3] highlighted the need for a coherent national strategy to reduce the burden of CHD on the Scottish population. On the initiative of the then Chief Medical Officer a group was convened with the following objective and remit (Table 4.3):

TABLE 4.3 Objective and Remit of the Coronary Heart Disease Task Force

Remit:
- Advise on all aspects of CHD from primary prevention through to cardiac rehabilitation
- Advise on strategic direction for organisation of adult cardiology services with particular emphasis on CHD
- Investigate and quantify the scope for increased intervention rates within the four current cardiac centres in Scotland and to address the issue of equity of access
- Build on existing work to develop a national database in conjunction with the Information and Statistics Division of the Common Services Agency
- Ensure implementation of relevant SIGN Guidelines
- Work with the Clinical Standards Board for Scotland to develop appropriate accreditation standards
- Examine existing, new and developing cardiological techniques

The Task Force reported in September 2001.[2] Overall, its report was very well received and had several important consequences for the prevention and management of CHD in Scotland (see below). To maintain momentum and build on the work of the Task Force, the Minister of Health for Scotland established an Implementation Group with a remit that included development of a CHD and Stroke Strategy for Scotland. This group, under the chairmanship of Dr N Boon, reported in October 2002.[4] The Minister (Mr Malcolm Chisholm) in accepting its recommendation, announced that £40million were to be made available over the next three years to ameliorate further the problems of CHD in our community. This is the first time that Scotland has had a comprehensive and coherent strategy for CHD and Stroke and includes important proposals for the prevention and treatment of CHD. A particular emphasis is placed on prevention and integrated service delivery, at local, regional and national levels.

Prevention of CHD

From the clinical point of view, the term primary prevention is used where the emphasis is on reducing the incidence of heart disease in the community. Secondary prevention aims to reduce the risk of a recurrent episode of CHD.

As indicated earlier, we now have a better understanding of risk factors. The significance of cigarette smoking has long been recognised and attention has focused recently on the role of cholesterol reduction. The relationship between clinical and experimental coronary artery disease and raised cholesterol levels has been known for many years but has been controversial. In the past 10 years evidence has accrued that a reduction in cholesterol levels reduces CHD risk. The West of Scotland Coronary Prevention Study (WOSCOPS)[5] was a landmark study indicating that, in those identified at screening as having a raised cholesterol, administration of the cholesterol-lowering drug pravastatin for five years led to a greater reduction in the death rate from CHD than placebo. Reductions were also found in the number of AMIs, the number of patients requiring coronary angiography and the number of revascularisation interventions. These results have subsequently been confirmed in worldwide studies. It is possible that the statin class of drugs have effects on CHD mortality and incidence other than those associated with cholesterol lowering and this remains the subject of further investigation.[6]

No one would suggest that cholesterol lowering is the only, or indeed the most important, factor in the prevention of CHD. Cigarette smoking, obesity, hypertension, lack of exercise, lack of dietary constituents, such as antioxidants from fresh fruit, are all factors that merit attention.

Capewell and his colleagues[7] have assessed the contribution of modern cardiovascular treatment and changes in risk factors to the decline in CHD deaths in Scotland between 1975 and 1994. There were 14 230 deaths from CHD in 1975; by 1994 the total number of deaths prevented or postponed was estimated at 6747. Forty per cent of the reduction was attributed to treatment and 51% to measurable risk factor reduction. Nine per cent appeared to be the result of other factors that could not as yet be defined.

Secondary prevention has also become well established. There is now good evidence that, after myocardial infarction, long-term treatment in appropriate patients with drugs such as aspirin or other platelet inhibitors, betablockers, the angiotensin converting enzyme inhibitor drugs (ACE inhibitors) and statins all have beneficial effects. These pharmacological agents are now often used in patients who have risk factors for CHD but who have not actually sustained a myocardial infarction. The HOPE study,[8] for example, showed that those who had hypertension or diabetes or symptoms of CHD did benefit from long-term therapy with an ACE inhibitor. There is also increasing appreciation of the fact that the prevention of CHD must address multiple risk factors. Lifestyle is of major importance and the community as a whole should be involved in healthy lifestyle measures. In this context, the Paisley project – *Have a Heart Paisley* – has now been underway for some three years as a major demonstration project funded by the Scottish Executive Health Department. This project seeks to involve the whole community, a range of partner organisations and the healthcare system in preventing CHD by lifestyle improvement involving enthusiastic education. Findings of this study are awaited with interest. It could well provide a template for the rest of Scotland.

One of the success stories of recent times in Scotland has been the reduction in cigarette smoking especially in males, although this has not been matched by a corresponding reduction in females. The incidence of AMI is three to six times higher in smokers of 20 cigarettes per day compared with non-smokers. The North Glasgow arm of the World Health Organisation MONICA (Monitoring

Trends and Determinants in Cardiovascular Disease)[9] study underlines the importance of smoking in this part of Scotland. Smoking prevalence in men in social classes IV and V is over twice that in social classes I and II (45% and 20% respectively) and the high smoking rates in women, notably in the least affluent sectors of society, are a particular cause for concern. Unhealthy diet and relative lack of physical activity also emerge as socially linked factors of importance in CHD in Scotland. It is important to emphasise that stopping smoking can allow the incidence of AMI to fall back to that found in non-smokers.

The identification of multiple risk factors has resulted in a shift of emphasis in health care delivery. It is increasingly recognised that risk factors are not specific to CHD; rather they are vascular risk factors. A multidisciplinary approach is, therefore, now being encouraged in which dieticians, physiotherapists, diabetologists, stroke physicians, nephrologists and cardiologists all work collaboratively.

Potential problems, however, remain. At present, large numbers of the population are becoming overweight and the incidence of clinical obesity is increasing. This affects the young, the middle-aged and the elderly. The incidence of CHD increases with age and it increases dramatically when diabetes is present. We are in danger of developing a growing population of obese, middle-aged diabetics and the favourable current trend in CHD mortality and morbidity may well come to a shuddering halt. This highlights the need for increased emphasis on a healthy lifestyle.

The Scottish Strategy for CHD[4] acknowledges the rate at which our knowledge of CHD continues to expand and the implications for preventative policy, by recommending that all local CHD preventative activities should be reviewed in the light of new evidence on prevention. More generally, the Strategy should bring fresh momentum to preventative efforts and recommends that local health plans developed by NHS Boards should adopt a, 'population approach to improving the health of the communities that they serve, complemented by a high-risk groups approach targeted at certain key groups, such as those with hypertension, hypercholesterolaemia or diabetes, as well as the most socially disadvantaged groups within the population.'

Treatment of CHD

Over the past few years our knowledge of the pathophysiology of CHD has increased and this has led to a change in diagnostic classification. We also have better methods of detecting myocardial damage. Troponin enzyme level increases are specific for myocardial cell damage and can be raised to diagnostic levels while other enzymes, such as the transaminases, long used in the diagnosis of acute infarction, remain negative. This has implications for long-term epidemiological studies since the diagnosis of myocardial infarction is now being made on criteria that differ from those of 15 years ago. If the diagnosis is made more frequently, this may well distort statistics. The term *acute coronary syndrome* (ACS) is now used to describe the spectrum ranging from unstable angina through to full-blown acute transmural myocardial infarction (AMI). This terminology is an attempt to recognise the unifying underlying pathology of the condition. It also allows the division of AMI into ST segment elevation-myocardial infarction (STEMI – which is the conventional classic AMI presentation) and non-ST segment elevation-myocardial infarction (NSTEMI) – a distinction that requires biochemical investigation as well as appropriate ECG changes.

The spectrum of disease described above has a common pathology in that coronary artery narrowing is a consequence of atherosclerosis. Initially, this was regarded as a relentlessly progressive process resistant to modification. It was believed that the severity of the resultant disease was a reflection of the degree of arterial obstruction. Coronary angiography, however, has changed our perception. A stenosis that appears modest at the time of angiography can be associated with a major clinical event. Atherosclerosis is now recognised to be a dynamic pathological process defined as a focal, inflammatory fibro-proliferative response to multiple forms of endothelial injury. Clinical events occur when coronary artery thrombosis follows acute plaque rupture. The coagulation cascade is activated by exposure to the thrombogenic contents of the plaque. Microscopy suggests that a thin fibrous cap, large volume of inflammatory cells and small number of smooth muscle cells and a large lipid core are all factors that contribute to an increased risk of rupture. In contrast, a stable plaque that is unlikely to rupture and cause an acute clinical incident is likely to have a thick fibrous cap enclosing the lipid core. This prevents exposure to the circulating blood. Attention is now being concentrated on measures to convert a vulnerable into a stable plaque. It is in this context that statins and ACE inhibitors may have a benefit other than that originally predicted.

Changes in Management

Recognition of the acute coronary syndrome has meant a change in management. It is now recognised that giving aspirin improves survival in the immediate as well as in the long term. In addition, the indications for early thrombolytic therapy have become established. Newer agents are also easier to administer. The use of thrombolytic therapy was initially confined to the coronary care unit but this no longer applies as speed of administration is critical. Thrombolytic therapy is being given in Accident and Emergency or indeed, in some situations, in the community. The work of Rawles and colleagues in Grampian[10] has been especially important in this regard. It is now recognised that administration of thrombolytic therapy is not the prerogative of the doctor. Nurses have been trained to administer it and it may well be that trained paramedical personnel (who are often the first on the scene after AMI) would be the appropriate administrators given that improvement in prognosis depends on time (see below for further consideration). Any delay may cause either loss of life or impairment of left ventricular function.

Interventional procedures

Coronary artery bypass grafting (CABG) by means of either saphenous vein conduits or arterial conduits using the internal mammary artery has been available for around 30 years. The number of operations in Scotland continues to increase and is currently around 650 per million of the population. Initial analysis in 1998–99 showed that rates of CABG and percutaneous transluminal coronary angiography (PTCA) for men and women aged 45–64 years had a broadly positive relationship with deprivation – that is, a trend for rates to rise as DEPCAT rose. The relationship was not maintained in older individuals. Intervention rates per 100 000 for men aged 65–74 years, for example, were much higher in DEPCAT 1 and 2 (693 and 389.5 respectively) than in DEPCAT 6 and 7 (372.2 and 262.2 respectively). This higher rate of intervention in more affluent areas does not sit comfortably alongside the fact that mortality rates from CHD are higher in deprived areas.

Whereas most of the mortality from CHD occurs in the over 65 year olds, proportionately more surgery is carried out in younger patients. The ratio of interventions performed to interventions expected, for example, (calculated by multiplying the Scottish age and sex-adjusted intervention rate by the population counts of the area being considered) in 1998–99 was approximately twice as high in affluent areas. It is clear that patients from more deprived areas do not have the same access to, uptake of, or supply of interventions for CHD as their counterparts in more affluent areas.

Pell and colleagues[11] have shown that in Scotland socioeconomically deprived patients may be further disadvantaged by having to wait longer for surgery because of being given lower priority. This situation has clinical significance since waiting list mortality has been shown to be 2.6% with a mortality risk of 0.28% per month of waiting.[12]

The technology used in treating CHD has changed in the past five years. The development of PTCA has had a particularly profound impact on the management of CHD. In this technique, the site of stenosis is identified by angiography. A small balloon at the distal end of the catheter is inflated. This compresses the atheromatous material against the wall of the coronary artery and enhances the lumen. The technique has been supplemented by the use of intra coronary stents, metal scaffolds that maintain the patency of the lumen of the dilated coronary artery. By these means the chance of re-stenosis has been considerably reduced and the need for urgent 'bail-out' cardiac coronary bypass surgery has been virtually abolished. Percutaneous transluminal coronary angioplasty is now well established in the management of stable angina when coronary angiography delineates suitable lesions. It is becoming increasingly used in the management of the ACS. Those patients whose symptoms fail to settle on medical treatment may well come to early investigation and, if appropriate, to PTCA. This would now be the procedure of choice rather than coronary bypass grafting. The major question is whether PTCA will become the primary treatment of acute myocardial infarction (AMI). If such interventions (rather than thrombolytic therapy) become the treatment of choice there will be profound resource implications in terms of the provision of cardiac catheterisation facilities and round-the-clock availability of trained personnel.

There have been changes also in the management of those who survive myocardial infarction. No longer are they wrapped in cotton wool. The role of pharmacological agents in prevention has already been discussed; active rehabilitation is increasingly recognised as conferring psychological benefit as well as improving prognosis. Rehabilitation is not solely a hospital function. It is increasingly being taken into the community. Many patients have set up self-help groups that have proved extremely valuable in the long-term management of the condition.

A recent development has been the increasing recognition of the importance of heart failure. With an ageing population and more survivors of myocardial infarction, the incidence of heart failure is rising and is likely to continue to so do. Echocardiography is now a standard and much employed investigation in all our hospitals. This non-invasive ultrasound technique can detect impaired ventricular function and has also allowed treatment to be based on investigative evidence rather than on symptoms. The improved diagnosis of heart failure has been associated with developments in management. We now have more powerful oral diuretics as well as recognition that betablockade can be beneficial rather than harmful.[13] A major advance has been the evidence that ACE inhibitors improve both symptoms and prognosis.[14] Treatment of heart failure is not now confined to the hospital setting and is being undertaken increasingly and successfully in the community. A nurse-led outreach heart failure service, for example, can reduce considerably the time spent in hospital and has been shown to be much more acceptable to patients.[15]

Potential advances in secondary prevention

New technology is also gradually being introduced to prevent the recurrence of cardiac events. The availability of portable cardiac defibrillators is a subject of much interest and emotion. We have still to establish whether or not the availability of defibrillators in community areas such as football grounds, railway stations and shopping centres will prove to be of benefit although recent evidence from Scotland indicates that any increase in survival will be marginal.[16] If defibrillation is to be widely available, there is an initial need to improve the training of the community in cardiopulmonary resuscitation. An adjunct to this development is that we know that a small number of patients are at risk from a catastrophic arrhythmia after myocardial infarction. Electrophysiological investigation has allowed the selection of patients for whom implantable cardiac defibrillators may be of benefit.

The number of ICD implantations may be greater than initially anticipated. In 1999, according to the National Institute for Clinical Exellence (NICE), 17 ICDs were implanted per million population. NICE recommended that ICDs should be considered for two groups of patients:[17] as secondary prevention in patients who have had a ventricular arrhythmia with haemodynamic compromise, and for primary prevention in patients at high risk of sudden cardiac death – most of whom are post-myocardial infarction with a left ventricular ejection fraction of less than 35%. NICE advocated that patients in the primary prevention group should be screened with ambulatory ECG and electrophysiological studies. NICE anticipated that implementation of their guidance would increase the implantation rate to 50 per million population. The MADIT 2 study[18] has shown that in patients after myocardial infarction with a left ventricular ejection fraction of less than 30%, ICDs confer a relative reduction in mortality of 31% compared to anti-arrhythmic therapy. As a recent editorial by McComb and Camm[19] highlights, this would increase the number of patients requiring ICDs by a factor of about five. The number of implantations would, therefore, increase from the current UK implantation rate of 17 per million to about 250 per million population. The NICE estimate of the cost per device was £25 000.

Current Developments

In terms of management of the clinical condition, there must be equity of access to services and deprived, remote and rural communities must not be neglected. It is disappointing that even in this era the death rate from myocardial infarction is seven times higher in women in the deprived East End of Glasgow than in the affluent suburb of Bearsden in the west of the city. The Arbuthnott report has defined the large unmet health need in deprived communities[20]. We have to ensure that appropriate and readily accessible facilities are provided and that communities are fully aware of what is available and the importance of using them.

Access to investigation and intervention must be improved further to ensure that long waiting lists are a thing of the past. There have been encouraging changes for the better in recent years. Scotland now has 70 cardiologists, which is one for every 73 000 people. A decade ago Scotland had only six cardiac catheterisation laboratories. It now has 11. Additional coronary angiography units have been set up in Inverness, Ayr, Dumfries, Lanarkshire and Inverclyde. These improved facilities will help to improve access for investigation. Ten years ago the waiting time for investigation by coronary angiography was more than one year. It currently stands at about three months.

Concomitantly, there has been increase in the number of cardiac interventions undertaken. There are two adult cardiac surgical centres in Glasgow, one in Edinburgh and one in Aberdeen. These units have expanded considerably and now more than 600 patients per million of the population have coronary bypass grafting annually. In addition, the angioplasty rate is increasing and currently stands at around 500 per million of the population. Waiting times for coronary bypass grafting are falling and guarantees are shortly to be given that the waiting time will not exceed six months for all patients. Around 50% of patients are investigated and managed on an urgent basis without necessarily appearing on a waiting list.

Scotland is unique in the United Kingdom in having databases that cover coronary angiography, coronary angioplasty and cardiac surgery. We are also well advanced in guideline production in the area of CHD. The Scottish Intercollegiate Guideline Network (SIGN – www.sign.ac.uk) has produced a number of excellent evidence-based guidelines covering primary prevention of CHD, secondary prevention of CHD, diagnosis and treatment of heart failure due to left ventricular systolic dysfunction, hypertension in older people and management of stable angina. A guideline on cardiac rehabilitation has also been published recently. Our knowledge of the implementation of these guidelines, however, is scanty and in this context the role of the Clinical Standards Board for Scotland (CSBS) and its successors will be crucial. This is a multiprofessional independent organisation with strong lay representation that has already prepared standards for myocardial infarction, especially with reference to secondary prevention. Every Acute Trust in Scotland dealing with patients with myocardial infarction has been visited and the existing standards assessed. Each Trust now knows what it has to do to improve its own performance to acceptable levels. As the CSBS report on secondary prevention has demonstrated,[21] there is a need to reduce delay in giving thrombolytic therapy and to provide appropriate facilities (that is, exercise testing and echocardiography) so that patients can be assessed before they go home after sustaining myocardial infarction. In future, the work of the Clinical Standards Board in relation to CHD should extend into primary care.

There remains a need for a massive investment to bring about sustained and significant improvement in information technology and data recording. A lack of central funding and direction has meant that committed and concerned clinicians have frequently had to establish their own networks and databases without regard to national coherence. The development of managed clinical networks provides an exciting way forward for the better management of CHD. In the past, cardiology services have been delivered by referral from primary care to secondary care to tertiary care. The term 'hub and spoke' has been applied to such a model of service delivery with the 'hub' representing a tertiary centre and the 'spoke' primary and secondary care. In future, it is hoped that managed clinical networks (MCNs) will allow better integration of care between primary, secondary and tertiary sectors and will also improve equity of access for the community. A pilot network in Dumfries and Galloway will provide much needed information. It aims to focus on improving the quality and responsiveness of services to patients who suffer a heart attack in the region. It will employ agreed protocols in both hospital and general practice (quality standards having been agreed beforehand with the Clinical Standards Board), use a partnership of GPs and ambulance staff to administer pre-hospital thrombolysis, and place emphasis on secondary prevention and the treatment of heart failure. The annual report (2001–2002) of the Dumfries and Galloway MCN for CHD, ably led by Dr Chris Baker from primary care, has shown that the network has succeeded in bringing together the public, patients, and primary and secondary care. The success to date may provide encouragement to the development of MCNs in many disciplines throughout the country.[22]

The new national CHD strategy[4] has adopted the approach piloted in Dumfries as a preferred model for local cardiac services and all NHS Boards are required to have established local cardiac MCNs by April 2004. In addition the strategy intends that a Scottish Cardiac Intervention Network (SCIN) should be fully operational by January 2004. This network will harness the expertise of existing high technology cardiac intervention centres and is designed to enable a co-ordinated approach to the equitable development of high quality services, and a managed process for the introduction of new technologies. The intention is that by building on existing clinical relationships through the development of common protocols for the referral and discharge of patients the local cardiac MCNs and SCIN will become effectively integrated. These are ambitious and exciting proposals that offer a basis for the future development of CHD services in Scotland, though the challenge of turning the vision into working reality should not be underestimated.

While the past 15 years in Scotland have seen a reduction in deaths from CHD, this does not necessarily mean that there is less CHD in the community. As more people survive an acute episode, the number of patients with CHD increases. The fall in death rate, though gratifying, is less than that seen in other countries and Scotland can have no grounds for complacency. For the community, the future lies in prevention. For the individual, success in the present hinges on the ready availability of appropriate health care facilities for all.

REFERENCES

1. Davidson LSD. *Principles and Practice of Medicine. Diseases of the Cardiovascular System.* Third edition. Edinburgh: Livingston; 1956.

2. Coronary Heart Disease/Stroke Task Force. Coronary Heart Disease/Stroke Task Force Report. Chairman: Professor AR Lorimer. Edinburgh: Scottish Executive Health Department. 2001.

3. *Acute Services Review Report.* Edinburgh: Scottish Office Department of Health, 1998.

4. *CHD and Stroke Strategy for Scotland.* Edinburgh: Scottish Executive Department of Health, 2002.

5. Shepherd J, Cobbe SM, Ford I, Isles CG, Lorimer AR, MacFarlane PW, McKillop JH, Packard CJ. Prevention of coronary heart disease with pravastatin in men with hypercholesterolemia. West of Scotland Coronary Prevention Study Group. *New England Journal of Medicine* 1995,333 (20):1301–7.

6. Aikawa M, Rabkin E, Okada Y, Voglic SJ, Clinton SK, Brinckerhoff CE, Sukhova GK, Libby P. Lipid lowering by diet reduces matrix metalloproteinase activity and increases collagen content of rabbit atheroma: a potential mechanism of lesion stabilisation. *Circulation* 1998,97:2433–44.

7. Capewell S, Morrison CE, McMurray JJ. Contribution of modern cardiovascular treatment and risk factor changes to the decline in coronary heart disease mortality in Scotland between 1975 and 1994. *Heart* 1999, 81:380–6.

8. Yusuf S, Sleight P, Pogue J, Bosch J, Davies R, Dagenais G. Effects of an angiotensin-converting-enzyme inhibitor, ramipril, on cardiovascular events in high-risk patients. The Heart Outcomes Prevention Evaluation Study Investigators. *New England Journal of Medicine* 2000, 342 (3):145–53.

9. Tunstall-Pedoe H, Morrison C, Woodward M, Fitzpatrick B, Watt G. Sex differences in myocardial infarction and coronary deaths in the Scottish MONICA population of Glasgow 1985 to 1991. Presentation, diagnosis, treatment, and 28-day case fatality of 3991 events in men and 1551 events in women. *Circulation* 1996, 93 (11):1981–92.

10. Rawles J, Sinclair C, Jennings K, Ritchie L, Waugh N. Audit of prehospital thrombolysis by general practioners in peripheral practices in Grampian. *Heart* 1998, 80:231–4.

11. Pell J, Pell AC, Norrie J, Ford I, Cobbe SM. Effect of socio-economic deprivation on waiting time for cardiac surgery: retrospective cohort study. *British Medical Journal* 2000, 320:15–19.

12. Seddon ME, French JK, Amos DJ, Ramanathan K, McLaughlin SC, White HD. Waiting times and prioritisation for coronary artery bypass surgery in New Zealand. *Heart* 1999, 81:586–592.

13. MERIT Study Group. Effect of metoprolol CR/XL in chronic heart failure: metoprolol CR/XL randomised intervention trial in congestive heart failure (MERIT-HF). *Lancet* 1999,353:2001–7.

14. The SOLVD investigators. Effect of enalapril on survival in patients with reduced left ventricular ejection fractions and congestive heart failure. *New England Journal of Medicine* 1991,325:293–302.

15. Blue L, Lang E, McMurray JJV, Davie AP, McDonagh TA, Murdoch DR, Petrie MC, Connolly E, Norrie J, Round CE, et al. Randomised controlled trial of specialist nurse intervention in heart failure. *British Medical Journal* 2001,323:715–8.

16. Pell JP, Sirel JM, Marsden AK, Ford I, Walker NL, Cobbe SM. Potential impact of public access defibrillators on survival after out of hospital cardiopulmonary arrest: retrospective cohort study. *British Medical Journal* 2002, 325 (7363):515.

17. National Institute for Clinical Excellence. Technology Appraisal Guidance No. 11: Guidance on the use of implantable cardioverter defibrillators for arrhythmias. www.nice.org.uk. 2000.

18. Moss AJ, Zareba W, Hall WJ, Klein H, Wilber DJ, Cannom DS, Daubert JP, Higgins SL, Brown MW, Andrews ML. Prophylactic implantation of a defibrillator in patients with myocardial infarction and reduced ejection fraction. *New England Journal of Medicine* 2002,346 (12):877–83.

19. McComb JM, Camm AJ. Primary prevention of sudden cardiac death using implantable cardioverter defibrillators.*British Medical Journal* 2002,325 (7372):1050–1051.

20. National Review of Resource Allocation for the NHS in Scotland. Fair shares for all: report of the National Review of Resource Allocation for the NHS in Scotland. Chairman: Professor Sir John Arbuthnott. Edinburgh: Scottish Executive Health Department. 1999.

21. Clinical Standards Board for Scotland. *Coronary Heart Disease. Heart Attack: Secondary Prevention*. Edinburgh:CSBS, 2002.

22. Dumfries and Galloway MCN. Managed Clinical Network for Coronary Heart Disease: Annual Report 2001–2002. www.show.scot.nhs.uk/mcn. 2002.

5. Cancer in Scotland

David Brewster and Anna Gregor

Cancer is a major cause of morbidity and mortality in Scotland, both in international terms[1,2] and in comparison with other diseases.[3] Currently, around 26 000 people are diagnosed with cancer in Scotland every year, and around 15 000 deaths are attributed directly to cancer as the primary underlying cause.[3] It is, therefore, appropriate that cancer and cancer services remain one of the main clinical priorities of the NHS in Scotland. It is encouraging that the target to reduce mortality from cancer in people aged less than 65 years in Scotland by 15% between 1986 and 2000 has been met. We go forward in this century with a more ambitious target, namely to reduce mortality from cancer by 20% in people under 75 years by 2010, taking 1995 as the base year. This will require a fall in age-standardised mortality from 188 to 150 deaths per 100 000 population, a much more difficult task.

One in three Scots will develop cancer during their lifetime; this means that almost everyone is exposed in one way or another to the effects of living with cancer and has interest in its management. Unfavourable comparisons with service provision and outcomes in countries outside the United Kingdom, particularly with respect to waiting times and access to modern technology, has been a major recent stimulus to debate and has helped to bring about fundamental change in the way we plan, monitor and organise cancer services within the Scottish NHS.

Burden of disease and epidemiology of cancer in Scotland

Age and sex distribution of cancer

Fortunately, cancer is a relatively rare disease in childhood. When children are affected, the incidence rates in the two sexes are largely comparable.

From young adulthood to middle age, the risk of cancer is higher in females than males, but thereafter age-specific incidence rates increase much more steeply in males (Figure 5.1). These differences reflect the generally earlier onset of breast and genital tract cancers in women, the later onset of prostate cancer in men, and the greater past exposure of men to tobacco and alcohol.

Figure 5.1   Age specific incidence rates for all malignant neoplasms combined (excluding non-melanoma skin cancer), 1998

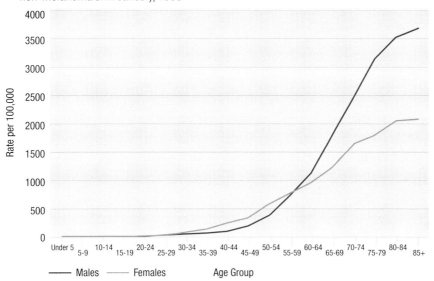

Males ——— Females ——— Age Group

Socioeconomic status and cancer

Socioeconomic status has a major impact on the risk of developing many types of cancer and on the probability of surviving the disease.[4] In general, the risk of developing cancer is higher among people living in deprived communities (Figure 5.2).

Notable exceptions are breast cancer, cutaneous malignant melanoma, and prostate cancer, all of which are more common among the affluent. Survival prospects, however, are almost without exception worse among patients from deprived communities, so that their risk of dying from cancer is higher (Figure 5.2).

Geographical distribution of cancer

Globally, there are major differences in the incidence of and mortality from cancer between countries.[1,2] These differences are unlikely to be explained by differences in data quality and completeness alone, and they are often used to generate hypotheses about the causation of cancer. Within Scotland, regional variations are less marked (Figures 5.3a and 5.3b) and are at least partly explained by socioeconomic status.

Figure 5.2   Incidence[1], mortality[1] and survival[2,3] by deprivation quintile. All malignant neoplasms combined, exluding non-melanoma skin cancer 1991–1995

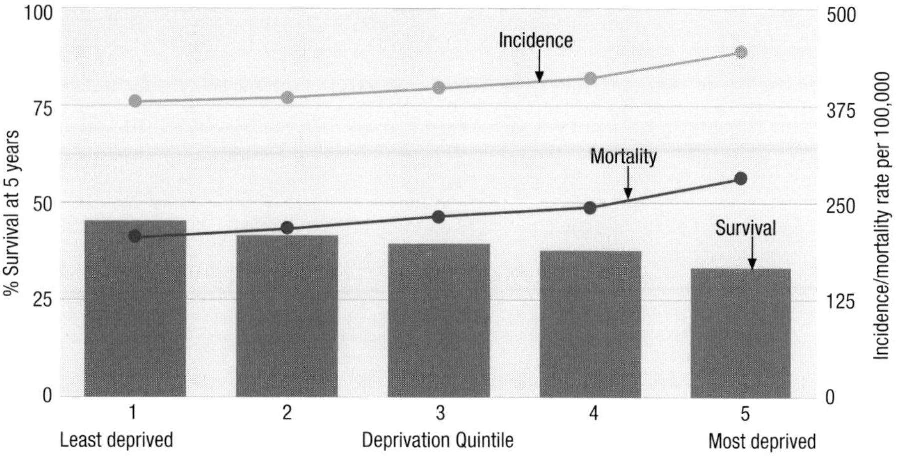

[1] Age-standardised rates per 100 000 person-years at risk (European standard population).
[2] Cause-specific survival adjusted for age and sex.
[3] Cases diagnosed in 1994 and 1995 do not have 5 years' follow up.

Figure 5.3a   Incidence of all malignant neoplasms combined (excluding non-melanoma skin cancer) by health board of residence, males, 1994–1998

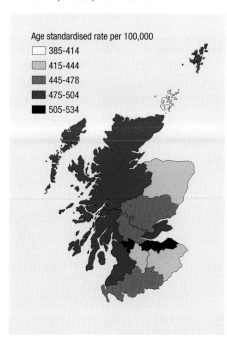

Figure 5.3b   Incidence of all malignant neoplasms combined (excluding non-melanoma skin cancer) by health board of residence, females, 1994–1998

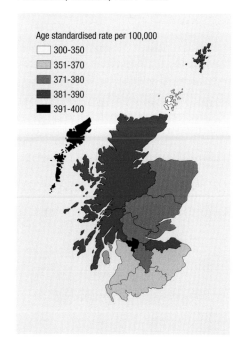

Most common cancers

The most commonly occurring cancers in males and females in Scotland in 1998 are shown in Figures 5.4a and 5.4b. The pattern is different at different ages: for example, leukaemia is the most common cancer in children, whereas cancers of the testis and cervix are respectively the most common cancers in

Figure 5.4a Top ten incident male cancers (excluding non-melanoma skin cancer), 1998

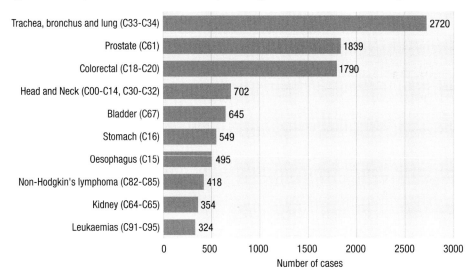

Figure 5.4b Top ten incident female cancers (excluding non-melanoma skin cancer), 1998

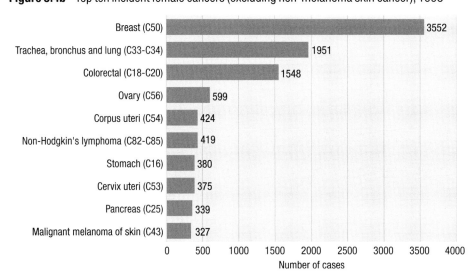

males and females aged 15–34 years.[5] Overall, cancers of the lung, large bowel, breast and prostate account for over 50% of all cancers (excluding non-melanoma skin cancer).[6]

Recent trends in incidence

Recent trends in incidence of the five most common cancers in males and females are plotted on a logarithmic scale in Figures 5.5a and 5.5b. The falling incidence of lung cancer in males is consistent with historic patterns of tobacco consumption.[7] Recent increases have been seen in the incidence of colorectal

Figure 5.5a   Secular trends in incidence of the five most common male cancers

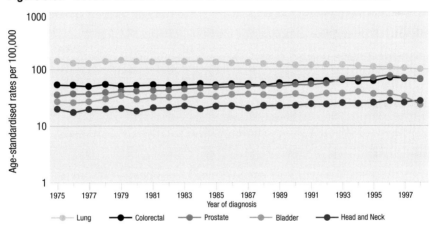

Figure 5.5b   Secular trends in incidence of the five most common female cancers

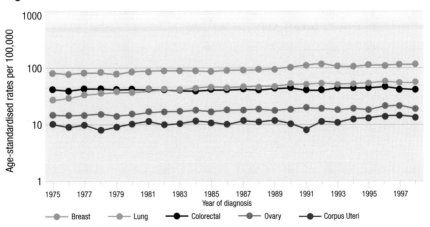

cancer,[8] head and neck cancer and prostate cancer, although it is unclear whether the increase in prostate cancer is the result of increased detection or a genuine increase in risk.[9] The very recent fall in incidence of bladder cancer is likely to reflect an internationally recommended change in classification and coding practice: if invasive tumours, carcinoma *in situ*, and 'neoplasms of uncertain or unknown behaviour' of the bladder are considered together, no substantial recent change in incidence is apparent.

In females, increases have been observed in lung cancer (again consistent with the historic pattern of tobacco consumption among women[7]), breast cancer (recently driven, at least in part, by the introduction of a national screening programme[10]) and cancer of the corpus uteri (largely endometrial cancers). Only a very modest increase has been observed in ovarian cancer. In contrast to the situation in males, the incidence of colorectal cancer in females has shown little change.[8]

Recent trends in survival

Over the last three decades, therapeutic advances have brought about remarkable improvements in survival from certain cancers. Observed five-year survival from cancer of the testis, for example, has increased from below 80% to more than 95%.[11] Improvements of a similar magnitude have been observed for some lympho-haematopoietic malignancies, notably acute lymphoblastic leukaemia in children. These successes must be tempered by the observation that gains in survival from the most common adult epithelial cancers have been more modest and, in some cases, for example lung cancer, virtually non-existent (Figures 5.6a and 5.6b). In the case of breast, cervical and prostate cancers, it is likely that part of the observed improvements in survival is a result of earlier diagnosis ('lead time bias').

Figure 5.6a Trends in survival at five years after diagnosis: five most common male cancers

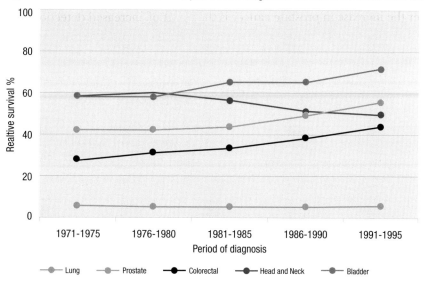

Figure 5.6b Trends in survival at five years after diagnosis: five most common female cancers

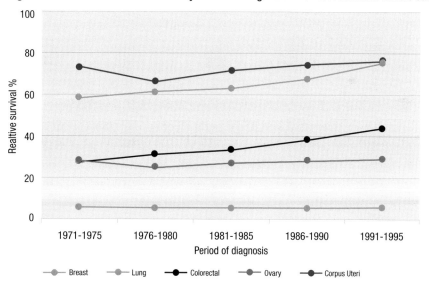

Recent trends in mortality

Recent trends in mortality for the five most common causes of death from cancer in males and females are plotted on a logarithmic scale in Figures 5.7a and 5.7b. It goes without saying that changes in mortality can reflect both changes in incidence and changes in survival rates. In males, the reduced mortality from lung cancer reflects the falling incidence, despite a lack of improvement in survival prospects. Although the incidence of colorectal cancer in males has increased, improvements in survival have meant that there has been little change in mortality.[8] Mortality from prostate cancer increased until 1993, but has remained relatively stable thereafter, despite an increasing incidence.[9] There has been little improvement in survival from cancers of the oesophagus and stomach so that trends in mortality are largely a reflection of trends in incidence. In Scotland, as in many other countries, there has been a striking decrease in the risk of developing distal stomach cancer and an increase in the risk of developing oesophageal cancer, especially adenocarcinoma of the lower oesophagus.[12]

In females, trends in mortality from lung cancer and stomach cancer are broadly in line with incidence trends. Despite increases in incidence, mortality from breast cancer is decreasing as a result of advances in therapy, although screening may also now be beginning to have an impact. Mortality from colorectal cancer is decreasing, in line with modest improvements in survival, and this presumably reflects advances in treatment and peri-operative care.[8] Mortality from ovarian cancer has remained relatively stable: in this respect, modest gains in survival have been largely cancelled out by increases in incidence.

Projected incidence and mortality

The Scottish Executive publication, *Cancer in Scotland: Action for Change*[13] was published in 2001. The supporting publication *Cancer Scenarios: an aid to planning cancer services in Scotland in the next decade* used statistical modelling to project the future incidence of and mortality from cancer.[14] Projected numbers are dependent on the risk of cancer in the population, the changing age structure of the population, and (for deaths) changes in survival from cancer. In addition, future numbers of cases and deaths may be influenced by changes in the prevalence of risk factors and any new interventions or circumstances that might have an impact on incidence or mortality. For all cancers combined (excluding

Figure 5.7a   Trends in mortality for the five most common cancers causing death in males

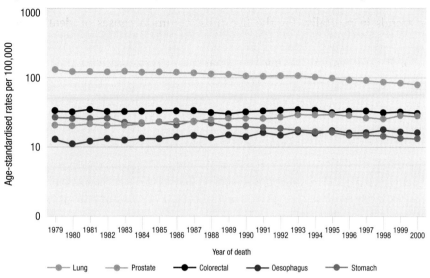

Figure 5.7b   Trends in mortality for the five most common cancers causing death in females

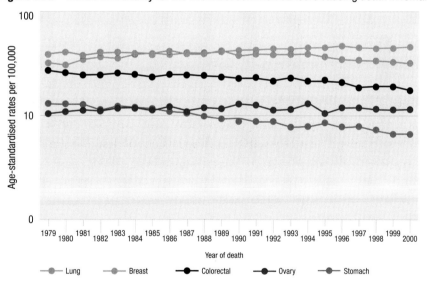

non-melanoma skin cancer), the projections of incidence and mortality (numbers and age-standardised rates) are summarised in Figure 5.8. For all age groups it is predicted that by 2010–2014, 33 000 cases of cancer will be diagnosed annually and that the number of cancer deaths will have increased to 16 300 a year. Figures for 1995–97 were 25 808 and 14 904 respectively. The projected increase in numbers of new cases, in part the result of ageing of the population, will have major implications for the planning and delivery of cancer services over the next decade.

Figure 5.8   Projections of incidence of and mortality from all malignant neoplasms combined (excluding non-melanoma skin cancer) in Scotland *Numbers of cases and deaths, and European age-standardised rates*

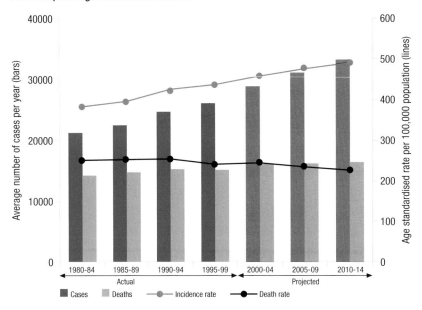

Screening for cancer in Scotland

Scotland currently has two established nationwide screening programmes that are the responsibility of the National Services Division. Cervical screening started in the 1960s in Scotland (when local programmes were initiated by enthusiastic clinicians) but it was not until the mid-1980s that the need for a national programme was recognised. A Scottish Office circular in 1988 charged all Health Boards with introducing computerised call and recall systems and required each Board to designate one individual who would be responsible for the organisation and effectiveness of each programme. In general, the programme has succeeded in reducing the incidence of invasive cancer. Imperfections in some Health Board call/recall programmes have been problematic, and a national system is now proposed. Uptake has been consistently good; assessment in 2002 showed that 81.7 % of eligible women in Scotland had been screened in the last 3.5 years; 86.5 % in the last five and a half years. Women in the age group 20–60 years are offered screening every five years, although screening is available on request to older women. Once the sixth most common site in women, the incidence and mortality of cervical cancer has fallen progressively; in 1998 there were 375 new cases in Scotland (making it the eighth most common cancer in women), and in 2001, 113 women died from the disease.

The UK is the first and only country to offer national population screening for breast cancer. The decision to introduce screening was based on the recommendation of a Working Party chaired by Sir Patrick Forrest, formerly Regius Professor of Clinical Surgery in the University of Edinburgh. The Scottish Breast Screening Programme was established in 1988 but national coverage was only achieved by 1991. Initially confined to women aged 50–64 years with screening every three to five years, *Our National Health* in 2000[15] announced the intention to increase the upper age limit to 70 years. The Programme continues to meet virtually all its targets – for example, detection rates for invasive cancer and small cancers, early recall rate – and attendance overall is steady at around 72.5 %. While early signs are encouraging, the long-term impact of national screening remains a controversial topic and only time will tell whether the Programme can reduce mortality by the 30 % suggested in the original Working Party deliberations.

In 2000 a demonstration project (*the Cancer Challenge*) offered screening for colorectal cancer to men and women aged 50–69 years in Grampian, Tayside and Fife Health Board areas. The Scottish project is one of two UK pilot studies that will assess the feasibility, public acceptability, safety and benefits of population screening for malignant and pre-malignant lesions of the large bowel. The first round of screening has now been completed, and evaluation by an independent expert team was generally favourable.

Organisation of Cancer Services in Scotland

Scotland has a well-trained and well-motivated clinical workforce, a tradition of excellence in cancer research and a long-standing and continuing ethos of public service. It has excellent cancer registration and collation of cancer statistics, with effective linkage between its data registries. As an example of integration and co-ordination, the Scottish Cancer Intelligence Unit (formed in 1993) brings together groups of ISD (Information and Statistics Division) staff working on cancer-related information in the Scottish Cancer Registry, Cancer Surveillance Group, Scottish Cancer Therapy Network and Epidemiological Studies Group. Given the advantages of this robust infrastructure, why is it that the clinical outcomes for cancer patients in Scotland are relatively unsatisfactory? It is clear that Scotland's burden of deprivation has a great deal to do with its high incidence of cancer and may explain in part some of the less desirable features of outcome. The remainder of this chapter will consider the way in which cancer services in Scotland are organised and delivered.

Commissioned Cancer Services

The influential Calman/Hine report on the organisation of cancer services in England was published by the Expert Advisory Group on Cancer in 1995. It recommended that cancer services should be based on a network of expertise reaching through primary care to Cancer Units in District General Hospitals, and from there to a small number of Cancer Centres equipped with a full range of resources. In 1995–96, the Commissioning of Cancer Services in Scotland was considered in the light of these proposals. In endorsing the Calman/Hine approach, five Scottish hospitals providing radiotherapy were designated as Cancer Centres (Western Infirmary, Glasgow; Western General Hospital, Edinburgh; Ninewells Hospital, Dundee; Aberdeen Royal Infirmary; and Raigmore Hospital, Inverness). Criteria were established for Cancer Units, and the provision of primary care and palliative care services was considered. It was recognised that the strategy might take many years to improve cancer care. In the event, the benefits of the approach were not realised, principally because of funding pressures (not least the difficulty of providing enough linear accelerators for radiotherapy) and the divisive nature of the internal market. The core proposal to develop networks for cancer services, however, has not been lost; indeed networking remains the basis of current arrangements for cancer (see below).

Developing a national policy framework

As outlined earlier, demographic changes are likely to lead to future increases in the number of patients with cancer and this together with reductions in mortality will increase the prevalence of cancer significantly.[14] The large numbers of people living with cancer and the availability of new treatments and interventions will make significant additional demands on the NHS. Patients and public are increasingly well informed about the progress and promise of research programmes and the potential advantages of new technologies and treatments. Information made available by the popular press, broadcasting media and the internet has meant that the relationship between patient and clinician is changing. Increasing numbers of patients are unwilling to accept the passive role of a recipient of treatment and rightly expect to participate in a more active and demanding partnership with their clinicians. These drivers of change are not unique to cancer medicine, indeed they apply to many chronic diseases. In an era of fundamental restructuring in which service provision will respond more readily to changing demands, Scottish cancer services are in the first wave and in many ways are serving as a pilot for other areas of complex chronic disease management. The model of managed clinical networks of care developed in the *Acute Services Review* has also been viewed favourably by other parts of the UK as a means of implementing cancer strategy.

Our National Health[15] set out the Scottish Executive's commitment to modernisation in 2001 and described the principles that will be used to achieve substantial service change. The emphasis is on patients and their needs, assuring standards of care, reducing waiting times, improved strategic planning and developing collaborative networks to deliver evidence-based care. These fundamentals have been developed further in *Cancer in Scotland: Action for Change.*[13]

Cancer networks

It is now widely recognised that cancer patients need multidisciplinary care and that the necessary expertise may not always be available on one site. Networking allows optimal care to be provided by a number of different organisations and individuals across a given geographical area. This has led to the adoption of managed clinical networks (MCNs) as the most appropriate model of care. The role of each network is to ensure both horizontal and vertical integration of services for a given patient population by bringing together the professions and disciplines involved in the care of patients with a particular cancer type. The West of Scotland has a MCN devoted to the treatment of colorectal cancer, for example, and the South East Scotland regional network (SCAN) has disease-specific groups (Figure 5.9) as well as generic networks for audit and pharmacy.

Figure 5.9   Summary of SCAN Structure

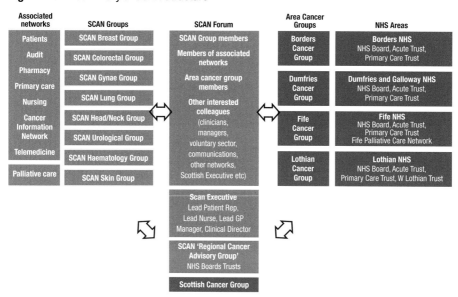

The principal function of MCNs is the delivery of effective care of a defined quality that is centred on patient needs. The networks are designed to make optimal use of available services and resources in supporting patient journeys of care across institutional and organisational boundaries.[16] The objective is to bring together the various multidisciplinary NHS components in a formal, coherent and managed grouping that links effectively with patient representatives and the voluntary sector.

Regional co-ordination of cancer services

In Scotland there are three regional organisations that co-ordinate cancer services in their area and contribute to the planning and implementation of new developments. These regional networks are not cancer site-specific and take an overview of the management of all types of cancer. The three networks are as follows:

- The **West of Scotland** network covers Argyll and Clyde, Ayrshire and Arran, Lanarkshire, Forth Valley and Greater Glasgow NHS Board areas and contains the West of Scotland Cancer Centre at the Beatson Oncology Centre in Glasgow.

- The **South East Scotland** network covers Lothian, Borders, Fife and Dumfries and Galloway NHS Board areas and contains the Edinburgh Cancer Centre at the Western General Hospital, Edinburgh.

- The **North of Scotland** network includes three cancer centres in Dundee, Inverness and Aberdeen and provides services for the people of Highland, Grampian, Tayside, Western Isles and Orkney and Shetland NHS Board areas.

The South-East Scotland Cancer Network (SCAN) is used in Figure 5.9 to illustrate network structure. Further details, including the constitution and summary of network activities, can be viewed on www.scan.scot.nhs.uk, but a traditional organogram is used merely to illustrate the complex relationships between the various components. It is the strength and effectiveness of these components that determines the overall effectiveness of the structure, although a great deal depends on the connectivity of the individual components. To paraphrase Don Berwick,[17] great health professionals 'interacting well with all of the other elements of the healthcare system make great health care'. To improve performance one needs to concentrate on such interactions and improve 'interdependency between individuals, professions and organisations'.

One key area of responsibility for each cancer network is ongoing and prospective data collection to support quality assurance of their services within a nationwide framework. Identified clinicians and managers have authority and responsibility for defined sections of service delivery and planning, and work with the multidisciplinary cancer specific groups using agreed and transparent rules, remits and criteria. The outcomes of this quality assurance process must be reported regularly to the clinical governance structure of the Trusts and NHS Boards concerned. Increasingly, the quality assurance work of MCNs is being linked to the quality assurance programme of the Clinical Standards Board for Scotland (CSBS) that is now incorporated in the NHSScotland Quality Improvement (NHSQIS) organisation. In its first wave, CSBS developed national standards, described their assessment by a self-report mechanism as well as external peer review, and introduced national reporting of the performance of all components of the NHS that were providing specified services. This comprehensive description of services for breast, colorectal, lung and ovarian cancer provide a baseline in 2001 against which networks can measure and report their own improvements.

Each of the three Scottish Cancer networks reports to a Regional Cancer Advisory Group (RCAG) which serves as a steering group to bring together representatives from all relevant stakeholders within that region. The RCAGs are responsible for annual monitoring of the work plan of the MCNs and in conjunction with their constituents for developing a prioritised investment plan. The RCAGs and their MCNs have a pivotal role in the implementation of *Cancer in Scotland* and are seen as the engine for change and service improvement.[18, 19] The three-year implementation programme of *Cancer in Scotland* is backed up by new, additional and recurring annual investment of £25 million which is available to the networks.

National co-ordination and advice – The Scottish Cancer Group

In 1998 the Scottish Cancer Group was established as the Scottish Executive's national advisory body on cancer services. Initially chaired by Dr Harry Burns (Director of Public Health, Greater Glasgow) and more recently by one of the authors of this chapter (AG), the Group reports to the Chief Medical Officer in Scotland. It brings together the three regional structures and is responsible for implementing and monitoring the service changes prescribed in *Cancer in Scotland*.

It reviews and ratifies regional investment plans, monitors progress, and uses subgroups to review specific issues such as Quality Improvement, Patient Information, Information Technology and Cancer Genetics.

This programme for the implementation of *Cancer in Scotland* has a number of unique features:

- The investment decisions are made by the regional networks (taking into account a national improvement framework developed by SIGN and CSBS, and according priority to reducing waiting times for diagnosis/treatment and to improving patients' experiences of services)

- Each investment proposal has specified improvement targets and timescales and names a lead individual who is responsible for the project

- The impact and progress of these plans are closely and regularly monitored

- The investment is ring fenced

- Both the investment plans and the monitoring reports are readily available in the public domain (www.show.scot.nhs.uk/sehd/cancerinscotland)

Potential advantages of these fundamental changes

Networks formalise pathways of care and referral arrangements, bring governance and stewardship in line with patient pathways and expectations, and engage clinical staff in managing the process. Networks are groups of individuals and/or teams whose activities are interdependent.[20] This arrangement appears to be a much more suitable and acceptable organisational model for the modern NHS than the traditional hierarchical organisation.

Networks can make optimal use of specialist services available within larger geographic areas and help to sustain services that would otherwise be vulnerable in their own right. Formal arrangements for referral and management improve equitable access for patients and standardise care, while at the same time reducing 'distance decay' – that is, the potential for results/outcomes to become less satisfactory with increasing distance from major centres.[21] By focusing on the needs of patients, MCNs can achieve immediate improvements in the experience of services by reducing delays and handover problems. By stimulating cross-specialty, cross-discipline and cross-sector dialogue, MCNs can foster innovative ways of improving services.

Barriers to change

By moving away from traditional vertical models, networks may appear to some to threaten the status quo. For some established clinical staff, the need to take an area-wide and multidisciplinary view of services may conflict with traditional narrow local views of service provision by a defined specialty. The need to develop MCNs may appear particularly problematic for a service struggling with challenging financial targets and externally imposed performance indicators. The pressures on management and key clinical staff may be such that the time available for strategic thinking and collaborative development is in short supply. Initial confusion over accountabilities and responsibilities of networks may compound the sense of frustration that some managers feel. It can appear as if the networks have all the 'fun' of new ways of working and modernisation without the 'pain' of accountability for overall financial or clinical governance. Some networks may appear messy with poorly defined and overlapping edges and/or multiple overlying layers,[22–24] although this may be exactly what is needed in some cases. Organisations based on relationships and function are much more liable to change with time, and we need to be able to manage this and anticipate necessary changes in shape, scope and behaviour of networks.

What can be done to allay fears, correct misapprehensions and minimise tensions between the various components as they try to work together more closely? Clarity of responsibilities and reporting arrangements is an essential first step and this is the task of the RCAGs. If established appropriately, networks should be seen as helpful by patients, clinicians and managers alike. Their role in audit will assure quality, underpin clinical governance, and inform the performance assessment framework of organisations and the appraisal and revalidation of clinicians. In times of increasing accountability for outcomes it may be comforting for individuals to know that they are functioning within the norms established by their peers and if they are not, that there is a mechanism that can help to improve performance and reduce variance. Managers are provided with ready-made regional peer review and with services that are more likely to be of high quality, consistent and sustainable. Training, continuing professional development, clinical research and service development can all be enhanced by successful networks.

The predominant peer-to-peer relationship of the networks needs to have a clearly agreed framework that will define the agenda and scope of the work being undertaken. Networks cannot rely on the vertical top-down reporting arrangements and objective setting used by traditional NHS organisations. The objectives of individual members of the network need to be aligned with those of the component organisations. This may challenge the behaviour and practice of some staff members and the introduction of MCNs needs to be managed without stifling innovation or imposing additional bureaucracy. The key recurring questions for all those involved in this process must be 'How does our service perform from the perspective of the patient?' and 'What can we do together to improve outcomes and the experience of our patients?' In the case of services as complex as those used by cancer patients, it can be argued that collaborative networks offer the only realistic prospect of achieving satisfactory responses to these questions.

Effective communication is essential for the development and support of teams and networks. Sustained success and momentum needs a foundation of trust and a shared philosophy of continuous learning and improvement. This will remain a particular challenge for network teams that are geographically dispersed.

What of the future?

Scottish cancer services are well on the way through a multistage process of major change. A sense of urgency has been established by international comparisons of outcomes, focus has been sustained by continuing public and political interest, and improvements are being supported by Government investment. An invaluable coalition of interests has been created that brings together patients (and their relatives, carers and representatives), clinicians, managers, politicians and the general public in a drive to improve cancer services. The signs are encouraging with growing acceptance of the need for new more effective forms of collaboration on the part of clinical leaders, the national quality improvement programme of the Clinical Standards Board for Scotland, politicians and NHS Boards and Trusts. It is anticipated that excellence in clinical care will be supported by excellence in biomedical research within Scotland's universities and medical schools, and by increasing recruitment to clinical trials.

Cancer in Scotland set out the strategy and vision for change and the Executive has started to remove obstacles by setting out regional structures, using national bodies to co-ordinate quality improvements and deploying evidence-based developments. The introduction of investment planning through regional networks has further strengthened the drive to improve services by ensuring wide clinical and managerial buy in. Patients and carers are fundamental partners in service change and a helpful and constant reminder of the overall purpose of the enterprise. Communication through websites, newsletters, road shows and forums is beginning to bring the changes designed by *Cancer in Scotland* to an increasingly wider audience. Novel technological solutions may further improve information sharing while new ways of tele-working and decision support may further enhance service provision.

The Scottish Cancer Group and its three regional networks are now beginning to achieve some early successes with visible improvements in performance. It will take time before changes now being set in train will translate into significant improvements in outcome. For the moment, we need to consolidate the early gains and anchor the new approaches in the culture of the NHS in Scotland. As the credibility of networks and the SCG grows, it should become easier to create further beneficial organisational changes and continue to support patient-focused care as a mechanism for the improved delivery of more effective services. Scotland has a unique opportunity to create cancer services that are among the best in the world.

REFERENCES

1. Parkin DM, Whelan SL, Ferlay J, Raymond L, Young J. *Cancer Incidence in Five Continents* (volume VII). IARC Scientific Publications No. 143. Lyon: International Agency for Research on Cancer, 1997.

2. World Health Organisation. *WHO Mortality Database*. http://www.who.int/whosis/ (accessed 28/05/02)

3. Information and Statistics Division. *Scottish Health Statistics 2000*. http://www.show.scot.nhs.uk/isd/Scottish_Health_Statistics/SHS2000/home.htm (accessed 28/05/02)

4. Kogevinas M, Pearce N, Susser M, Boffetta P (eds). *Social Inequalities and Cancer*. IARC Scientific Publications No. 138. Lyon: International Agency for Research on Cancer, 1997.

5. Harris V, Sandridge A, Black RJ, Brewster DH, Gould A. *Cancer Registration Statistics Scotland, 1986–1995*. Edinburgh: ISD Publications, 1998.

6. http://www.show.scot.nhs.uk/isd/cancer/facts_figures/facts_figures.htm (accessed 28/5/02)

7. Sharp L, Brewster D. The epidemiology of lung cancer in Scotland: a review of trends in incidence, survival and mortality and prospects for prevention. *Health Bulletin* (Edinburgh) 1999; 57: 318–331.

8. Gray RF, Brewster DH, Kidd J, Burns H. Colorectal Cancer in Scotland: Recent Trends in Incidence and Mortality. *Gastrointestinal Oncology* 2002, 4: 213–222.

9. Brewster DH, Fraser LA, Harris V, Black RJ. Rising incidence of prostate cancer in Scotland: increased risk or increased detection? *BJU International* 2000; 85: 463–472.

10. Brewster D, Everington D, Harkness E, Gould A, Warner J, Dewar JA, Arrundale J. Incidence of and mortality from breast cancer since introduction of screening. *British Medical Journal* 1996; 312: 639–40.

11. Scottish Cancer Intelligence Unit. *Trends in Cancer Survival in Scotland, 1971–1995*. Edinburgh: Information & Statistics Division, 2000. http://www.show.scot.nhs.uk/isd/Scottish_Health_Statistics/subject/Cancer_survival/trends_1971–95.pdf (accessed 28/05/02)

12. Brewster DH, Fraser LA, McKinney PA, Black RJ. Socioeconomic status and risk of adenocarcinoma of the oesophagus and cancer of the gastric cardia in Scotland. *British Journal of Cancer* 2000; 83: 387–390.

13. Scottish Executive Health Department. *Cancer in Scotland: Action for Change*. Edinburgh: The Scottish Executive, 2001. http://www.scotland.gov.uk/library3/health/csac.pdf (accessed 28/5/02)

14. Scottish Executive Health Department. *Cancer Scenarios: an aid to planning cancer services in Scotland in the next decade*. Edinburgh: The Scottish Executive, 2001. http://www.show.scot.nhs.uk/sehd/publications/csatp/csatp-01.htm

15. Scottish Executive Health Department. *Our National Health: A plan for action, a plan for change*. Edinburgh: The Scottish Executive, 2001

16. Management Executive Letter. Introduction of Managed Clinical Networks within the NHS in Scotland. MEL (1999) 10.

17. Berwick, DM. Medical associations: guilds or leaders. *British Medical Journal* 1997; 314: 1564–65.

18. Health Department Letter. Managed Clinical Networks in Palliative Care HDL (2000) 10.

19. Health Department Letter. Regional Cancer Advisory Groups. HDL (2001) 71.

20. Mullins LJ. *Management and organisational behaviour*. London: Prentice Hall, 1999.

21. Campbell NC, Elliott AM, Sharp L, Ritchie LD, Cassidy J, Little J. Rural factors and survival from cancer- analysis of Scottish cancer registrations. *British Journal of Cancer* 2000; 82: 1863–66.

22. Conner M. Developing network based services in the NHS. *International Journal of Health Care Quality Assurance*. 2001; 14: 237–244.

23. Fisher FE, Sharp A. *Lateral Leadership*. London: Harper-Collins Business, 1999.

24. Ostroff F. *The Horizontal Organisation*.Oxford: Open University Press, 1999.

6. Mental Health in Scotland

Angus Mackay

Introduction

Powerful levers for change have been felt by mental health services throughout the UK over the past 15 years, some internal, many external. By the year 2002 the process of replacing Scotland's large asylums has come a long way (see chapter 7), largely through a process of evolution from within the service itself as the need for large numbers of in-patient beds for those with chronic disability has manifestly become unnecessary. The Scottish process stands in some contrast to that in England and Wales, where de-institutionalisation tended, in many instances, to be forced rather than facilitated, resulting in unhelpful extremes and the eventual recognition in some quarters that the contraction of in-patient resources had gone too far. To some extent the resettlement and care of people with mental illness into the community has been enabled by improved treatments, but the main ingredients in this change have been attitudinal. External levers are always the most uncomfortable to feel, and here the most potent have been the expectations of an increasingly well-informed public, expectations for involvement in decision-making (about both resource use and personal treatment plans), quick and direct access to information and to specialist services at all times, and the blurring of the reference point of definable mental illness into 'mental health problems'. The involvement, or 'inclusiveness', principle has become an imperative not only for patients and potential patients but also for service providers. This has led to various forms of joint planning, joint commissioning and joint provision of services between NHS agencies, local authorities, voluntary organisations and patient representative groups. That attitudes have changed, both within and outside the mental health service, is not in doubt. There is, however, a gap between aspirations and actualities that is diminishing only slowly in Scotland. To some extent this reflects the inevitable time required in which to manage change and redeploy resources, but it also reflects a sincere, and perhaps typically Scottish, caution that comes from a perception of the risks associated with the possible benefits. The following sections consider these issues in greater detail. From the standpoint of a practising psychiatrist in rural Scotland, the chapter attempts to provide an honest and balanced consideration of risks and benefits, idealism and pragmatism, political aspirations and safe solutions.

Service Management and Structure

The early 1980s saw the eventual demise, generally, of Physicians Superintendent, a reaction to a succession of dismal special enquiries in England and Wales, and crystallised by the Nodder Report.[1] This report, by a wise senior civil servant in Whitehall, drew attention to the inherent risk in power being held by one individual within the relatively closed system of the mental institution. Nodder recommended a multidisciplinary management group comprising medical, nursing and administrative representation, the tri-partite Hospital Management Team. This approach was adopted in some services in Scotland, and rapidly moved on to the creation of increasingly larger and more inclusive management teams, sometimes distinct from, but linking to, professional Divisions of Psychiatry. This was healthy, but greeted with some suspicion by medical professionals who saw a dilution of their status.

Even more convulsive changes were to happen with successive reorganisations of local health services; moving from Districts, through Units and multi-service Trusts to Primary Care Trusts and Local Healthcare Co-operatives (LHCCs). At each stage the mental health service worked alongside and linked with other services within a geographical catchment area. In most Districts and Units the mental health service was one of a number of specialties serving a catchment population and, by and large, mental health services managed to retain integrity as a managed entity. Into this increasingly confusing organisational merry-go-round, the further ingredient of the internal market was introduced during the Thatcher years. The free market principles had probably least relevance to mental health services, and least direct impact, but the resultant complications felt by neighbouring specialties inflicted collateral damage. The ball to which eyes became fixed was not the development of services for the mentally ill, a perennially low priority in any case, and the result was a frustrating (albeit unintended) moratorium on progress in mental health service development in many parts of Scotland.

Integration between specialist mental health services and primary care was given impetus through the inclusion of mental health services within Primary Care Trusts in the NHS reorganisation of 1999. This relationship is being further encouraged through policy statements such as *Mental Health: Moving the Agenda Forward* [2] that seek to dismantle any boundaries still existing between general practice and psychiatry. This may be a dangerous, potentially disastrous path down which psychiatry is being pushed, one which is being mapped out in the context of health service reorganisation, but which reflects a philosophical view that mental health services can better serve the mental health needs of the population by de-specialising and becoming a branch of primary care. Fuelling the risk in all of this is the associated trend towards an emphasis on the softer, more social aspects of mental health at the expense of knowledge about, and expertise around, the biological aspects of mental illness and the established evidence base from which clinical behaviour should be derived. The inevitable result could be the dumbing down of the specialty to a lowest shared denominator, with psychiatry soon ceasing to be a specialty at all.

The shift of the focus of treatment and care from centralised institutions to treatment in or close to the patient's home is now the central plank of mental health policy, associated with the recognition that Local Authority Social Work Departments have much to offer within the overall care package, and that co-ordination between NHS and Local Authority is essential. 'Jointness' has now become the operational goal, both in terms of planning and execution of services. Potential benefits from such a partnership include gains in efficiency and seamlessness. Jointness is an attractive property in the delivery of any complex health care system, and can probably be achieved successfully where there is a shared sense of necessity and respect for judgement and common sense. If forced as an ideology on systems which are inherently widely disparate in their training, philosophy and executive structures, however, the imperative of jointness can become paralysing, characterised by power competitions and decision blight.

The round the clock mental health service has also become an expectation, but it is arguable whether this is, indeed, a sensible way to go. In Scotland, as in the rest of the UK, the primary care service is the absolute cornerstone of the NHS; community and family-orientated and not only the first line in emergency situations but also a vital collection and integration point at which all of the patients needs and services are recorded and co-ordinated. The desire for direct access to specialist mental health services at any time of day or night runs the risk of subjecting the patient to 'primary care bypass', with many associated disadvantages. Encouraging the development of specialist mental health services as an alternative to, or even a separate wing of, primary care for mental health issues may actually increase the risk of compartmentalisation, and perhaps even greater stigma associated with the use of the mental health service.

Within LHCCs there is the really good opportunity for sensible integration and division of labour between specialist mental health services and primary care teams. Success or failure is, as usual, very much dependent upon local personality mix and the strength of longstanding prejudices. In some cases there appears to be a genuine and productive willingness to work together in mutual respect; in other instances there appears to be pressure from primary care to engulf, asset-strip and manage the mental health service; and in others a reluctance on the part of psychiatrists to accept that the effective delivery of many aspects of a comprehensive mental health service is properly positioned within primary care.

Achieving a Sensible Community/Hospital Balance

This has been one of the perennial issues facing clinicians and health service planners for many decades.[3-6] The mental health service in Scotland has never leapt before it looked and nowhere is this more important than in achieving a safe and satisfactory balance between the provision of specialist hospital services and the distribution of community resources throughout a catchment area. The philosophy governing the need for hospital services is the guarantee of a safe, caring and clinically effective environment for any person suffering from mental illness in situations where either the speed of deterioration overtakes other provisions or where, despite best efforts, more ambitious or organisationally more complex solutions suddenly fail.

In some countries the move to community care has assumed the dimensions of a crusade, often with frank political overtones.[7] In Italy and the United States, political decisions, backed up by statutory force, brought about the widespread closure of mental illness hospitals, encouraged by the belief (dubbed 'the new simplicity' by Finzin in 1981[8]) that all mental illness could be managed in the community. In the United States the dismal experience of the Community Mental Health Centre Programme set up by President Kennedy has been amply catalogued in the Report of the Group on American Psychiatry, and the Italian experience is another cautionary tale which includes a catalogue of clinical risks such as the dangerous over-prescription of antipsychotic drugs in order to achieve speedy hospital discharge. In Scotland, the production of the Framework for Mental Health Services has been a significant milestone, a generally respected recipe for the form and content of comprehensive local mental health services in which there is recognition of the future need for modestly proportioned, purpose-designed hospital services.[9] The Framework, an impressive document upon which there has been the widest consultation, continues to evolve and be extended, and specifies the sort of specialist hospital facilities which should be available in any comprehensive mental health service for the diagnosis and treatment of that very small but important percentage of people requiring such facilities at certain times. This is a logical and appropriate reflection of the explicit focus of the Framework, people with severe and enduring mental illness. Thus, while every effort must be given to the delivery of help as close as possible to the person's natural environment, and to minimising the social disruption for the patient and his/her family, the safety net must always be there. The mental hospital will be seen as but one component of a comprehensive community-orientated mental health service rather than a nucleus whose mass greatly exceeds that of the resources in its surrounding catchment area. Although huge investment is still required in order to put such models into practice, the signs are good that Scotland will eventually see the re-provision of hospital services within relatively small, purpose-designed buildings of domestic appearance. It is to be hoped that they will also enjoy a protected surrounding environment of high amenity in which patients can enjoy the open air, walk and enjoy recreational facilities in an environment in which they are protected from ridicule.[4] While perhaps having the ring of paternalism, this recognises the reality of the needs of some people at some times. This is hardly rocket science, more an area in which balanced judgement must prevail alongside the art of reconciling the needs and wishes of people emotionally tethered to either end of the community-hospital spectrum.

The question of the future of psychiatric units placed within district general hospitals arises. Their success has undoubtedly been highly variable, but it is the opinion of this writer that more often than not they represent an uncomfortable attempt to reduce the stigma and neglect of mental health services by placing such facilities in the midst of popular clinical specialties. This seems to be misguided and not offset by any advantage coming from proximity to specialist investigation and professional liaison. On the contrary, it often seems to be the case that the psychiatric ward is a victim of even greater stigma and its patients exposed to ridicule and restriction to an extent that is greater than that which was ever experienced in a discrete mental health facility.

The Patient-Professional Relationship

Part and parcel of the reality of a better informed public has been an increasing unwillingness by people simply to accept, without question, advice from health professionals. Caricatured as the need for a role reversal from obedience to assertiveness, a high-profile semantic expression of this has been to prohibit use of the term 'patient' and to substitute terms such as 'user' or 'consumer'. The term user enjoys the dictionary definition of someone who 'employs, exploits, exhausts or consumes'. Although in many respects an understandable reaction to the position of passivity often inflicted upon recipients of health care, the term user is for many both unattractive and inappropriate. Ironically, most users dislike the term just as much as the people who are seen as being used. The term serves only to discourage any recognition of the value that can be derived from the patient-professional relationship in terms of trust and mutual respect.[10, 11]

There has been a simultaneous growth of realistic and quite justifiable expectations of involvement by patients and their families in service planning and delivery. This has sometimes led, however, to a degree of overstatement based on dogma rather than sensible practice. An example of the latter is the expectation that everyone should have equal say in the detail of planning decisions, a practice seen to be politically correct, but one which neglects the fact that experts have special knowledge and experience to bring to such issues – an expertise which, ironically, is often recognised more by patients than by policy-makers. On the other hand, involvement in decisions about personal care is entirely appropriate, albeit tempered by the sad fact that, for some people, at some stages of illness, insight, comprehension and judgement may be impaired. Here, there has been the helpful introduction of advocacy services designed to offer ready access by patients to personal help with understanding and voicing opinions on issues affecting their treatment and care.

Quality Assurance

The past 15 years have seen a gradual erosion of simple trust in health professionals. This has, to a large extent, been earned through a succession of revelations, most recently the Bristol Inquiry and Harold Shipman. In response to public disquiet the professions have set about creating mechanisms through which to reassure the public and Parliament that practitioners are behaving properly and according to best current knowledge. The CRAG Working Group on Mental Illness was established in 1992, charged by the Chief Medical Officer with the task of identifying areas in which national initiatives were likely to encourage better standards of care with optimal use of resources. Over a four-year period the Group published 11 Good Practice Statements on areas of controversy (such as ECT and neurosurgery for mental disorder) or in which practice was highly variable across the country.[12] Around the same time the Scottish Intercollegiate Guideline Network (SIGN) was gathering speed and producing Clinical Guidelines on a wide range of clinical issues, but relatively few devoted to mental health issues. With the emergence of the Framework for Mental Health Services in Scotland in 1997,[9] a successor to the Working Group, the Mental Health and Well Being Support Group, was charged with auditing and overseeing the implementation of the Framework. The term 'clinical governance' gained prominence during the mid-1990s, embodying few new concepts; but serving as a symbol for quality assurance, eventually resulting in Chief Executives of Trusts being held responsible for the quality of clinical services, specifically the responsibility to show that mechanisms were in place to audit and assure standards of service delivery. Audit requires standards, and a complex network of organisations (see chapter 10) has arisen which are either concerned with the formulation of standards of good practice, or with their implementation and/or audit. They have all jostled for elbow room with long-established and respected guardians of standards such as the Scottish Health Advisory Service (SHAS) and the Mental Welfare Commission for Scotland (MWC). Not only did local health services feel confused about which priority to address (with little or no new resources) but they were made to incur substantial and increasing opportunity costs due to time devoted to accreditation visits from these various organisations.[13] There was also tension between belief in 'box ticking' and more discursive forms of service evaluation. The creation of NHS Quality Improvement Scotland, as the bold remedy for diseconomy and confusion caused by so many organisations, is dealt with in chapter 10.

Alongside these developments has grown the concept of risk assessment and risk management, both clinical and fiscal. The ingredients in this category of organisational introspection include the need to be seen to avoid untoward incidents (either from mistakes, wilful violence or accident) and the need to minimise the probability of accusations of negligence and associated claims for damages. Awareness of risk and the establishment of procedures to identify and manage risk is an undeniably good thing in principle. For physical health interventions there have been statutory elements of the British establishment in place for some 30 years in the form of the Medicines Control Agency and the Medical Devices Agency, the former being responsible for a safety vigilance system that is the envy of the world and through which the risks from medications are continuously scrutinised. The newly formed National Patient Safety Agency (NPSA) represents an extension of the existing agencies, charged with encouraging a no-blame culture in which professionals admit to, and record, mistakes and shortcomings, and with the establishment of a national information gathering system for clinical mishaps and near misses. The NPSA was established in England and Wales in 2001 and the intention is to include a Scottish equivalent in a UK-wide safety database. This is one example where national boundaries are decidedly unhelpful, the larger the database the more likely it is that sufficient data will be collected to generate important safety signals. While the highlighting of risk is beneficial, there is also a danger, especially in the area of clinical risk management in mental health. Any reliance on numbers coming from non-validated risk scales (such as many of those purporting to predict the risk of suicide) may be misleading and exert greater weight than global clinical judgement based on knowledge of the patient.

Clinical Effectiveness and Value

Being clinically effective, and demonstrating it, is a vital part of the powerful concept of clinical governance, which has already been referred to. In the absence of anything approaching a comprehensive set of valid clinical outcome measures the Health Service has tended to rely on an expectation that if practitioners are adhering to guidelines describing good practice then clinical outcomes (both in terms of benefits and safety) will improve. In Scotland, SIGN has produced an impressive array of clinical guidelines, the adoption of which is auditable. So, enormous pressure is being exerted to require health service professionals to show that they are practising according to officially approved guidelines based on the best of current evidence. In psychiatry, the top priority for a national standard was, quite appropriately, felt to be one describing good quality services for people who suffer from schizophrenic illness.

The Clinical Standards Board for Scotland conducted an all-inclusive audit of mental health services throughout Scotland to measure their performance against explicit standards relating to the management of schizophrenic illness. While much of value was identified, perhaps the most striking cause for concern was the wide variation between local services in meeting these standards. The major deficiencies were in the need for life and social skills training, the need to provide information to patients and carers, the absence of standardised clinical documentation, patchy implementation of guidelines and clinical audit, widely variable composition of community mental health teams and their links to primary care, and poorly resourced training.[14] Much food for thought, a positive stimulus to clinicians and NHS Board planners.

The concept of cost-effectiveness, linked to clinical effectiveness, is a vitally important one for the efficient distribution of resources within a capped health budget. Value for money is a concept with which most people are familiar, but its association with the term rationing has always tended to make politicians uncomfortable. Prioritisation is a generally more acceptable term, and it is precisely what has to happen at all levels of the health service given the finite and limited nature of resources. The decision about how to invest any affordable resource must be guided by information on cost-effectiveness, or in other words the amount of benefit that can be derived from a given amount of investment. The assessment of clinical and cost effectiveness, as well as the associated implications for health service organisation and for the patients' experience, is the business of Health Technology Assessment (HTA). Hard on the heels of the creation of the National Institute for Clinical Excellence (NICE) in England and Wales, the Health Technology Board for Scotland (HTBS) was created in 2000. Its job has been to advise NHS Scotland on the clinical and cost effectiveness of new and existing health interventions, and also to consider outputs from NICE with regard to their implications for Scotland. NICE have produced several items of guidance on psychiatric interventions, including anti-dementia drugs, the newer antipsychotic agents, and ECT. HTBS has produced a comprehensive and detailed health technology assessment on interventions to reduce the risk of relapse in alcohol dependence in Scotland. So a very useful start has been made on the provision of guidance to clinicians, and advice to Scottish Trusts and Health Boards on what is effective, and moreover what is cost-effective.[15] Sadly, the topics in mental health which have been tackled by these various organisations have been hampered probably more than in any other specialty by a relative lack of valid outcome data through which to measure effectiveness, and therefore cost-effectiveness.

Mental Health Interventions

Before considering certain specific forms of intervention it is important to review the evolving service context in which these interventions are being delivered. Increasingly more interventions are being delivered in the community, either through various forms of day-care, outpatient clinics, or in peoples' homes. The value of Community Mental Health Teams (CMHTs) has been widely recognised but the composition and operational behaviour of such teams vary widely. Some of this variation is justifiable in terms of the geographical nature of catchment areas, but some is not. Value is maximised through multidisciplinary and multi-agency membership of CMHTs but inadequate resourcing often limits both their size and composition. The community psychiatric nurse has always been the irreducible common factor, but the clinical burden on CPNs can be overwhelming if they are unsupported by a properly resourced group. The Care Programme Approach (CPA) is an operational initiative introduced in 1992 and consolidated in 1996.[16] The purpose of the CPA is to focus multi-agency planning on people with severe and enduring mental illness who also have complex health and social care needs. While this official requirement can act as a valuable catalyst for multi-agency collaboration, in some services the procedure has become over-inclusive and weighed down with bureaucracy. A simple test should always be applied; 'will the use of the formal CPA actually make a difference to the care of this person?', and the answer regularly tested against results.

Advances in physical interventions have occurred over the past 20 years, but it has to be said that none has produced the sort of quantum leap in benefit that followed the discovery of chlorpromazine in 1951. Chlorpromazine has many descendants that are used in the treatment of the schizophrenias and mania, but the success with which these psychoses are treated has increased only modestly. The pharmaceutical development of depot antipsychotic agents has been a positive factor in the satisfactory resettlement and maintenance of patients in the community, but only a minority of patients receive a depot, and medication concordance apart, the active ingredients are no more effective than their oral counterparts. In many ways the 'atypical' antipsychotics represent the most significant recent development in the treatment of the schizophrenias and mania. These agents are much less liable to induce the traditionally troublesome side-effects on movement, many have an adequate evidence base, but they are considerably more expensive and are not completely free of potentially dangerous side-effects such as cardiac dysrhythmia. For only one, clozapine, does good evidence exist for superior efficacy but, sadly, this unique benefit co-exists with an appreciable risk of potentially fatal blood disorder, and so its use is tightly restricted. The cost of the newer antipsychotics is generally an order of magnitude higher than their older antecedents, and the question of whether this increased cost is balanced by increased benefit is unclear.[17] The whole question of the clinical and cost effectiveness of the newer atypical antipsychotics is currently the subject of debate and structured evaluation. One very welcome product of the scrutiny of clinical practice associated with guidelines and algorithms, has been the explicit discouragement of the use of high-dose antipsychotic medication and polypharmacy. The evidence base is quite clear, that in the vast majority of cases there is no justification for the prescription of doses greater than those defined in the medicines' product licence or BNF, and indeed while there is a ceiling on benefit there is a greatly increasing risk of adverse effects as doses rise.[18] To that extent, there has been real advance in recent years in that patients are now much less likely to be toxically overdosed without any off-setting benefit.

The newer antidepressants are generally as effective as the older generation and are not only considerably safer in overdose, but associated with less distressing and concordance-limiting side-effects. As with the antipsychotic agents, however, it remains a matter of debate whether these advantages can be justified against the considerably greater costs of the new generation antidepressants, except in those few cases where the proprietary agent has outlived its patent and a cheap generic equivalent is available. The familiar theme of a paucity of reliable and useful outcome data is again evident. Sceptics point to the inexorable increase in global suicide rates in the face of the introduction of new antidepressants but this is to ignore the simple fact that most suicides are not associated with depressive illness.[19] So in order to demonstrate an impact on this crude outcome measure, any intervention for depressive illness would have to exert a dramatic effect. While it may be unclear from the available data whether these newer drugs have led to general improvements in mental health, it would be reasonable to assume that they have in the light of evidence suggesting greater concordance with prescriptions and more sensible dosing decisions by those prescribing them. There has been further refinement of the target clinical syndromes for the new generation antidepressants, such as generalised anxiety disorder, social phobia, obsessional compulsive disorder and bulimia nervosa. This broadening of the potential use of these drugs has brought with it a public concern about their safety. The introduction of Prozac (fluoxetine), with its apparently improved safety profile, led to huge overprescribing in North America and a tendency for it to be seen as an antidote to unhappiness and dissatisfaction. A counter-movement arose, originally from the Church of Scientology, but latterly joined by several other vocal and high profile critics. Currently in the UK the concern centres on a claimed tendency for people to become addicted to the newer antidepressants, and the alleged failure by the regulatory authorities to warn patients of this danger. These extremes of opinion have been less obvious in Scotland and here, as elsewhere, the uptake of the new agents has overtaken the older ones.

Another excellent consequence of standards and guidelines has been the scrutiny of ECT practice in Scotland. Based on best available evidence, the Working Group on Mental Illness and the Royal College of Psychiatrists produced an evolving set of standards that were audited in both England and Wales and in Scotland. The Scottish audit was particularly thorough and looked not only at process but also at clinical outcome through a series of on-site visits to all services delivering ECT throughout Scotland. Successive audits have demonstrated rising standards and this process is on-going.[20] The Scottish Audit of ECT represents a gold standard for the rest of the world in quality assurance.

The so-called anti-dementia agents emerged through the licensing process during the late 1990s. Although certainly no magic wand in the management of dementia, these agents do offer some patients the prospect of something like a six-month 'hold' on the progression of their disorder. Given this prospect and in the absence of convincing alternatives, current judgement is that these agents are both clinically and cost-effective. This was the opinion of NICE, and in its recognition of problems of access to specialists in rural areas of Scotland, the

HTBS modified this guidance to allow experienced general practitioners to initiate and monitor the treatment.[21]

Psychosurgery is an emotive term associated with evil connotations and often poor clinical outcomes. Assessing the place of 'neurosurgery for mental disorder', as it was renamed, by the Working Group on Mental Illness led to the publication of a Good Practice Statement in which the clinical indications were specified for which there was reasonable evidence of effectiveness. This is guidance unique to Scotland and it was associated with a series of recommendations about the process of choosing and delivering such a rare intervention for individual patients, including the designation of a single specialist centre in Dundee to which all eligible cases would be referred for surgery and detailed follow-up.[22] Associated ethical and legal issues were to become the subject of intense debate.

Highly structured and 'manualised' psychotherapies have grown in popularity and availability. Although still somewhat less than for pharmacological interventions, the evidence base for such psychological interventions is substantial and growing. Among the many advantages of structured and explicit techniques is their potential for adoption by a whole range of professionals who simply have to follow the manual. Another advantage is the greater possibility of subjecting such tightly described techniques to traditional randomised and controlled clinical trials. A further welcome development has been the meeting of biological and psychological paradigms in the territory of cognitive-behavioural therapy, with intense interest in the association between disordered limbic function, and even structure, and the targets for some of these therapies such as post-traumatic stress disorder (PTSD).[23] Two particular psychotherapies for refractory distress arising in the context of PTSD and severe personality disorder, dialectical behaviour therapy (DBT) and eye movement desensitisation and reprocessing (EMDR), have been pioneered in Lochgilphead.

The period spanning 1990 to 2000 was christened 'the decade of the brain', signifying concerted effort by neurobiologists and neuropharmacologists on the aetiopathology and treatment of the major psychiatric illnesses. Some advances were made during these years, but altogether these could only be described as marginal, and certainly less dramatic than the advances of the 1950s that were the result of serendipity rather than design.

Thorny Issues and Gaps in Service

Forensic Services

Alongside a detailed reconsideration of policy relating to offenders with mental disorder in recent years, there has been an important shift in the policy regarding where such people should be treated and rehabilitated. The intention is to reduce, drastically, the size and role of the State Hospital, accompanied by a corresponding provision of locally based medium-secure forensic units within the major Scottish regions. These regional units will function in tandem with amplified community forensic teams that, in turn, will link to local general mental health services. A nice idea if properly resourced, but two major problems have already been encountered with, as yet, no ready solution. The first is the presence of 'not in my back yard' antibodies to the introduction of forensic units, the titre of which rises dramatically during the course of consultation and planning applications. The second problem is one of capacity. There is a mismatch between rising demand fuelled by the increasing reluctance of local mental health services to manage high risk offenders and the increased demands of legislation on sex offenders on the one hand, and inadequate numbers of places in secure accommodation provided by a contracting State Hospital and slowly developing community services on the other. It is the perennial problem of achieving a safe and satisfactory balance, and recognition that existing provision should not be lost before the alternative is in place.

Child and Adolescent Services

Mental health services for young people across Scotland have generally become examples of good practice with regard to multidisciplinary and multiagency co-operation, despite shoestring budgets from the health service purse. Firm links between childhood disorder and subsequent mental health problems in adulthood are now well established, and society pays a high price in terms of social disruption, educational failure, ill health and anti-social behaviour for failing to tackle these problems effectively. The adage of penny wise, pound foolish, is particularly apt in this area. The publication in 1995 of the NHS Health Advisory Service Thematic Review made important statements about principles and practice in the delivery of mental health services for young people, including multiagency involvement, planning services on the basis of assessed needs, auditing and evidence-based activity.[24] The review, popularly known as *Together We Stand* recommended a four-tier framework as a basis for a comprehensive provision. Tiers one to three describe increasing levels of team-based specialisation but it is at Tier Four that the most obvious deficiencies still exist. This most specialised element is the availability of accessible residential NHS units for young people where they can be assessed, treated and rehabilitated by expert staff. Local Authority social work departments have, for too long, had to provide the safety net for insoluble crises in which the family and the community can no longer cope. The NHS in Scotland really must address this need if the seeds of problems in the future are to be prevented from germinating.

Abuse of Substances

There are numerous elements in this topic, including the assessment and management of people with dual diagnoses (mental illness and substance abuse), where best to put the primary responsibility for substance abuse, and whether services for drug abuse and alcohol abuse should be unified or separate. One thing is clear – the incidence of drug-associated psychotic illness in relatively young people is exerting an escalating pressure on general psychiatric services and revealing an inadequate hospital capacity, particularly in intensive care beds. In the absence of evidence for effectiveness of psychiatric techniques in reducing drug-addictive behaviour, there seems little logic in psychiatric staff being involved in first-line services for people abusing drugs in the absence of mental illness. Of course, the involvement of psychiatry in alcohol services may therefore appear illogical, but the association of mental illness with alcohol abuse is strong, and there is a good evidence base for the clinical and cost-effectiveness of both psychotherapies and pharmacotherapy in reducing the risk of relapse in alcohol abuse.[25] One particularly difficult practical issue stands in need of urgent guidance; the management of individuals who express suicidal ideation while intoxicated with alcohol. Some 80% of individuals who complete suicide are believed to have consumed alcohol before the act, and a similar percentage is associated with self-harm. An accurate examination of the mental state is often impossible, however, in the setting of alcohol intoxication. Current legal advice suggests that the patient, when drunk, is the responsibility of whichever clinician in whose care the patient finds himself, although a psychiatrist would have to establish firm grounds for refusing to assess a patient in that state. There is a lack of consensus among Scottish psychiatrists about what best to do,[26] and the Royal College of Psychiatrists has issued no specific guidance on how to manage this common and often difficult combination.

Repeated Deliberate Self-Harm

This is a growing problem for the individual, for families, and for a wide spectrum of health service components, including general practice, accident and emergency departments and mental health services. The overall cost to the NHS services is considerable, not to mention social work departments and the Police, and yet we have no consistent nor tested response to the problem. Although the contexts in which self-harm occurs are numerous, including typical depressive disorder, a substantial proportion of repeated self-harm occurs in girls who have been sexually abused in childhood. For particularly difficult cases, only one therapeutic technique has been shown through randomised controlled trials to be effective, that of dialectical behaviour therapy (DBT).[27, 28] There is a need for a large multi-centre pragmatic trial of the clinical and cost-effectiveness of DBT or related techniques in repeated self-harm in the Scottish setting.

Rights and Dignity

Mental health services have been responsible for some very good things and some very bad things in relation to respect for individuals who were within their power to affect. In probably the majority of services in Scotland there has been a traditional sensitivity to individual rights and dignity, possibly to some extent due to the absence of gargantuan institutions such as those in certain parts of England. There has also been bad practice, through both omission and commission. The neglect of the needs of mentally ill people in sparsely populated and remote areas of the country has perhaps been greater than elsewhere in the UK, and the neglect of these needs in inner cities possibly slightly less. Bad things can happen in institutions, and while Scotland is not innocent, the extent of any abuses of human rights has at least been limited by the thoroughly excellent work carried out by the Scottish Health Advisory Service (previously Scottish Hospitals Advisory Service) and the Mental Welfare Commission for Scotland. These organisations have been staffed by people with whom health professionals could identify and for whom they felt respect. The result, over the past 20 years, has been that their reports, after visits to a service, have generally been received as valid and credible. It is to be hoped that the current tendency towards box-ticking will not hold sway over discussion and in-depth exploration, and thus avoid any resultant distrust between the observed and the observers.

The arrival of the Adults With Incapacity Act and the prospect of a new Mental Health Act for Scotland will see a consolidation, development and strengthening of the statutory safeguards against unwarranted assumptions and dominance by mental health professionals over those who may be disadvantaged through mental illness. The right of patients and their important others to have their opinions heard and respected will be given greater statutory place, and this is all to the good. There is another right that people with mental disorder require to have protected, and that is the right to treatment. As often, this seems likely to happen in Scotland as a result of plain common sense; for example, in the case of the statutory ability to continue involuntary but appropriate treatment for a person living in the community (see below). A most important element to emerge in recent years has been the increasingly influential and sophisticated activities of various voluntary organisations with an interest in mental health. The Scottish Association for Mental Health, the National Schizophrenia Fellowship (Scotland), Scottish Action on Dementia, the Manic Depression Fellowship Scotland, and the Scottish Users Network have all contributed helpfully to the furtherance of modernisation and investment in mental health services in Scotland. Sometimes their views can be perceived as extreme and even threatening by those working in the service, but using the old Titanic metaphor, it usually takes a powerful force to alter even slightly the course of a bulky giant.

Legislation

The Adults with Incapacity (Scotland) Act (2000) made it imperative that all decisions made on behalf of an adult with impaired decision-making capacity (because of either mental disorder or inability to communicate) must benefit that adult, take account of the adult's wishes (both past and present) and those of relevant others, minimise any restriction of freedom and encourage the person to use and develop existing skills. Medical practitioners are given new explicit duties to assess capacity for specific purposes – for example, consent to medical treatment, Guardianship Orders – and to certify incapacity if appropriate.

During the course of 2002 a highly significant legislative milestone was under development, the Mental Health (Scotland) Bill, destined through its anticipated enactment to replace the 1984 Act. Much of the intention and detailed content of the Bill has been informed by the recommendations of the Millan Committee.[29] The draft Bill reflects the Millan Committee's recommendation that, as in the existing 1984 Act, mental disorder should be defined to include mental illness, learning disability, and personality disorder. The issue of how to deal most appropriately with the disordered personality associated with the risk of aggression is one which has caused considerable disquiet among clinicians and others in England and Wales, where the corresponding new legislation proposes what amounts to preventive detention. The Royal College of Psychiatrists believes that the English proposals represent 'little more than a Public Order Bill dressed up as mental health legislation.'[30] Traditionally the Scottish legislation has always followed, by about a year, that for England and Wales and it is generally perceived that this has enabled Scotland to identify and learn from the problems (not to say mistakes) of our neighbours. It seems highly likely that important lessons will again be applied – both over the issue of personality disorder and that of treatment adherence in the community, although the latter reflects the inadequacy of the current Section 18 of the Scottish Act through which treatment adherence outwith hospital can only be ensured for up to one year. The new Bill will introduce Compulsory Treatment Orders to replace long-term detention and Community Care Orders, which will allow treatment to be continued in the absence of valid, informed consent in any defined setting, but with ample safeguards of review and appeal. Balancing restrictions with regard to public safety against the human rights of the individual is nowhere more complex than in the field of mental health. A recent case involving the appeal against continued detention by a person in the State Hospital led to the hurried enactment of the Mental Health (Public Safety and Appeals) (Scotland) Act 1999. This Act introduced a new test, to be applied by Scottish Ministers and Sheriffs, in determining whether a restricted patient should be denied discharge, if deemed necessary to protect the public from serious harm, and continue to be detained in hospital, whether for treatment or not. At the same time, the MacLean Committee was established (in March 1999) to come forward with proposals for Scotland on how best to deal with dangerous people with severe personality disorder.[31] There are many positive aspects of the new Mental Health Bill, such as removing responsibility for approving anything but emergency detention from the sole person of a Sheriff and making it the responsibility of a multidisciplinary Mental Health Tribunal. Emergency, short-term (72 hours) detention will be discouraged and the usual routes to hospital detention will be by means of a four-week detention order, followed, if necessary, by a Compulsory Treatment Order which can specify hospital care as part of the treatment plan. Additional new benefits include requirements to involve interested parties, other than family members, in decisions concerning treatment and detention. The difficult problem will be accommodating the associated processes within the resources available, on the part of workers in both the Health Service and Local Authorities.

Service Identity

Psychiatry in Scotland, as in many developed countries, has to sort out what it wants to be. The dismantling of psychiatric institutions, with the consequent loss of focus on serious mental illness, has created an increasing and unresolved identity crisis for mental health services. Put crudely, there are two cultures which, at their poles, are as different as brain surgery and religion. On the one hand, there are practitioners who are comfortable with the physical aspects of mental illness, who therefore concern themselves predominantly with those disorders for which there is demonstrable physical cause, and for which certain proven physical remedies can be prescribed. On the other, there are those more comfortable with feelings, talking and social issues for which any interventions tend to be interpersonal and targeted at a range of problems, many of which cannot be formulated as illnesses according to accepted diagnostic rules. Since the evidence for beneficial outcome from interventions at the physical end of the spectrum tends to be considerably better than for psychosocial interventions, the former domain tends to be more fact-intensive and evidence-based. Neither is right or wrong, they are simply different, and a question arises as to whether these two streams should reconcile their differences into productive eclecticism, or should separate. Tension exists, and for some the increasing encouragement to allocate the conduct and management of mental health care to general practice represents a threat to the specialist knowledge base and the practice dependent upon it. The dichotomy described above is, of course, crude and simplistic. Talking therapies are accumulating a growing evidence base, and this includes evidence of effectiveness in the serious and long-term mental illnesses. It is, however, arguable that the specialty of psychiatry (in its multidisciplinary form) might best be served by retracting and consolidating its boundaries in order to concentrate on specialist advice and intensive treatment and care. Clinical activity could in that context be more rigorously evidence-influenced, subject to continuous audit, and provide a setting conducive to structured research. The service would have to relinquish some of its current resource to primary care where it could profitably be used to support the general practice teams in the initial assessment of those with any form of mental disorder, and to support them in the delivery of straightforward psychosocial and pharmacological interventions. The 'tier' metaphor might be appropriate, with initial tiers being firmly embedded in primary care, and secondary tiers of reduced size but greater intensity concentrating on illnesses of a type or severity which required specialism. The issue has been raised many times in the literature in recent years, including the suggestion of aligning clinical neurology with clinical psychiatry. In Scotland at present , there are 10 times as many consultant psychiatrists as there are consultant neurologists and it is certainly arguable that this is disproportionate to the excess of serious mental illness requiring specialist attention over neurological illnesses. Perhaps fewer consultant psychiatrists, working with neurologists in a neuropsychiatry service is not too fantastic, and any liberated resources could be reinvested in primary care. Psychiatry really has to get its act together if it is not to be lost in the network of primary care and local authority services, a joint future in which the gains may not be as great as the losses. Scottish psychiatry has a history of which it can be proud, and a lot to lose.

The Research Agenda

Evidence, evidence, evidence. There is an urgent need for mental health services to re-focus on the generation of an evidence base. Ironically, psychiatry led the way in the 1950s and 60s through the conduct of structured clinical research. The large multi-centre, randomised, blinded clinical trial was almost unheard of before the studies conducted (mainly in North America) to evaluate chlorpromazine and related antipsychotics. Likewise, the impressive work by Wing, Kendell and others on diagnostic discipline was at least as good as anything happening in other branches of clinical practice. In Scotland there was a firm tradition of locally based clinical research, and certainly not confined to University centres, the work of Willy Maeyer-Gross at the Crichton Royal in Dumfries in the 1940s being an example in point. Examples of these types are hard to identify in recent years (with notable exceptions such as Robin McCreadie, again in Dumfries) and the clinical specialty has been largely overtaken by structured research and audit in other specialties. The Scottish Audit of Surgical Outcomes, for example, leaves psychiatry looking rather impoverished. One other notable exception, already referred to, is the National Audit of ECT, but in no other area in mental health is there a standard, nationally co-ordinated mechanism for generating, collecting and analysing such data. The value of such databases is several-fold, including the ability to demonstrate work done, pressure on resources and so on. Outcome data are currently crude, at best, including data on admission and discharge rates in terms of activity, and suicide in terms of outcome. The whole area of clinical effectiveness and the need to collect data on both clinical and cost-effectiveness requires simple and manageable outcome data to be recorded as part of everyday clinical life. This dictates the form and content of such data, which must put a premium on simplicity and patient-relevance.[32, 33] This area has recently been helpfully reviewed.[34] For reasons already suggested, the attention and energy of mental health professionals has become increasingly divided and uncertain. Research is considerably easier if problems can be clearly formulated and it will only be useful if the clinical material is defined, 'diagnosed', in such a way as to allow generalisable conclusions.

The specific areas which would appear to deserve research effort in terms of clinical and cost-effectiveness are:

- The clinical and cost-effectiveness of new and expensive medications, as distinct from efficacy data of the sort on which marketing authorisation is based. This requires extensive and continuing research effort, with input from health economists and including the measurement of quality of life.

- Identifying the 'active ingredients' of talking therapies, and their target clinical syndromes.

- The evaluation of interventions with severe personality disorder; their appropriateness based on their clinical and cost-effectiveness, and their medical and legal status.[35]

- The effectiveness and cost-effectiveness of the whole area of standard setting and national audit, such as those associated with the Framework, SIGN Guidelines and CSBS standards. What impact do they have on clinical outcomes (as distinct from processes), and what is their value in relation to the resources invested?

- The critical evaluation of mental health promotional activities.

- The encouragement of basic research into the biological aspects of mental illness.

- The whole area of pharmacogenomics (the targeting of chemical interventions to individuals whose susceptibility to benefits or adverse effects can be predicted from their genetic profile) which offers huge promise for maximising clinical and cost-effectiveness in medicine in general, and perhaps particularly within psychiatry given the soft definition of phenotypes.

To look at itself, and to broaden its evidence base, a specialty must be comfortable with its role and identity. Unless Scottish psychiatry can rediscover its sense of purpose then the prospects of any of these research themes being taken up are threatened.

Scottishness

Frequent reference has been made to the wisdom, quality and respect for values which have characterised Scottish psychiatry for many decades. The creation of the Scottish Parliament in 1999 provides a unique and exciting opportunity for the devolved authority for health to proceed in sensible directions unfettered by perceptions of what should be done in the rest of the UK. Already there have been several examples of separate, but measured, evolution – the Framework for Mental Health Services, the Clinical Standards Board for Scotland, the Health Technology Board for Scotland, and so on. So far, these and various other aspects of devolved evolution have managed to avoid any unwarranted and unhelpful discrepancies between Scotland and England and Wales and Northern Ireland.[36] This is a delicate path to tread – on one side the risk of silly post-code variability in healthcare provision, and on the other the risk of missing the opportunity to do what is best for the Scottish people. Thus the political context for which John Smith and Donald Dewar fought so hard is now a reality full of potential.[37] What is required is a combination of courage and clarity of purpose with which to seize the initiative and recover the lead position of Scottish mental health services, not only in a European but in a global context. Considerable courage will be required on the political benches to conduct a public debate about the triad of cost-effectiveness, affordability and health priorities for health services in general, within which those for mental health will always be vulnerable. The window of opportunity for Scottish psychiatry to re-establish its reputation for excellence is there; mental health has been re-affirmed as one of the major health priorities for the NHS in Scotland.[38] It is, therefore, vital that Scottish psychiatry seizes the opportunity with a clarity of purpose which is unlikely to be expressed without resolution of the issues relating to its identity which have been laid out in this chapter.

Conclusions

Much that is good has happened in Scottish mental health services in recent years. The political framework is conducive to an accelerating development of mental health services that are responsive to the needs of the Scottish people without the need for deference to models from elsewhere. However, this will only happen if psychiatry can decide what it should be doing, can advise the Scottish Parliament accordingly with clear and compelling arguments, and be willing to work hard to make up lost ground.

ACKNOWLEDGEMENT

Grateful thanks to Fiona Broderick for manuscript preparation.

REFERENCES

1.   Department of Health and Social Security. *Organisational and management problems of mental illness hospitals*. (The Nodder Report). London: DHSS, 1980.

2.   Scottish Executive. *Mental Health: Moving the Agenda Forward*. Edinburgh: Scottish Executive Health Department, 2002.

3.   1. World Health Organisation. *The future of mental hospitals: report on a Working Group*. Mannheim 1976. ICP MNHO 19 R2. Geneva: WHO, 1978.

4.   Scottish Home and Health Department. *Mental Hospitals in Focus*. Edinburgh. HMSO, 1989.

5.   The need for asylum for the mentally ill. *Lancet* 1987, 2: 546-547.

6.   Thornicroft G, Tensella M. Balancing community-based and hospital-based mental health care. *World Psychiatry* 2002, 1 (2): 84.

7.   Tonsella M, Williams P. The Italian experience and its implications. *Psychological Medicine* 1987, 17: 283-289.

8.   Finzin A. Die neue einfachheit oder die entprofessionalisierung der psychiatrie. *Socialpsychiatrische Informationen* 1981, 63-64: 5-20.

9.   Scottish Office. *A Framework for Mental Health Services in Scotland*. Edinburgh. Scottish Office,1997.

10.   Swift G, Zacariah M, Casey PR. A rose by any other name: Psychiatric out-patients' views on dress and address. *Irish Journal of Psychological Medicine* 2000, 17 (4): 132-134.

11.   Lancet. What's in a name? *Lancet*; 2000, 356 (9248): 2111.

12.   CRAG. *The Final Report of the Working Group on Mental Illness*. Edinburgh: HMSO,1996.

13.   Goldberg D. The Benefits and Costs of Continuous Inspections – at what point does patient care suffer? *Psychiatric Bulletin* 2002, 26 (10): 361-362.

14.   Clinical Standards Board for Scotland. *National Overview: Schizophrenia*. Edinburgh: CSBS, 2002.

15.   Mackay AVP. Health Technology Assessment and Mental Health. *Psychiatric Bulletin* 2002, 26 (7): 243-245.

16.   Social Work Service Group. *Community Care: Care Programme Approach for People with severe and enduring mental illness including dementia*. Circular No SWSG, 1996.

17.   Stark C, Jones J, Agnew J. Antipsychotic drug prescribing trends in primary care in Scotland 1994-1997. *Health Bulletin* 2000, 58 (2): 96-101.

18.   Royal College of Psychiatrists. *Consensus Statement on the use of high dose antipsychotic medication*. Council Report CR 26. London: Royal College of Psychiatrists, 1993.

19.   Bertolote JM, Fleischmann A. Suicide and Psychiatric Diagnosis: A Worldwide Perspective. *World Psychiatry* 2002,1 (3): 181-185.

20.   Fergusson G, Hendry J, Freeman C. Do patients who receive electroconvulsive therapy (ECT) in Scotland get better? Results of a National audit. *Psychiatric Bulletin*, in press, 2003.

21.   Health Technology Board for Scotland.*Comment on National Institute for Clinical Excellence Technology Appraisal Guidance on the use of donepezil, , rivastigmine and galantamine for the treatment of Alzheimer's Disease. Glasgow*: HTBS, 2001.

22.   CRAG. *Neurosurgery for Mental Disorder*. Report of a Working Group on Mental Illness. Edinburgh: HMSO, 1996.

23.   Hull AM. Neuroimaging findings in post-traumatic stress disorder. Systematic Review. *British Journal of Psychiatry* 2002, 181: 102-110.

24.   NHS Health Advisory Service. The NHS HAS Thematic Review: *Child and adolescent mental health services: together we stand: the commissioning, role and management of child and adolescent mental health services*. London: HMSO, 1995.

25.   Health Technology Board for Scotland. Health Technology Assessment Report 3. *Prevention of Relapse in Alcohol Dependence*. NHS Quality Improvement Scotland. Glasgow: HTBS, 2002.

26.   McCaffery R, Lee A, Jauhar P, Scott J. A survey of opinions on the management of individuals who express suicidal ideation while intoxicated with alcohol. *Psychiatric Bulletin* 2002, 26 (9): 332.

27.   Linehan MM, Tuteck DA, Heard HL, Armstrong HE. Interpersonal outcome of cognitive behavioural treatment for chronically suicidal borderline patients. *American Journal of Psychiatry* 1994, 151 (12): 1771-1776.

28.   Verheul R, Van den Bosch LMC, Koeter WJ, De Ridder MAJ, Stijnen T, Van den Brinck. Dialectical behaviour therapy for women with borderline personality disorder. *British Journal of Psychiatry* 2003,182: 135-140.

29.   Scottish Executive. *New Directions.A Report on the Review of the Mental Health (Scotland) Act 1984*. Edinburgh: Scottish Executive, 2001.

30.   Shooter M, Zigmond T. Personal communication, 2002.

31.   Darjee R., Crichton JHM. The MacLean Committee: Scotland's answer to the 'dangerous people with severe personality disorder' proposals. *Psychiatric Bulletin* 2002, 26: 6-8.

32.   Bilsbury CD, Richmann A. A staging approach to measuring patient-centred subjective outcomes. *Acta Psychiatrica Scandinavica* 2002, Supplement 414, 106: 5-40.

33.   CRAG. Outcome indicators in acute psychiatry. Edinburgh: HMSO, 1996.

34.   Gilbody SM, House AO, Sheldon TA. Outcomes research in mental health. Systematic Review. *British Journal of Psychiatry* 2002, 181: 8-16.

35.   Kendell RE. The distinction between personality disorder and mental illness. *British Journal of Psychiatry* 2002, 180: 110-115.

36.   Loudon J, Coia D. The Scottish Scene. *Psychiatric Bulletin* 2002, 26 (3): 84-86.

37.   Smith M. Devolution and 'public psychiatry' in Scotland. Psychiatric Bulletin 2003,27 (2) 41-43.

38.   Scottish Executive. *Our National Health: A plan for action, a plan for change.* Edinburgh: Scottish Executive Health Department, 2000.

7. The Scottish Approach to Community Care

Alison Petch

Introduction

If the relative importance of an issue were to be measured by terminology, community care in Scotland is in the ascendancy, boasting within the last couple of years a committee presence in the Scottish Parliament (the Health and Community Care Committee), a Minister (of Health and Community Care) and a Division within the Health Department. At the same time, however, there is an argument that much of the language routinely associated with community care is heavily redolent with notions of dependency and traditional models of dispensing care, inappropriate to the principles of choice, independence and empowerment which sit more comfortably with current perspectives on disability.[1]

Nonetheless, both for generic issues such as inter-agency working or commissioning and for policy and practice specific to particular user groups, the last 10 years have been characterised by accelerating activity both at strategic and local level. There has been increasing differentiation of the range and variation in needs, both within and across different groups, and increasing recognition of the significance of community care within the political arena. This chapter will seek to balance an account of the more important landmarks from this period with a distillation of those issues which are emerging as critical to immediate and future development.

Historical perspectives on community care can assume either a macro or a micro approach. The macro approach often presumes an institutional focus, mapping the transition from workhouse to specialist psychiatric and learning disability hospitals, noting the decline in institutional numbers from a peak in the 1950s, and speculating on why, in comparison with the rest of the United Kingdom, Scotland has traditionally favoured institutional solutions.[2] The micro focus tends to set as its initial landmark the NHS and Community Care Act, 1990, seeking the extent to which the promised shifts prefaced by the Audit Commission,[3] the Griffiths Report[4] and the White Paper, Caring for People,[5] have been achieved. Core to the agenda emerging from these reports were the shifts from an institutional to a community base, from a single provider to a mixed economy with the local authority becoming an enabler rather than a provider, from a service-led to a needs-led response, from central to devolved budgets, from a single service to a multiple choice, and from a professional to a user-led perspective. In this more recent focus also there is evidence of differences in Scotland, in particular no requirement as there was in England for 85% of the monies transferred from the DSS to local authorities (on their assumption of responsibility for residential care funding) to be spent in the independent sector.

Hospital closure

The resettlement of individuals from long-stay beds, particularly from psychiatric hospitals, is often characterised by the media as the essence of community care, despite affecting only a small proportion of those who may be characterised as the users of community care services. To a certain extent this emphasis has also been sustained, at least until recent years, in the policy arena. Mental health policy had for some time been castigated for its uncertainty and lack of coherence,[6] and in 1994 the Closure of Psychiatric Hospitals in Scotland was selected by the Scottish Affairs Committee of the Westminster Parliament as the focus for an Inquiry. The Report of the Inquiry[7] highlighted a number of key issues which were emerging as the balance of care shifted from long-stay beds to community-based options: the appropriate models for provision for respite and crisis, the logic of jointly planned mental health strategies, the need for transparency in resource transfer arrangements and in the bridging funds designed to establish community infrastructure in advance of bed closure, the pressure for a fully costed strategy for the closure of long-stay beds and the development of community-based alternatives.

In its response to the Inquiry,[8] the Scottish Office accepted the need for a national strategy document to guide the production of local mental health strategies and in 1997 the Framework for Mental Health Services in Scotland was published,[9] detailing templates for the production by health boards of six-year mental health strategies. In 1993 there had been a clear statement from the Scottish Office that they expected 600 discharges per year from long-stay psychiatric hospitals,[10] with the creation of 8000 additional community care places by the end of the decade. Subsequently, however, attention has focused on the wider development of the service framework for meeting the needs of individuals with severe and/or enduring mental health problems, supported by a Mental Health Development Fund, while the major target for more recent activity in the mental health field has been around legislation, culminating in proposals for the impending new Mental Health Act (see chapter 6).

A critical overview of the policy for resettlement from learning disability hospitals has been presented by Stalker and Hunter.[11] They concluded, from interviews with health and social care managers for all but one of the 15 long-stay hospitals, that 'resettlement is largely in disarray' (p177); moreover they asserted that 'the resettlement process has not only lost momentum over recent years but that some reversal of direction is taking place' (p182–3).

TABLE 7.1 Long-stay beds in Scotland

	1980	1990	1995	1998	2001
Learning disability	7139	5021	3468	2888	1907
Geriatric long stay	7899	9277	7729	5488	4089
*Mental health**	17 168	14 407	11 034	9076	7760

*NB includes all beds for general psychiatry and psychiatry of old age

SOURCE: Scottish Community Care Statistics 2001

Nonetheless, as Table 7.1 demonstrates, there has been a considerable reduction in bed numbers over the last 20 years, most markedly in respect of learning disability.

Parliamentary Inquiries into Community Care

Following its inquiry into psychiatric hospital closure, the Scottish Affairs Committee broadened its scrutiny to the implementation of community care as a whole. In response to its call for evidence in 1996, it received over 150 written submissions and took oral evidence from 20 groups of witnesses.[12] A key element of the Report[13] was the detailed scrutiny of the resource base for community care, seeking to distil a coherent picture from the disparate funding streams. While acknowledging there will always be demands for enhanced resources, the Committee highlighted both absolute and organisational shortfalls.

> 'We have concluded that community care is, at present, under-resourced in that the funding has proved inadequate to meet the Government's original aims as set out in the 1990 Act. But the problem is not simply the global size of resources, it concerns also their best use … When arranging care packages, health and social work tend to take into account only the costs to their own respective budgets. As joint strategic agreements are reached between health and social work, we expect to see the development of a single fund from which services could be jointly commissioned.' (para 121)

At this date the levels of resource transfer from health boards to local authorities in recognition of transferred responsibility for particular community support needs continued to be a major source of discontent, with resource transfer the focus for an investigation by the Accounts Commission in 1997.[14] The Scottish Affairs Committee also expressed concern on grounds of equity over the distribution of bridging finance for hospital closure, two-thirds of expenditure in 1996–97 having gone to Greater Glasgow Health Board, and recommended a form of weighted capitation, including particular allowance for the Royal Scottish National Hospital. A further recommendation sought to address the totality of the community care £.

> 'We recommend that, as part of a more fundamental review of the financing arrangements for community care, consideration be given to mechanisms for the integration and pooling of resources to avoid beds being blocked because appropriate budget heads cannot be accessed.' (para 47)

A range of other issues featured among the recommendations from the Inquiry. A particular interest was whether the balance of care between residential and domiciliary settings had changed, including whether perverse incentives bolstering residential care had been eroded. The potential for more intensive home support was explored, together with the validity of cost thresholds for individual care packages. An innovative recommendation was that 'the DSS residential care allowance be diverted into home care schemes where the level of care is such that the alternative to augmented care would be continuing, nursing, or residential care' (para 57). Initial promotion of local integration of health and social care through the six pilot schemes of the Local Care Partnerships[15] was commended. Contemporary developments were also prefaced: 'we recommend the development of an agreed set of minimum national standards of community care and wish to encourage a shift in emphasis to examine the outcomes of community care delivery' (para 95).

The Government response to the Inquiry[16] accepted, inter alia, the need to improve the transparency of care package costs, confirmed the continuation of the Mental Illness Specific Grant and a comprehensive review of the funding of community care housing, endorsed the development of integrated intensive home care, and indicated that an independent registration and inspection system would be established, to include domiciliary support. There was a tentative acceptance of the need for national standards, but a reluctance to impose from the centre – 'whatever approach is developed, the Government agree that standards should relate to outcomes'. Uncertainty in respect of entitlement to assessment by young carers was acknowledged and corrective action promised.

Despite this detailed scrutiny, when the Scottish Parliament established its Health and Community Care Committee in 1999, it too selected community care as the focus for its first major investigation. The initial remit focused on issues arising from the Sutherland Report, resource transfer, service co-ordination between health and local authorities, and views on the optimal means for delivery of care, and targeted provision for older people and for individuals with mental health problems, but inevitably the scrutiny extended more broadly. The Report which was published late in 2000[17] included 45 recommendations, a detailed blueprint for enhancing community care practice. It made explicit its underlying values of fairness and equity, of viewing service provision from the perspective of the service user, and of adopting a broader perspective on community care than the narrow remit of health and social care. Concern at the resource commitment for community care was reiterated – 'an insurmountable barrier in realising service ambitions'. The inefficiency of short-term project funding, 'projectitis', was also highlighted, and pooled budgets were deemed essential, not least to transcend the inefficiencies of resource transfer identified earlier. There was criticism of wide variation in local authority charging policies on the grounds of equity, and renewed calls for a transparent specification of funding streams. Current developments prefaced by the Inquiry include the development of a single, multidisciplinary assessment (linked to the specification of unmet need), the implementation of pooled or aligned budgets, the promotion of Direct Payments, and wider availability of augmented home care.

The timing of the Committee Inquiry in the wake of the Sutherland report from the Royal Commission on Long Term Care has inevitably led to an emphasis on the recommendations from the Inquiry which chimed with those of the Commission, in particular an overwhelming endorsement from witnesses of the principle of personal care on the basis of assessed need free at the point of delivery – 'the redistribution of wealth from rich to poor is the function not of a health care system, but of a taxation system. The function of a health care system is the redistribution of health from the well to the sick' (para 23). By the time of the response to the Inquiry Report by the Scottish Executive,[18] the political profile of the personal and nursing care debate led, as with the Sutherland Report, to a focus on these elements at the expense of other detail. This detail included a number of significant elements, including three-year budgeting for local authorities in line with NHSScotland financial cycles and in the context of a National Planning and Financial Framework, and an expectation that local authorities would contract with voluntary sector providers on a three-year basis. Moves to reduce inconsistencies in charging policies between authorities were endorsed, while the need for close working between Local Health Care Co-operatives (LHCCs) and social work departments to ensure local care solutions was acknowledged. Much of the response cited recommendations from the Joint Future Group, an indication of the extent to which community care at this stage was under multiple scrutiny.

Implementation following the 1990 Act

Outwith the parliamentary arena, much of the more detailed scrutiny of the development of community care over the last decade has focused on the extent to which the desired procedures have been put in place. Care management, including the core component of assessment, was to be the 'cornerstone' of the new system; key studies both in England[3] and in Scotland[20, 21] have highlighted the variety of practice that has emerged. Most areas stop short both of a distinct post for the role of care manager and of budgets devolved to the individual care manager for purchase of the tailored care package, elements prescribed as key after evaluation of the initial demonstration projects which were influential to the adoption of care management.[22] Studies have also questioned the extent to which assessment and provison has been transformed from service-led to needs-led[23] and whether key elements of choice and empowerment have been more than rhetoric.[24]

More generally there has been an emerging awareness of the disparities in community care provision and distribution across Scotland. In 1997, the Accounts Commission[25] highlighted the variation in expenditure; across Scotland as a whole expenditure on residential care is 37% of community care expenditure but this ranges from 10% to 60% between different local authorities. Nursing home care ranges from 13% to 32% (overall 18%), while the variation for home care (overall 27%) is more than eight-fold, 6% to 47%. These figures illustrate also the skew to institutional expenditure compared to the numbers involved: 84% of service users in the community with 45% of the expenditure, 55% of the funds in care homes but only 16% of service users. Linking this differential in provision to wide variation in charging policies for day, domiciliary and respite care, has generated increasing unease.

The political focus on community care was renewed in 1998, five years after the initial implementation, with the publication of *Modernising Community Care: An Action Plan*[26] 'We have made progress in the five years since the community care policy came fully into force. But there are still many concerns about the way we manage and deliver services and whether the services we provide are the services people need' (p6). The twin aims of the Action Plan were to secure 'better and faster results for people by focusing on them and their needs; and more effective and efficient joint working based on partnership' (p2). A 'can-do' approach was advocated, with financial leverage offered by way of funds targeted towards shifting the balance of care, developing more flexible home care services, and working in partnerships – 'we cannot emphasise strongly enough that joint working across all organisations is one of the most important themes of the new agenda for community care' (p7).

The Action Plan signified a shift towards a more concerted and decisive assault on the goals of community care. Initial community care plans had been lacking in detailed strategy, targets and timetables;[27] this level of detail needed to be provided, while coherence was necessary across the proliferation of health improvement plans (HIPs), trust improvement plans (TIPs), local authority and (then) Scottish Homes housing strategies, proposals for community planning. Likewise, it was acknowledged that detailed care and housing strategies had to focus on all the needs within an area, not merely the traditional response to hospital closure. The overriding importance of the total resource function, the 'community care £', was also highlighted, a recognition that cost shunting does not achieve efficiency savings. Reference was made to the need for speedier decision-making, for example in assessment and care management, to the importance of well developed information systems, and to the facilitation of flexibility and choice through delegation of budgets.

There has been a somewhat ambivalent stance in Scotland towards what has been variously termed intermediate care or rehabilitation provision ('step up'/ 'step down'), characterised by the designation of premises designed either to permit convalescence or to avert the need for hospital admission. The Audit Commission has highlighted a range of innovative provision in England[28] but the preference in Scotland has been to support an individual wherever possible in their own home rather than introduce further moves within the system.

Integrated working

Of major significance in the evolution of the community care agenda has been the recent emphasis on the pursuit of cross-agency working, most particularly across health and social care. The report of the Joint Future Group,[29] chaired by the then Deputy Minister for Community Care, marked a renewed attempt to shift the balance of care, particularly for older people, from institutional to domiciliary settings. It focused on the potential of joint initiatives and marked a shift (in terms of Scotland) from a permissive to a more directive approach. It sought to promote early assessment and intervention, to remove barriers within care pathways, to facilitate single points of access to services, and to deploy joint resources closer to individual needs. Each authority was required to establish a joint rapid response team and a joint intensive home support team, with a requirement to specify in local outcome agreements[30] the targets for each of the areas of investment. The Report also paved the way for the introduction of joint resourcing and management of services for older people[31] and of a single, shared assessment process from April 2002.[32] Local Partnership Agreements (LPAs) had to be produced by local partners for April 2002, specifying for older people's services over five years the arrangements for joint management, for resourcing, for development priorities, for joint governance and accountability, and for joint performance management. Six of the 20 recommendations of the Joint Future Group had already been anticipated in a Ministerial statement on older people, 'a step change in care to older people in Scotland', delivered in October 2000 at the same time as the publication of the response to the recommendations of the Sutherland Report.[33] Investment of an additional £48 million by 2003 was to provide, in addition to the rapid response and intensive home support teams identified above, free home care for up to four weeks on leaving hospital, 1000 additional long-term home care packages, 22 000 additional weeks of respite care, and a local service for shopping, laundry and household maintenance. A further £5 million was to be available for equipment and adaptations and an annual £10 million for delayed discharge. Most recently attention has turned to the specification of the performance criteria by which progress on the components of the Joint Future agenda can be assessed,[34] 'bottom line' requirements being specified for April 2002, with full implementation of joint resourcing and management and of the single shared assessment by April 2003.

Integrated working has assumed a range of meanings within the health sphere,[35] but in respect of community care refers to working across both agency and professional boundaries, most commonly health and social care but also housing, education, transport and others. In order to remove any real or perceived legislative barriers to joint working between the NHS and local authorities, the Community Care and Health (Scotland) Act 2002 sets out arrangements to allow pooling of budgets between the two bodies, the delegation of functions from one agency to the other, and the transfer of payments between the two agencies. The Act did not, however, unlike the Health and Social Care Act 2001, include the possibility of a single agency as prefaced in England by the Care Trusts proposed in their NHS Plan,[36] and the provisions of the 1999 Health Act following the Discussion Paper *Partnership in Action*.[37]

The possibility of merging health and social care provision has been aired on a number of occasions in recent years and was given careful consideration by the

Health and Community Care Committee Inquiry into Community Care. Although they concluded that 'a single body must be given lead responsibility in every location, with control over a single, integrated budget' (para 66), they remained agnostic on the organisation which should take the lead. Moreover, sensitive to the experience in Northern Ireland, they did not believe 'that a single body with a single budget will in itself solve the problems associated with current arrangements' (para 70). The Ministerial statement of 5 October 2000 however marked a withdrawal from substantive organisational change: 'we do not believe that imposed structural change or forced integration of NHS and social work services would be in the best interest of those who depend on care or those who deliver it'.

Much of the emphasis has been on joint working between health and social work, but equally critical, indeed a prerequisite, for the successful achievement of community care is the contribution of housing.[38] A succession of circulars and guidance have sought to ensure inclusion of the third key partner,[39-42] but the Scottish Affairs Committee Report in 1997[43] highlighted major deficiencies.

> 'The vital contribution of housing to Community Care is being seriously compromised. This is due to a number of factors including: a complex combination of a tight financial environment for both capital and revenue, with associated problems of harmonising these funding timescales; some unhelpful responses to the environment created by the mixed economy of care; inherent defects and risks in the funding mechanisms which are too great for housing associations to bear; and a degree of co-operation required which is difficult to achieve given the other pressures on the various participants in community care housing.' (para 116)

The 1999 guidance reiterated the importance of equal participation of the range of housing agencies both in strategic and locality planning, with contribution as appropriate to needs assessment at the individual level. The need to integrate individuals within communities and to embrace community care needs within allocation policies was emphasised. Particular concerns were raised in respect of hospital discharge programmes:

- insufficient recognition of housing's role in the process with housing agencies being involved too late

- lack of co-ordination between agencies including delays in assessment

- housing provision for discharged long-stay patients was too often 'mini institutions' or group homes rather than houses promoting independent living

- uncertainty over long-term revenue funding arrangements in supported housing for discharged patients.

There were also concerns, which continue, that discharge programmes dominate the community care programme, strategically, financially and individually, to the expense of those already based within the community.

Nonetheless, the role of housing as catalyst in the discharge process is demonstrated by the impact of *Home Link*, a co-ordinating agency critical to the achievement of the closure of Lennox Castle, the major learning disability hospital in Glasgow.[44] The agency was significant also in co-ordinating the key elements of housing and care, a reflection of the shift over the last decade from a traditional single agency supported accommodation model to the separate provision of the two components of housing and of support. Most recently, the emerging implementation of *Supporting People,* financing support elements necessary to maintain a tenancy, has introduced new twists to the interface between housing and support.

Housing alone, however, is not sufficient. Of major concern must be the extent to which a change of location is associated with other positive indicators;[45] individuals are not merely in the community but more substantively a part of it. There have been doubts as to the extent to which the current rhetoric on social inclusion[46] embraces those with community care needs; nonetheless the availability of opportunities for participation by individuals across the broad spectrum of education, training, employment, transport, recreation and friendship must be a key marker for the achievement of community care.[44] This does not necessarily however equate with a standardised model of integrated provision. Optimum provision, for example, for the health needs of individuals with learning disability, traditionally neglected,[47] may require specialist input for particular needs in addition to the provisions made in local community health services.

Unpaid carers

This chapter has focused to this point on the formal provision for individuals with community support needs. The *Carers (Recognition and Services) Act 1995* gave legislative acknowledgement to the role of the informal care provided by family members or others on an unpaid basis. In practical terms it provided for unpaid carers 'providing substantial care on a regular basis' to receive an independent assessment of their needs from the local authority. Subsequent developments have produced some interesting divergence from policy in England. Following the publication of the UK *National Strategy for Carers,*[48] a *Strategy for Carers in Scotland*[49] was launched in November 1999. Six areas were prioritised for action:

- promotion of new and more flexible services for carers, including respite care, at a local level

- introduction of national standards for such services

- need for monitoring by the Scottish Executive of the performance of health and social services in supporting carers

- introduction of carers' legislation to allow carers' needs to be met more directly

- provision of better and more targeted information for carers at national level

- attention to the specific needs of young carers.

From 2000–01, £10 million of Grant Aided Expenditure (GAE) was identified for distribution to local authorities to fund carers' services, including respite care. Authorities were required to consult with health boards and local carers' organisations on the allocation of these resources and to report to the Scottish Executive on the decisions made.

To prepare for legislation, a Carers' Legislation Working Group was established which reported in January 2001.[50] A key philosophy underpinning the 31 recommendations of the Report, seven of them requiring legislative change, was that the unpaid carer should be acknowledged as a partner in care provision rather than a person with 'needs' to whom services are provided. Any needs of the unpaid carer stemmed from those of the cared for person and should be treated as such, most particularly in respect of charging. Whereas in England the Carers and Disabled Children Act 2000 provided for carers to receive services or other support in their own right as an alternative form of support to community care services and allowed local authorities to charge carers for such services, in Scotland it was considered that the broader provisions of the Social Work (Scotland) Act already allowed for carers' needs to be met – 'we do not envisage carers as direct recipients of services in so far as their caring role goes, and thus we do not see a case for carers being asked to contribute to the cost of services or support' (p40).

A consultation paper was issued in April 2001 to assist with the framing of legislative proposals, posing 15 specific questions. Among the 203 responses there was particular support for a right to assessment for all unpaid carers, irrespective of whether the cared for person is being assessed, a right subsequently achieved by the Community Care and Health (Scotland) Act 2002. Considerable discussion was generated in the final debate on the Bill around the role of the NHS in identifying unpaid carers. Consideration of a statutory duty on NHSScotland to identify carers had been recommended by the Working Group; the ensuing wrangle focused on whether NHSScotland should be required to implement a carer *identification* strategy or a carer *information* strategy, the latter, less directive, option being adopted.

Community Care and Health (Scotland) Act 2002

The Community Care and Health (Scotland) Act 2002 was significant on a number of fronts. For older people in Scotland it finally delivered after the political roundabouts on the promise of free personal care for people aged 65 years and over on the basis of assessed need. The recommendation from the Royal Commission on Long Term Care[51] had initially been rejected, in line with south of the Border, but after a change of First Minister and pressure from the minority party (Liberal Democrats) within the coalition, it was given the green light (and implemented from July 2002) and hailed by many as the first significant evidence of the potential for divergence within the Scottish Parliament. The likely cost and impact of funding free personal care was examined in detail by the Care Development Group under the then Deputy Minister for Health and Community Care, Malcolm Chisholm. It should be noted that the Report of the Group[52] gave considerable emphasis to the development of initiatives designed to shift the balance of care for older people, stubbornly resistant to policy goals in the decade since the 1990 Act. In resource terms it allocated £50 million from a total of £125 million to this end. In order to ensure its use for older people, the additional resource allocation was to be ring-fenced until robust outcome agreements were in place, a response to the shortfall in expenditure of £63 million from the GAE allocation of £603 million for older people.

The Act also provided the legislative directive for joint resourcing and management and expands the provisions for Direct Payments (see below). Whereas five years earlier *Modernising Community Care* had tentatively consulted on whether extra powers were necessary to encourage joint working – for example, removing perceived barriers to pooling budgets, promoting lead commissioning, enabling the transfer of resources between local authorities and NHS boards or allowing NHS trusts to provide social care – the adoption of the legislative route indicated a more robust directive. The Act permits payments from NHS Scotland to local authorities and vice versa, allows for the delegation of functions between the two bodies, removes any doubt as to the facility to pool budgets, and protects staff transferring between the agencies. Significantly it has also specified the power to enforce joint working where services or systems are deemed to be failing, the focus of some speculation at the committee stage. The practical guidance specifies alternative models for partnership working and for pooled or aligned budgets.[53] Analysis of the key drivers and barriers to joint working[54] highlighted the negative impact of differing pay and conditions of employment, areas examined in detail by a group charged with detailing the Human Resource issues.[55]

Direct Payments

The 2002 Act also offers a significant opportunity for the development of Direct Payments. Direct Payments, the provision of a monetary payment to an individual in place of service provision in response to assessed need, were originally introduced through the Community Care (Direct Payments) Act 1996.

Local authorities were given a discretionary power to introduce a scheme for such payments, initially from April 1997 to people with disabilities aged 18–64 years, and from July 2000 to those 65 years and over.[56] Amendments through the Regulation of Care (Scotland) Act 2001 also enabled 16 and 17 year olds and the parents of disabled children to access Direct Payments for the purchase of children's services.

Local authorities were slow to implement Direct Payments, with a review published in 2000 [57] reporting only 13 of the 32 authorities with full or pilot schemes and only 143 individuals in receipt of a payment (303 at August 2002). The importance of Direct Payments relates to the argument that it is a more empowering strategy for meeting the support needs of individuals, promoted by the disability movement and offering greater autonomy to individuals to determine the nature of their support mechanisms.[58] Much of the initial development of Direct Payments has focused on the promotion of independent living schemes through the employment of personal assistants. The 2002 Act strengthens the provision for Direct Payments by transforming the discretionary power into a statutory duty and extending eligibility to all those assessed as requiring community care services. It follows detailed proposals first outlined for consultation in *Better Care for all our futures*.[59] Specifically, from June 2003 local authorities will have a duty to offer Direct Payments to disabled people, and from April 2004 to all those assessed as needing care. Where an individual is unable to give consent, regulations will allow attorneys or guardians to receive a payment on their behalf. As a concession to local authorities, whose past reluctance has in part been ascribed to protection of in-house provision, the Act relaxes the provision prohibiting the purchase of services from a local authority. The Scottish Executive has also funded Direct Payments Scotland to promote uptake across Scotland.

Service reviews

Major service reviews for both mental health[9] and for learning disability[60] have been carried out in recent years, both predating their English equivalents.[61] For older people, however, there has not been a parallel to the National Service Framework for Older People[62] south of the border, with its detailed specification of eight core standards.

The Same as You?, developed with the active involvement of both individuals with learning disabilities and family members, set a blueprint for action over 10 years. Among its 29 recommendations a number of key features were proposed:

- 'partnership in practice' agreements (PIPs) between health boards and local authorities to be in place by June 2001

- 'local area co-ordinators' for learning disability to be established in each local authority

- a 'personal life plan' for all those with learning disability who wish to have one

- a national network for people with autistic spectrum disorder (ASD)

- establishment of local registers

- closure of all remaining long-stay hospitals for learning disability by 2005

- development of a range of employment and training opportunities

- provision of integrated community health care

- Scottish Executive to establish a 'change fund' to help achieve the recommendations

The implementation of *The Same as You?* is being monitored closely. There is interest in the extent to which these developments for people with learning disability and parallel work on joint resourcing and management of services for older people are usurping to some extent earlier generic arrangements. Partnership in practice agreements (PIPs) and LPAs detail the arrangements for partnership working, while local area co-ordination, initially developed in Western Australia and based on core principles of self-determination, partnership and inclusion, vies for definition with care management, despite assertions that the role is distinctly different.

Key issues

This account of emerging policy and practice in community care in recent years suggests a number of core issues, themes which are likely to endure over the next decade.

• At the organisational level, the pursuit of integrated activity will continue, with an assumption that systems for single assessment and joint resourcing and management will extend outwards from older people to embrace the majority of community care activity. Political will in Scotland will dictate whether more radical organisation restructuring occurs, but among health, social care and housing there may well be a more critical examination of the effectiveness of particular models of integrated activity, including scrutiny of the impact on outcomes for individual service users. Recent evidence from the integrated care trust in Somerset suggests the situation may be more complex – and perhaps less optimistic – than initially envisaged.[65] The development of the Care Together initiative in Perth and Kinross, a single agency model for community care services backed by Treasury funding, will be monitored with interest.

• At policy and practice levels, there needs to be an acknowledgement of perceived and actual limits on the achievement of community-based care, or perhaps more precisely on the particular models of care which can be sustained. Are there, for example, a small number of people with learning disabilities for whom the closure of all long-stay hospital places will produce challenges for the development of alternative placements. For individuals with dementia, there has already, with the redefinition of entitlement to NHS continuing care,[64] been a radical shift for those supported outwith their own homes from NHS hospital provision to care homes, particularly nursing homes. Much of the provision, however, remains institutional in size and there is considerable potential for alternative housing and support models, with the advent of *Supporting People* offering both opportunities and challenges. For individuals with complex physical needs, the capacity to meet health needs outside hospital settings, for example for ventilation or for aspiration, has grown considerably in recent years. In many instances it is not the type but the amount of care that differentiates between domiciliary and institutional settings, with considerable potential, for example for frail older people, for larger numbers to be sustained in their own homes.[65] Many, though not all, of these debates have at their heart issues of resource allocation, of spending priorities, and of equity across different sets of needs, age groups and localities. In respect of drug treatment for Alzheimer's disease, for example, there has been an attempt to remove inequity in prescription.[66] Across much of community care, however, the legacy of traditional practice still resonates. Cost thresholds operate, implicitly or explicitly, for community-based support packages for older people which are not applied to those under 65 years of age; care homes for older people have bed numbers which would be deemed totally inappropriate for individuals with learning disabilities or mental health needs. At the same time, resources are finite and costings and analysis are required which recognise both the totality of the community care £ and the implications of alternative potential spending scenarios. Significant in such scenarios will be the opportunities advanced by increasingly sophisticated technology to facilitate home-based care.[67]

- Shifting the balance of care, particularly for older people, is not, however, solely related to resources. It is a complex product of professional and lay expectations, of information flows, of building community capacity, of creating flexible and responsive services, and of promoting early and preventative intervention. It is intricately woven with current concerns with delayed discharge and may start to succumb under the onslaught of rapid response and early discharge schemes, intensive home care, joint resourcing and similar strategies.

- The recent years of community care have seen considerable emphasis in both strategic and local policy statements on elements of choice, of participation and of empowerment. User-led provision has been promoted (and debated), the role of advocacy sharpened, and within the disability movement there has been a recognition of the demands extended by individuals with impairments different to those of the initial activists. Direct Payments are being promoted by a range of different interests as a mechanism for achieving the choice and empowerment that is sought. With more directive legislation in place to ensure compliance by local authorities, the next five years will demonstrate whether there is indeed capacity within the Direct Payments mechanism to transform service delivery.

- This may be one, but not the only, route through which the principles of person-centred support are more closely achieved. Working out the ways in which the goals of social inclusion can be operationalised and the strategies by which a holistic community support system which extends more broadly than the three components of health, social care and housing can be attained will require concerted energy and resource input.

- Whatever the mechanism for the provision of support, of major concern is whether there is a sufficient work force to meet support requirements. The Inquiry into Care and Support for the King's Fund[68] underlined the serious challenges which exist in providing a workforce of sufficient size and skill. 'The recruitment and retention of staff in care and support services is a major and growing challenge that demands imaginative and creative solutions to avoid a crisis. Improved pay and conditions must be at the heart of the solution, while other ways of raising the status of care workers are also crucial'. While technological developments may facilitate more intensive home-based support, any reduction in workforce demand is difficult to predict. Moreover reduction in the need for certain tasks may be offset by the demand for services such as befriending designed to enhance quality of life.

An appraisal of community care elsewhere in the United Kingdom would no doubt predict similar features for scrutiny over the next decade, although some of the detail might differ. Of key interest, however, will be the extent to which policy and practice in Scotland increasingly diverges from that of its partners as the impact of devolution unfolds. For political scientists, the adoption of a universal funding model for personal care by the Scottish Parliament signified that devolution might constitute more than symbolic structures. For community care it opens up a range of possibilities, as yet embryonic, for further differentiation, including the logical extension of the personal care provision to individuals under 65 years of age. The development of the Care Standards for Scotland adopted a very different approach to that in England, prioritising the achievement of outcomes for service users and avoiding specification, for example, of space standards (interestingly England has subsequently retreated from its initial prescriptive approach). It may be, however, that the impact of other developments, such as accelerated shifts in the balance of care or increased partnership working, could lead to convergence between the nations as past disparities are reduced. As with other areas of health policy, the preference in Scotland has been for organisational and cultural development rather than structural change and prescription. Both north and south of the border, however, the future trajectory for community care is not entirely predictable.

REFERENCES

1.   Priestley M. *Disability Politics and Community Care*. London: Jessica Kingsley, 1999.

2.   Petch A. Social care across Great Britain: consolidation or fragmentation. In Hudson B (ed) *The Changing Role of Social Care*. London: Jessica Kingsley, 2000.

3.   Audit Commission. *Making a Reality of Community Care*. London: HMSO, 1986.

4.   Community Care: *Agenda for Action* (Griffiths Report). London: HMSO, 1988.

5.   Department of Health. *Caring for People*. London: HMSO, 1989.

6.   Drucker N. Lost in the haar: a critique of Mental Health in Focus, in D McCrone (ed) *Scottish Government Yearbook 1986*. Edinburgh: Unit for the Study of Government in Scotland, 1986.

7.   House of Commons Scottish Affairs Committee Session 1994–95. Third Report. *Closure of Psychiatric Hospitals in Scotland*, Volumes I and II. London: HMSO, 1995.

8.   House of Commons Scottish Affairs Committee Session 1995–96. First Special Report. *Government Observations on the Third Report from the Committee (Session 1994–96) on Closure of Psychiatric Hospitals in Scotland*. London: HMSO, 1996.

9.   Scottish Office. *A Framework for Mental Health Services in Scotland*. Edinburgh: Scottish Office, 1997.

10.   NHS MEL 67. Edinburgh: Scottish Office Management Executive, 1993.

11.   Stalker K, Hunter S. To close or not to close? The future of learning disability hospitals in Scotland. *Critical Social Policy* 1999; 19: 177–194

12.   House of Commons Scottish Affairs Committee Session 1996–97. Second Report. *The Implementation of Community Care in Scotland*, Volumes ll and lll. London: HMSO, 1997.

13.   House of Commons Scottish Affairs Committee Session 1996–97. Second Report. *The Implementation of Community Care in Scotland*, Volume l. London: HMSO, 1997.

14. Accounts Commission. *Shifting the Balance: Resource transfer for community care*. Edinburgh: Accounts Commission for Scotland, 1997.

15. Scottish Office. *Ready for the Future*. Cm 5331. Edinburgh: HMSO,1997.

16. House of Commons Scottish Affairs Committee Session 1997–98. Second Special Report. *Government Observations on the Second Report of the Committee (Session 1996–97) on The Implementation of Community Care in Scotland*. London: HMSO, 1997.

17. Scottish Parliament. *Inquiry into the Delivery of Community Care*. Health and Community Care Committee, 2000.

18. Scottish Executive. Health and Community Care Committee 16th Report 2000. *Inquiry into the Delivery of Community Care in Scotland*. Response by the Scottish Executive, 2001.

19. Lewis J, Glennerster H. *Implementing the New Community Care*. Buckingham: Open University Press, 1996.

20. Petch A, Cheetham J, Fuller R, MacDonald C, Myers F with Hallam A, Knapp M. *Delivering Community Care: Initial Implementation of Care Management in Scotland*. Edinburgh: The Stationery Office, 1996.

21. Stalker K, Campbell I. *Review of Care Management in Scotland*. Edinburgh: Scottish Executive Central Research Unit, 2002.

22. Challis D. Case Management: A Review of UK Developments and Issues. In Titterton M (ed). *Caring for People in the Community: The New Welfare*. London: Jessica Kingsley, 1994.

23. Myers F, MacDonald C. Power to the people? Involving users and carers in needs assessments and care planning – the views from the practitioner. *Health and Social Care in the Community* 1996; 4: 86–95.

24. Myers F, MacDonald C. 'I was given options not choices': Involving older users and carers in assessment and care planning, in R Bland (ed) *Developing Services for Older People and their Families*. London: Jessica Kingsley, 1996.

25. Accounts Commission. *The Commissioning Maze*. Edinburgh: The Accounts Commission for Scotland, 1997.

26. Scottish Office. *Modernising Community Care: An Action Plan*. Edinburgh: The Stationery Office, 1998.

27. Scottish Office. *Community Care Planning*. Circular SW14. 1994.

28. Audit Commission. *The Way to Go Home: Rehabilitation and Remedial Services for Older People*. London: HMSO, 2000.

29.   Scottish Executive. *Community Care: A Joint Future* – Report by the Joint Future Group. Edinburgh: The Stationery Office, 2000.

30.   Scottish Executive Health Department. *Developing Services for Older People: Local Outcome Agreements*. CCD 6/2001.

31.   Scottish Executive Health Department. *Joint Resourcing and Joint Management of Community Care Services*. CCD 7/2001.

32.   Scottish Executive Health Department. *Single Shared Assessment of Community Care Needs*. CCD 8/2001.

33.   Scottish Executive. *Response to the Royal Commission on Long Term Care*. Edinburgh: Scottish Executive, 2000.

34.   Scottish Executive Joint Future Unit. *Consultation on Developing a Joint Performance Information and Assessment Framework (JPIAF) for Joint Working*. 2002.

35.   Woods K. The development of integrated health care models in Scotland. *International Journal of Integrated Care* 2001; 1 (April–June) www.ijic.org

36.   Department of Health. *The NHS Plan: A Plan for Investment, A Plan for Reform*. London: The Stationery Office, 2000.

37.   Department of Health. *Partnership in Action: New Opportunities for Joint Working between Health and Social Services – A Discussion Document*. London: The Stationery Office, 1998.

38.   Bochel C, Bochel H, Page D. Housing: the foundation of community care. *Health and Social Care in the Community* 1999; 7: 494–501.

39.   Scottish Office. Housing and Community Care Env8/1991.

40.   Scottish Office. *Community Care: The Housing Dimension* (Env 27/1994; SW7/1994; NHS MEL 79. 1994.

41.   Scottish Homes. *Care in the Community: Scottish Homes Policy Statement*. Edinburgh: Scottish Homes, 1998.

42.   Scottish Executive Development Department. *Modernising Community Care: The Housing Contribution – A Guidance Note*. 1999.

43.   House of Commons Scottish Affairs Committee Session 1996–97. Second Report. *The Implementation of Community Care in Scotland*, Volume 1. London: HMSO, 1997.

44.   Petch A, Rosengard A, Naumann L, Dean J. *'Help Me Out, Let Me In': Reprovisioning, Resettlement and the Scope for Social Inclusion in Scotland*. Edinburgh: Scottish Homes, 2000.

45. Emerson E, Hatton C. *Moving Out: The impact of relocation from hospital to community on the quality of life for people with learning disabilities.* London: HMSO, 1994.

46. Scottish Office. *Social Exclusion in Scotland.* A Consultation Paper. Edinburgh: Scottish Office, 1998.

47. Thompson J, Pickering S. *Meeting the Health Needs of People who have a Learning Disability.* London: Bailliere Tindall, 2001.

48. Department of Health. *Caring about Carers: A National Strategy for Carers.* London: Department of Health, 1999.

49. Scottish Executive. *Strategy for Carers in Scotland.* 1999
http://www.scotland.gov.uk/library2/doc10/carerstrategy.asp

50. Scottish Executive. *Report of the Scottish Carers' Legislation Working Group.* Edinburgh: Scottish Executive, 2001.

51. Royal Commission on Long Term Care. *With Respect to Old Age.* London: The Stationery Office, 1999.

52. Care Development Group. *Fair Care for Older People.* Edinburgh: The Stationery Office, 2001.

53. Scottish Executive Joint Future Unit. *Practical Advice on Joint Resourcing and Joint Management.* Edinburgh: Scottish Executive, 2002.

54. www.integratedworking.org.

55. Report of the Integrated Human Resource Working Group on the Human Resource Implications of the Joint Future Agenda, 2002.

56. Community Care (Direct Payments) (Scotland) Regulations 19977 (SI 1997/693); Community Care (Direct Payments) (Scotland) Amendment Regulations 2000 (SI 2000/183)

57. Witcher S, Stalker K, Roadburg M, Jones C. *Direct Payments: The Impact on Choice and Control for Disabled People.* Edinburgh: Scottish Executive Central Research Unit, 2000.

58. Pearson C. Money talks? Competing discourses in the implementation of direct payments. *Critical Social Policy* 2000; 20: 459–477.

59. Scottish Executive Health Department. *Better Care for all our futures.* Edinburgh: Scottish Executive, 2001.

60.   Scottish Executive. *The Same as You? A review of services for people with learning disabilities.*
       Edinburgh: HMSO, 2000.

61.   Department of Health. *Valuing People: A New Strategy for Learning Disability for the 21st Century.*
       London: HMSO, 2001.

62.   Department of Health. *National Service Framework for Older People.* London: The Stationery
       Office, 2001.

63.   Peck E, Towell D, Gulliver P. The meanings of culture in health and social care: a study of
       the combined Trust in Somerset. *Journal of Interprofessional Care* 2001;15: 319–327.

64.   *NHS Responsibility for Continuing Health Care.* NHS MEL (1996) 22, 1996.

65.   Curtice L, Petch A with Hallam A, Knapp M. *Over the Threshold? An Exploration of Intensive
       Domiciliary Support for Older People.* Edinburgh: Scottish Executive Central Research Unit,
       2002.

66.   Health Technology Board for Scotland. Comment on the National Institute for Clinical
       Excellence Technology Appraisal Guidance on the use of donepezil, rivastigmine and
       galantamine for the treatment of Alzheimer's disease. Comment 1. 2001.

67.   Cowan D, Turner-Smith A. The Role of Assistive Technology in Alternative Models of
       Care for Older People. Appendix Four in Royal Commission on Long Term Care. *With
       Respect to Old Age*: Research Volume Two. London: The Stationery Office, 1999.

68.   Henwood M. *Future Imperfect?* Report of the King's Fund Care and Support Inquiry.
       London: King's Fund, 2001.

8. Developing Primary Care in Scotland

Lewis Ritchie

General Practice and Primary Care in Context

Over the last 20 years general practice has undergone remarkable and relentless change as part of an increased prominence for primary care services.[1] The patient consultation remains at the hub of clinical practice but is now being delivered in different ways, in new settings and by a growing team of health professionals. In donning the wider mantle of primary care it is important that the values and contribution of general practice are not lost sight of in a view of primary care that is multidisciplinary, multidimensional and evolving rapidly.[2]

Principles and Values

Early concepts of the health care encounter were medically led – dominated by a compartmentalised view of the individual patient – in time (the present), in space (usually a hospital bed) and in priority (immediate).[3] This limited perspective, sometimes dubbed the 'patient/doctor/illness triangle' was episodic, reactive and problem based, with the patient occupying an essentially passive role. Missing from this equation was due recognition of the need for greater patient autonomy and participation in the therapeutic relationship and the impact of life circumstances on illness and disability. The dimension of disease prevention was notably absent and the carer role focused on the doctor, excluding other health professionals.[2]

To address these flaws, alternative models for primary care have evolved, where the patient is the main focal point. Patient-centred care embraces health promotion as well as illness management,[4] values the supportive role of family and friends,[5] includes continuity of care and requires a multidisciplinary team approach.[4] Additionally, the community or public health dimension of primary care acknowledges a responsibility beyond the care of individuals and the need to monitor and systematically improve the health of all patients.[6] Such proactive care builds on the great advantage of the registered general practitioner patient list in the UK and is complimentary to the traditional reactive role of caring for those who are sick and seeking help. Another fundamental value of primary care is an equity imperative for patients,[7, 8] recognising the adverse effects of deprivation on health,[9] the continuing paradox of the 'inverse care law'[10] and the variability of service provision.[11]

A further, economic dimension includes an increasing appreciation of both costs and benefits in relation to health care interventions – as our understanding of disease and illness behaviour continues to accrue so does our view of the most clinically effective and cost-effective treatments and prevention programmes.[2] The rising expectations of patients as consumers or participants[6] and patient empowerment[12] also need to be accommodated, with a potential tension between patients' rights and responsibilities.[2]

Many of these guiding principles and values are not exclusive to primary care – but primary care is unique in embracing them all. They need to be set in the context of our ageing Scottish population which faces many socio-economic challenges, is ethnically diverse and geographically disparate. Assimilation of all of the complexity and richness of primary care thus amounts to a considerable task for our policy- makers, health professionals, administrators and support staff alike – in order to deliver and demonstrate effective, high quality patient-centred care.[8, 13, 14]

Consideration of the evolving remit of primary care cannot be undertaken in isolation. There are many care relationships within and beyond primary care – including health service, local authority social care and voluntary provision. Of particular interest are the interfaces between self-care and primary care and in turn, primary care and secondary care. In the UK some 85% of all episodes of ill health are self-treated without seeking further help.[11] Of the remainder 90% are dealt with entirely by primary care teams and only 10% or 1% of the total, are referred for secondary care. By contrast it has been estimated that self-care accounts for 5% of the costs (including over the counter medicines and allied treatments); primary care accounts for 30% of the total (including community nursing costs and the majority of all spending on prescribed medicines) and secondary care, 65% (including outpatient activity).[11]

As the role of primary care has evolved over the last 20 years, acute hospital (secondary and tertiary) care has moved in tandem towards the delivery of progressively more high-cost, high technology interventions involving shorter inpatient stays, with increasing specialisation,[15] as described in Chapter 9. In turn, this impacts on the expanding remit and responsibilities for primary care – and on the quality of the 'journey of care' for the individual patient.[16]

Primary Care – Place and Worth

Successive UK and Scottish government discussion papers, White Papers and policy documents have carolled the importance of primary care over the last 20 years.[17–33] This reflects a growing international evidence base supporting the worth of health services which are underpinned by a substantive primary care foundation. International comparisons have demonstrated the importance of primary care as the key to an effective and efficient health service.[8, 34–38]

Perception of the value of primary care is not only about available evidence from ecological studies but is also supported by the perceptions of patients. There are consistent findings from surveys that primary care in its various guises is valued highly by Scottish patients.[39, 40]

Recent Evolution of Primary Care in Scotland

Putting Quality on the Map

In the late 1970s and throughout the 1980s a *'ferment of ideas'*[41] took place on the improvement of primary health care in the UK. The General Medical Services Committee of the BMA proposed a new GP contract,[42] and the Royal College of General Practitioners (RCGP) sighted on the importance of quality and the unacceptability of variable standards of care.[43] In 1986 the Green Paper, *Primary Care – an Agenda for Discussion* was published,[17] which emphasised a commitment to comprehensive primary health care and a willingness to negotiate on the development of new patient services. The proposals, which included a 'good practice allowance,' directly linked remuneration and quality for the first time. In the absence of agreed quality standards for primary care, many of these ideas, including the good practice allowance, were abandoned in 1987, when the White Paper, *Promoting Better Health*,[18] was published.

Visible changes arising from this paper included financial incentives – target payments to encourage immunisation and cervical cytology, practice payments for working in deprived areas, based on a modified Jarman Index,[44] and the advent of practice based audit activity. Around this time a review of community nursing also took place and the recommendations were published in 1986 as the Cumberlege Report: *Neighbourhood Nursing: a Focus for Care*,[45] which advocated a switch of resources from hospital into the community, nurse prescribing and a new nurse practitioner role.[46] A key plank of this particular report, was the establishment of locality or neighbourhood based nursing services actively promoting the concept of the primary care team.[47] As for some aspects of *Promoting Better Health*,[18] these proposals were not formally implemented but were clearly influential for the subsequent organisation of nursing services in Scotland and the rest of the UK.

The 1990 Contract and a Primary Care Led NHS

In 1989, the White Paper, *Working for Patients*,[19] paved the way for dramatic reforms (see chapter 1). The scene was set for the NHS internal market and the epithets of a primary care led NHS and the purchaser-provider split. Initially GPs involved in large practices (>11000 patient lists, approximately 5% of the total) were encouraged to apply for their own budgets or funds. Fundholding GPs would be able to agree contracts and to purchase a defined range of services direct from hospitals.[20]

In the absence of significant new funding, however, the provisions of *Working for Patients*[19] pivoted upon redistribution of existing monies, which translated to many GPs as more work for the same money. As such, most grassroots doctors did not welcome the new reforms, and the new 1990 Contract was imposed in the absence of agreement by the profession's negotiators. Unlike the original 1965 GP Charter[48] – implemented at a time when the self-esteem of general practice was at a low ebb, premises and organisation poor and recruits dwindling – the 1990 Contract was introduced at a relative high point for GP morale, infrastructure, and manpower.

In Scotland, in the wake of *Working for Patients*,[19] a series of papers to facilitate implementation were produced, including one on the implications for primary care.[21] The proposed changes included: introduction of an associate scheme for GPs practising in isolated areas; a reduction in the maximum retirement age of GPs from 70 to 65; the offer of annual health checks for elderly people aged 75 years and over; minor surgery payments; deprivation payments, and payments for structured child health surveillance. The proposed introduction of indicative prescribing budgets for the first time recognised an uncontrolled annual 5–6 per cent growth in drug spending above inflation with a three-fold increase in the previous decade and a 50% variation in prescribing costs (net ingredient cost per patient) between the lowest and highest Health Board Areas.[49] To facilitate this, Medical Prescribing Advisers were recruited to set and monitor indicative prescribing budgets, with support from pharmacist colleagues. Improved information systems[50] and prescribing information were also flagged. Scottish Prescribing Analysis (SPA) was introduced in 1990,[51] providing quarterly updates to individual GPs of their prescribing habits and allowing peer group comparison with practice colleagues and local Health Board averages.

At the outset, these reforms were viewed by many as conceived by the few and long on direction but short on detail.[52] In Scotland, this criticism could be regarded as unfair: the Scottish Home and Health Department prepared detailed guidance on fundholding,[22, 25] with a flurry of advice on other specific issues for primary care services. In response to the widespread scepticism about fundholding, the Scottish Home and Health Department agreed to a shadow pilot scheme of six practices and also embraced an evaluation programme of this initiative which was undertaken by the Department of General Practice at the University of Edinburgh.[53–58] In due course, primary care purchasing was introduced in 1995, intended principally for GPs working in small practices. This enabled purchasing of community-based services, including those provided by district nurses, health visitors and allied health professionals (AHPs) and responsibility for their practice and prescribing budgets. Total purchasing was also introduced in pilot form, allowing groups of GPs to buy all health care services for patients. A further objective of this initiative was to explore closer working with social care services and to assess its feasibility for optimising future health purchasing.[28] As time passed, progressively more GPs embraced fundholding, rising to a high of 530 practices, covering 56% of Scottish patients, by the time the initiative was discontinued in 1998.[59]

Impact of the 1990 Contract

Detailed discussion of the impact of *Working for Patients*[19] and the 1990 GP Contract[20] is outwith the scope of this chapter but numerous articles and analyses have been published seeking to confirm or refute the benefits of the fundholding initiative. Overall, there is minimal evidence that fundholding had a beneficial effect on patient outcomes and while GP fundholders had a greater repertoire of secondary providers, little progress was made for patient choice and autonomy.[54-63] In essence, funding-enabled primary care teams did not translate directly to empowered patients with better clinical outcomes. Moreover, the generic cry of a 'two-tier service' remained plausible and the fundholding initiative produced greater inequality between practices.[64] This reduced the capacity of the NHS to plan strategically and threatened patient equity[7, 8] – one of the key pillars of health care in general and primary care in particular.

The 1990 Contract was not just about fundholding, however, and other aspects included the introduction of target payments for childhood immunisations and for cervical cytology. Initial controversy about targets notwithstanding, Scottish uptake levels reached new highs in the wake of the 1990 Contract for established childhood immunisation[65] and cervical cytology programmes in primary care.[28, 66] Another far-reaching and beneficial reform occurred in 1995, perhaps in spite of, rather than because of the 1990 Contract. After sharp rises in GP night visits, the introduction of new out-of-hours arrangements spawned the establishment of out-of-hours co-operatives throughout Scotland and the creation of primary care emergency centres leading to significant improvements in the quality of GPs' lives coupled with high levels of patient satisfaction.[67] By the end of 1997, 75% of the Scottish population was covered by GP out-of-hours co-operatives and this figure has continued to escalate since. As at end December 2002, 85% of the Scottish population were covered by 29 separate out-of-hours co-operatives.[*]

The Primary Care Development Fund (PCDF) was a further initiative in the lee of *Working for Patients*.[19] PCDF was first established in 1993 as a challenge fund to stimulate innovation and new models of working in primary care, providing an annual sum to be distributed for individual projects.[28] Although the impact and the legacy of the Primary Care Development Fund has not been formally appraised, it has facilitated many initiatives since its inception which otherwise would have languished without support.

---

[*] Source: Mallinson E, 2003, NHS24 Integration Plan (personal communication)

Beyond the 1990 Contract: Moving On

Since 1990 Government policy had concentrated on a 'primary care led' NHS which was seen as building on the established strengths of various independent contractors working in primary care.[28] To reinforce this approach, a slew of government papers appeared in 1996 and 1997. In the van came the Scottish discussion paper: *Primary Care – the Way Ahead*.[26] It garnered a desire for greater flexibility to meet local needs and built on the earlier proposals for developing a strategic framework for primary care.[24] The UK White Paper: *Primary Care: the Future – Choice and Opportunity* was also published in 1996,[27] containing proposals for legislative change which would create local flexibility, allowing different models of delivery of primary medical and dental services to be piloted and evaluated. New options offered in *Choice and Opportunity*[27] embraced:

- Salaried option for GPs within independent partnerships or with NHS Trusts

- Single budget for general medical services including prescribing and community health services (total purchasing)

- Practice based contracts, including contracts for non–medical staff: nurses, managers and allied health professionals

- Similar flexibility within general dental services for salaried options and practice-base contracts and for developing community pharmacy services

These were encapsulated in the NHS (Primary Care) Act 1997,[68–70] following two further White Papers – *The Scottish Health Service: Ready for the Future*[30] and *Primary Care: Agenda for Action*.[29] Both signalled a more co-ordinated approach and that:

- Flexible primary care arrangements must address local needs

- Primary care services were at different stages of development throughout Scotland requiring support to develop capacity and standards across the board

- Multiprofessional skills were required for primary care and needed to be valued and nurtured

To facilitate this, further funding was earmarked, including provision for extra monies for supporting undergraduate medical teaching (ACT – additional costs of teaching funds) and for research and development in primary care. A commitment was also made to extending roles for nurses (including prescribing), community pharmacists, skill-mix in dental teams, developing managerial skills and addressing recruitment alongside other workforce issues.

The proposals contained in *Primary Care: Agenda for Action*[29] were supported with additional resources and widely regarded as a signal for more collaborative working and less competition. As a result, they received broad multi-professional support at a time when many organisations and individual voices were contributing to the debate on the future of primary care.[71–74]

PMS Pilots – Policy into Practice

Further innovation came in the form of proposals for Personal Medical Services (PMS) Pilots. Fuelled by the provisions of the NHS (Primary Care) Act 1997, PMS Pilots afforded the opportunity for a new range of contractual options for GPs and other primary care staff to engage and evaluate new models of care. PMS Pilots were required to improve access and quality of services.

The accent was on flexibility and experiment, with models that were appropriate for local circumstances and needs, both for patients and for health professionals.[75] While some saw PMS as a threat to general medical services (GMS) and the thin end of the wedge for independent contractor status, others were much more enthusiastic and embraced the opportunity to break the mould.[76]

Although a change of government from Conservative to Labour in the summer of 1997 heralded the demise of fundholding and the scrapping of the internal market, the PMS concept survived and first round pilots were introduced in 1998 with a second round in 1999.[77] A positive Ministerial review was published in 2000,[78] supported by a further evaluation undertaken by the University of Southampton which provided evidence compatible with improved quality of care.[79–81] Since inception, uptake of PMS gradually gathered momentum[82] and by the end of December 2002 more than 100 schemes were in operation throughout Scotland.

Designed to Care: Partnership and a Patient Centred NHS

The incoming Labour administration in Scotland moved quickly to publish the White Paper, *Designed to Care*,[31] in late 1997. While the primacy of the needs and expectations of patients had been signalled originally with the publication of the *Patient's Charter* in 1991,[83] *Designed to Care*[31] markedly raised the stakes for meaningful patient and public engagement in health services, as did the equivalent White Paper south of the border.[84] There was also an emphasis on collaboration – not competition – and renewed support for the pivotal role of primary care, shorn of the fragmentary effects and bureaucracy of fundholding. Innovation and collaborative working would be stimulated by new Primary Care Trusts (PCTs).

Although the departure from fundholding was a radical change from previous policy, the primary care provisions of *Designed to Care*,[31] built further on earlier proposals contained in *Primary Care: Agenda for Action*[29] – including local needs assessment, capacity building, clinical effectiveness and multiprofessional working.

In addition to their responsibilities for primary care services, PCTs were also to be accountable for the running of community hospitals,[85, 86] developing local comprehensive mental health services (building on a *Framework for Mental Health Services in Scotland*)[87, 88] and promoting networks of general practices in Local Health Care Co-operatives (LHCCs). In contrast to England, where Primary Care Groups with commissioning powers were created,[84] LHCCs were established in Scotland with the following objectives:[31]

- Providing services to patients within an identified level of resources including expenditure on prescribing

- Working with the support of public health medicine to develop plans which reflect the clinical priorities of the area, while taking into account specific needs of the registered population covered by the co-operative

- Supporting the development of population-wide approaches to health improvement and disease prevention which require lifestyle and behavioural change

- Improving the quality and standards of clinical care within practices and
  to support clinical and professional development through education,
  training, research and audit

- Supporting the development of extended primary care teams to be
  formed around the practice structure and promote the development of
  specialisms within primary care.

Many of the provisions of *Designed to Care*[31] also map onto the principles and
values of primary care articulated at the outset of this chapter. For many
frontline staff these outline proposals proved welcome but some concerns were
expressed about the loss of practice-based control of resource allocation for
purchasing, without compensatory powers of commissioning care.[40, 89]

Quality and Accountability – the Advent of Clinical Governance

One of the most important aspects of *Designed to Care*[31] was a desire for
demonstrable quality of care coupled to 'accountability', which began to appear
more frequently in the lexicon of primary care. In Scotland, the RCGP took an
early lead in synthesising advice on promoting clinical governance[90] in 1998 and
pursued this with widely endorsed guidance on implementing clinical
governance in primary care.[91] In turn, this spawned SPICE-PC in 1999, the
Scottish Programme for Improving Clinical Effectiveness in Primary Care
under the aegis of the RCGP and supported by the Scottish General
Practitioners Committee (SGPC).[92] Publication of the Acute Services Review[93]
in 1998 also provided a stimulus for improved quality of care with specific
resonance for primary care[94–104] – see also chapter 9.

Towards a Healthier Scotland – Assessing Needs, Addressing Inequalities

The year 1999 marked the publication of the White Paper: *Towards a Healthier
Scotland*,[105.] following on from the Green Paper: *Working Together for a Healthier
Scotland*[106] – see also chapters 2 and 3. A dominant theme of this White Paper
was health improvement and primary care services – LHCCs in particular, were
seen as playing a key role in trying to secure this aim.

This agenda played into the public health dimension of primary care: addressing the needs of communities without losing sight of the needs of individuals.[2] For many primary care professionals, used to the care of individual patients, the concepts and methods of needs assessment for communities were unfamiliar. This deficit was recognised by the Scottish Needs Assessment Programme (SNAP)[107] which published helpful guidance on needs assessment, building on successful primary care projects that had been undertaken in Scotland.[108, 109] The partnership between primary care and public health was also reinforced by the publication in 1999 of the Chief Medical Officer's *Review of the Public Health Function*.[110] This Review again emphasised the key role of LHCCs in improving community health and promulgated a major role for Health Boards and public health specialists in helping acquisition of the relevant skills.

Our National Health: A Plan for Action, a Plan for Change

In 2001, the first White Paper on Health was published after the establishment of the devolved Scottish Parliament –*Our National Health – A Plan for Action, a Plan for Change*.[32] This signalled a renewed commitment to health improvement, modernisation of the NHS and patient engagement to be underpinned by a substantial and sustained injection of new resources into the health budget, aligned to re-allocation of existing funds via a new needs-based formula published in *Fair Shares for All*.[111–112] Endorsement for enhanced partnership working was emphasised as was the particular need for effective working between health and social care services, crystallised in *A Joint Future*.[33] Specific commitments for primary care included:

- Maximum 48 hour patient access time for an appropriate primary care team member

- Development and investment in new contractual arrangements, building on PMS pilots, to allow NHS Trusts to employ GPs to work in socially deprived and remote areas[82]

- Support for expansion of roles and responsibilities of primary care members, building integrated teams and freeing up GPs to spend more time with those requiring their skills[113]

- Increase in numbers of nurses trained to prescribe and widening the range of medications prescribed[114]

- Extension of model schemes to allow pharmacists to prescribe a broader range of medicines, conduct medication reviews and monitor certain treatments[115, 116]

- Enhanced training and leadership programmes for primary care nurses including public health practitioners[117, 118]

- Workforce planning, training and job content implications of changing roles in primary and intermediate care[118–125]

- Extension of occupational health services to staff working in general medical and dental practices[126]

- Introduction of NHS24 to provide 24 hour access to health advice and healthcare services by telephone from trained health professionals[127]

Of great importance in this context was *Making the Connections: Developing Best Practice into Common Practice,*[113] published by the Primary Care Modernisation Group in 2002 and which offered strategic priorities and actions for the development of primary care. The Group had been tasked to develop a coherent framework programme for primary care modernisation, a three year timetable of priorities and to provide delivery mechanisms taking account of the enhanced role of LHCCs.

Making the Connections was issued with a warm endorsement by the Scottish Executive, which tasked NHS Boards to take lead responsibility for implementation of the required actions in their local areas.[128] While the focus of the report was on developing capacity within the primary care sector, the recommended actions impinged on the whole of the NHS and also acknowledged the important inter-relationship with other agencies, particularly local authorities (see also chapter 7).

Partnership for Care

The Health White Paper for the NHS in Scotland – *Partnership for Care*[129] – published in March 2003, just as this chapter was being finalised, consolidated many of the recommendations in *Making the Connections*,[113] emphasising again the pivotal role of primary care and reasserting the role of LHCCs. They were to be strengthened and to evolve into 'Community Health Partnerships,' in concert with local authorities for the planning and delivery of high quality, accessible care. Without rushing to premature judgement, *Partnership for Care* signalled a further shift along the axis of enhanced, integrated primary care services, attuned to local circumstances and predicated on balancing the needs of individuals and communities.[2,6]

Key Trends in Primary Care

The next section of this chapter discusses key trends in primary care in the past 20 years, including resources, workforce and contemporary issues for health professionals working in primary care. Data are sourced from the Information and Statistics Division of the Common Services Agency (ISD)** or from the Scottish Executive Health Department (SEHD).

Primary Care Funding

Changes in health resources allocated to primary care services are listed in Table 8.1. Overall, resources allocated to primary care increased from £246M in 1980–81 to £666M (by 170%) in 1990–91 and again to £1343M (by a further 101%) in 2000–01. As a percentage of overall NHS expenditure the percentage allocated to primary care (family health) services increased significantly from 19% in 1980–81 to 22% in 1990–91 and by a smaller amount in the 1990s to 24% in 2000–01. Within primary care funding, between 1980–81 and 1990–91, percentage expenditure on pharmaceutical services (GPS) remained fairly constant at ~48%, with a rapidly rising share to 55% of the total by 2000–01. Much of the increased expenditure on primary care services in the 1990s can, therefore, be attributed to rising prescribing costs, which are discussed separately. In contrast, percentage expenditure on general medical services (GMS) increased slightly from 31% to 33% between 1980–81 and 1990–91,

---

** www.show.scot.nhs.uk/isd/Scottish_Health_Statistics/SHS2000/home.htm

falling back to just less than 30% by 2000–01. General dental services (GDS) followed a similar trajectory to GMS, while the proportion of funds allocated to general ophthalmic services (GOS) halved between 1980–81 and 1990–91 with a marginal increase by 2000–01.

TABLE 8.1 Trends in Primary Care Funding 1980–2000

NHS funding allocations (£M – Millions)	1980–81	1990–91	2000–01
NHS Total	1324	2970	5615
Primary Care Total	246	666	1342
Primary Care percentage of NHS Total	**18.6%**	**22.4%**	**23.9%**
Primary Care percentage allocation by service			
Medical (GMS)	31.4%	32.9%	29.8%
Pharmaceutical (GPS)	48.3%	48.2%	55.0%
Dental (GDS)	16.1%	16.8%	12.8%
Ophthalmic (GOS)	4.2%	2.1%	2.4%
Primary Care Total	**100.0%**	**100.0%**	**100.0%**

Notes: Primary Care Total includes general medical (GMS), general pharmaceutical (GPS), general dental (GDS) and general ophthalmic services (GOS); Years end 31 March; Source: SEHD.

Prescribing Trends

Reference was made earlier to a three-fold increase in prescribing costs in the 1980s comprising a 5–6% annualised growth above inflation and a variation in prescribing costs of 50% between the lowest and highest Health Board areas.[49] In the 1990s drug costs continued to escalate with an overall growth of £393M, a greater than two-fold increase between 1990–91 and 2000–01 (to £694M) with a similar level of increase in annual net ingredient cost per patient (to £119). Over the same period the variation in prescribing costs declined, with a ~30% discrepancy between the lowest and the highest Health Board areas.

These changes emphasise the relentless upward pressures on prescribing costs but also show a narrowing of the variation between Boards. This occurred in a decade of indicative prescribing budgets, regular prescribing adviser input, dissemination of SPA analysis[50] and increasing use of generic drugs. These data also demonstrate the continuing challenge of optimal prescribing and the importance of matching patient need with evidence-based treatments. This challenge broadens with increasing polypharmacy in an ageing population and the incorporation of extended prescribing roles for nurses and pharmacists.[114, 115]

GP Lists and Partnership Size

The change in average list size by GP headcount continued to decline between 1980 and 2000, with an overall decrease of 22% from 1831 to 1425. Since 1990 list sizes have been monitored both by headcount and whole time equivalent (wte) numbers – the 1990 wte list size was 1620, decreasing to 1510 (by 6.8%) in 2000. Between 1985[†] and 2000 the average partnership size steadily increased from 2.8 to 3.5 with a decline in overall numbers of practices from 1139 to 1055 (by 7.4%). There was also a concomitant fall in the proportion of single-handed practitioners from 29% to 18% of all practices. As new models of primary care evolve, including PMS and LHCC developments, it is likely that this trend of consolidation will continue.

Primary Care – Changing Workforce

In 1980, Scotland had a workforce of 2959 GP principals rising during the decade by 13% to 3359 in 1990, with a more modest increase in the 1990s of 10% to 3706 in 2000 (overall headcount increase 1980–2000 = 25%, whole time equivalent increase = 19%). These raw figures conceal further significant changes. In 1980, 18% of the GP workforce was female, rising to 26% in 1990 and continuing to increase to 37% by 2000. As well as constituting a smaller percentage of the workforce, overall numbers of male GPs declined by 8% from the peak year of 1985 (2541) to 2000 (2338). Another major difference was the increasing number of part-time GPs. In 1990[††] of the 3350 whole time equivalent (wte) GPs in Scotland, 4% were part-time; by 2000 of the 3503 wte, 11% were part-time. Interestingly, of the 604 part-time principals in 2000, the vast majority

---

[†]   No data available from ISD before 1985
[††] No detailed wte statistics available from ISD for part-time GP workers prior to 1990

(81%) were female, but that proportion remained virtually static throughout the nineties, demonstrating no changing gender bias in seeking part-time work.

As far as the future medical workforce is concerned, there were 248 GP registrars (trainees) in post in 1980 (44% female), rising to a zenith of 330 in 1990 (52% female), coinciding with the publication of the 1990 GP Contract.[19, 20] During the 1990s numbers of registrars declined, reaching a nadir of 236 in 1996 (72% of peak figure) but regaining ground to 261 in 2000 (79% of peak). The decline in GP registrars, therefore, ran counter-current to the increasing prominence of primary care in government policy. By 2000, the proportion of female registrars had increased to 63% of the total, pointing to a future GP workforce where females will be in the majority, with a significant proportion of part-time workers.

A further comparison of note is illustrated in Figure 8.1, which examines the trend in numbers of GPs compared to hospital consultants over the period 1980–2000:

Figure 8.1   Trends in Medical Manpower 1980–2000

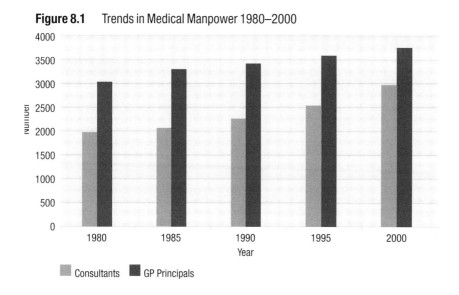

This shows a narrowing of the gap between GPs and hospital consultants. In 1980 there were 1.6 GPs for each consultant, by 1990 this ratio had dropped marginally to 1.5:1. In the 1990s the ratio narrowed more sharply to 1.2:1 by 2000, accelerating between 1995 and 2000, when consultant headcount numbers increased by 19%, compared to 5% for GPs. The differential for the latter period is more marked for changes in wte: consultants increased by 18% compared to 3% for GPs, reflecting the more marked trend to part-time working in general practice. Paradoxically, these workforce changes again coincided with government policies that sought to promote a primary care-led NHS – when the converse might have been expected.

The picture, however, is more complex than a simple comparison of medical workforce trends conveys. Figure 8.2 illustrates the contrasting picture for GP practice nurses. In the early 1980s there were slight increases in the employment of practice nurses with a striking change towards the end of the decade, with a virtual doubling in the year between 1989 (505 headcount, 295 wte), and 1990 (974 headcount, 584 wte). This dramatic increase coincided with the publication of *Working for Patients*,[19] the 1990 GP Contract and increasing health promotion activity. Although the rate of increase then moderated, there were still marked year-on-year increments since 1990, and by year 2000, 1746 (1065 wte) practice nurses were employed. Over the period 1982 [§]–2000 the total number of GP

Figure 8.2   Trends in GP Practice Nurses 1982–2000

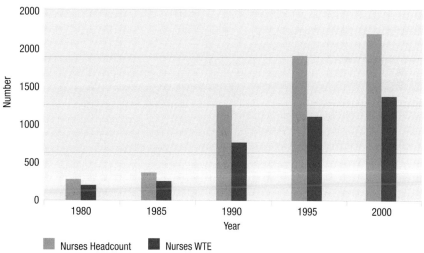

practice nurses increased more than nine-fold while the ratio of headcount to wte number remained remarkably steady at ~1.6:1. The significance of the fundamental change in the practice nursing workforce is perhaps best illustrated

---

[§]   1982 was the first year baseline data were recorded

by examining the GP:practice nurse ratio by wte. In 1982 this ratio was 26:1, by
1990 it had fallen to just under 6:1 and by 2000 the GP : practice nurse ratio
declined further to just over 3:1.

In Table 8.2, relevant workforce numbers and changes occurring between 1980
and 2000 are listed, allowing comparisons to be made:

TABLE 8.2 Changes in NHS Staff Categories 1980–2000 by Whole Time
Equivalent (wte)

	1980	2000	
Staff Category	Number	Number	Change
All Hospital Doctors	5173	7354	+ 42 %
Hospital Consultants	1907	2884	+ 51%
GP Principals	2980	3503	+ 19 %
GP Registrars[1]	248	261	+ 5 %
GP Practice Nurses	2 116	1065	+ 818 %
GP Administration Staff[2]	2521	5642	+ 123 %
Dentists (GDPs)	1277	2069	+ 62 %
Community Dental Practitioners	333	246	− 26 %
Community Health Doctors	455	341	− 25 %
Pharmacists[3]	367	643	+ 75 %
Clinical Psychologists[4]	133	360	+ 170%
Ophthalmic Opticians	1 503	1252	+ 149 %
Allied Health Professionals[4]	3352	7013	+ 109 %

[1] Headcount as wte not available;
[2] Baseline 1982;
[3] All NHS sectors excluding community pharmacies;
[4] All NHS sectors. Source: Scottish Health Statistics 2000.

Over this period, general practice administrative staff time also grew steadily
and significantly by 123%. As far as the wider primary care team is concerned,

general dental practitioners (GDPs) increased in wte by 62%, compared to a 19% increase for general medical practitioners(GPs). In contrast, the numbers of community dental practitioners employed by the NHS fell by 26%, mirrored by the same order of decline for community health doctors – 25%. Qualified pharmacists employed by the NHS increased by 75%. Of those, 76% were employed in Acute NHS Trusts, 22% in Primary Care Trusts (PCTs) and 2% in NHS Boards in the year 2000. In the 1990s overall numbers of registered pharmacists in Scotland increased by 20% (to 3841 in year 2000), but this did not translate into more community pharmacy outlets where the numbers remained remarkably steady throughout the decade (1144 in year 2000). Qualified clinical psychologists also increased in numbers by 170%, most of whom were employed in PCTs (87% in year 2000). Numbers of ophthalmic opticians also rose significantly over the period by 149%, as did allied health professionals (AHPs) – by 109%. In 2000, 55% of AHPs were employed in Acute NHS Trusts compared with 45% in PCTs. As for pharmacists, it will be interesting to note future trends in the deployment of AHPs in hospital and community settings.

Primary Care – Changing Patterns of Activity

The Continuous Morbidity Recording Project (CMR)[130–131] was established as part of the national core data set in 1998 following development work at the University of Aberdeen.[132] The main purpose of the CMR database is the provision of a national resource for the study of morbidity and related workload in primary care using face-to-face clinical contacts in primary care. Originally confined to GP-patient contacts, CMR was extended to begin to include nursing and health visitor clinical encounters. National CMR data became available from 1997 onwards and therefore trend data cover a narrow time window. The annual average GP consultation rate was just over 3.1 per patient in 1999, covering a range of 1.5 per annum in males aged 15–24, to 5.1 in females aged ≥ 75 years. At all ages with the exception of 0–4 years female consultations exceeded male – in the age ranges 15–24 and 24–44 years the rate for females was more than double that for males. Further analyses are available by diagnostic category – upper respiratory tract infection being the most common reason for GP consultation in 1999, followed by depression and then hypertension. It will be important to monitor variation in these patterns, in the light of demographic change and newer models of care delivery, which embrace more extended roles for nurses and pharmacists working in primary care.

While GP home visits have declined steadily over the past 20 years during normal working hours,[133] estimates of demand for out-of-hours care, including home visits, are more difficult to assess, given the move to co-operatives. Representative survey work undertaken in 1997/98 gave an average standardised out-of-hours rate of 221 calls per 1000 patients/year in Scotland compared to 145 in England and was much higher in deprived areas.[134] These findings provide a useful baseline for assessing the effect of further changes in service organisation, particularly the advent of NHS24. They should also be set in the context of research on out-of-hours care that underpins the importance of meeting patients' expectations,[135, 136] and for improved communications with patients.[137]

Significant changes also occurred for health visitors between 1980 and 2000 with a steady decline in home visits by 40%. District nurse home visits fluctuated over the same period but finished overall slightly lower by 6%. In those aged 75 years and over, however, district nurses actually increased home visitation by about 75%. This latter trend coincided with the GP contractual requirement for the provision of systematic annual health checks in this age group. A number of other changes of activity are reported in Scottish Health Statistics,[§§] demonstrating significantly higher levels of activity for general dental practitioners, ophthalmic opticians, pharmacists and AHPs, between 1980 and 2000.

Explaining Changing Trends in Primary Care

Many of the observed changes in resources, workforce and patterns of activity have been clearly influenced by government policy – for example, the dramatic increase in GP practice nurses, primarily engaged in health promotion and chronic disease management, triggered by the 1990 GP Contract.[19, 20] This trend is likely to continue as more nurses adopt the nurse practitioner role,[138] engaging in care and triage of acute illnesses.[139, 140] Some changes, such as the very modest increase in the GP workforce compared to the growth in numbers of hospital consultants, appear at first sight to question the principle of a primary care led NHS and are not supported by available research evidence.[8, 34, 37, 38] It is clear that delegation and role substitution will continue for many of the current clinical activities in primary care with a differing skill-mix, including nurses, pharmacists and AHPs. While GPs are not an endangered species, the statistical

---

[§§] See: www.show.scot.nhs/uk/isd/Scottish_Health_Statistics/SHS2000/home.htm

message is plain: all other healthcare professional groups have numerically prospered in comparison, excepting community doctors and dentists. Government policies have influenced change, but they are not sufficient to explain away all of the observed differences. Other significant drivers have been: a rapidly ageing population,[33, 141] with increasing co-morbidity,[8] the availability of new treatments and technologies, a heightened awareness of health promotion and the pursuit of unmet need. In turn, all of these are underpinned by increasing patient expectations. Finally, the crucial role and aspirations of health professionals in determining the changing shape and substance of primary care should not be overlooked.

GP Issues

Secular changes in the GP workforce have not been confined to issues of number or gender. Many young doctors have indicated that they do not wish to follow the standard independent principal route - coupled as it is to a small-business ethos - and also expect less demanding hours of work. The workforce is also ageing significantly (average age just over 44 years in 2000), with survey evidence of lower morale and with increasing numbers expressing an interest in premature retirement.[142–144] Reasons cited for low morale and rising unfilled GP vacancies included: perceptions of insufficient resources for improved staffing, shorter consultation times than desirable, too much bureaucracy and insufficient engagement in a rapidly changing NHS.[142, 143] As such, GP supply came under additional pressure because of reduced training numbers, diminished commitment to full-time work after training and increased levels of early retirement – a trend that became firmly established throughout the 1990s, following the introduction of the 1990 GP Contract.[19, 20] These sobering data were tempered by more encouraging findings from one study which reported that the most recently qualified doctors in the late 1990s regarded general practice as a more attractive career than hospital medicine.[145] The results of this lone study found an echo in the upswing of GP registrars in training in Scotland, over the same period. This should also be set in the context of competing claims from acute hospital services, however, with an increasing demand for junior hospital medical staff, in response to European legislation on working hours restrictions (see also *Unfinished Business*[146] and additional references to reappraisal and revalidation).[147–149]

The New GP Contract – Addressing Needs, Pursuing Quality

Many of the outstanding workforce and morale issues for GPs are intimately tied up with contractual matters. The way forward for many existing GPs will be substantially determined by the outcome of negotiations on their radical new contract[150, 151] which was ratified in 2003 for implementation in 2004. Under the terms of the general medical services contract framework document,[150] a new UK weighted capitation formula replaces the 'Red Book of Fees and Allowances', as the main method of remunerating GPs. The UK formula is a resource allocation model that in principle provides money to GP practices on the basis of the relative need of their patients. In effect the current system of remuneration where money mostly follows doctors will be superseded by a new system where money follows patients. Other funding streams available under the contract include: infrastructural funding for premises and IM&T, and a new quality framework. The latter is designed to reward GPs for the quality of care provided and a range of enhanced services over and above those deemed to be essential or additional. This aspect of the proposed new contract revisits history: as discussed earlier, a 'good practice allowance' was first proposed in 1986,[17] but foundered in the absence of agreed definitions for quality practice.[18]

Another fundamental aspect of the new contract is a division of responsibilities for normal hours and out-of-hours cover, allowing GPs formally to opt out of the latter for the first time, with a resulting trade-off in income. The likely adverse impact on the availability of GPs for out-of-hours cover may well be substantial, putting further pressure on the rapid development and refinement of robust multiprofessional alternatives, including NHS24.[127, 134, 152] Whether the new contract will stimulate additional recruitment and enhance retention of GPs, remains to be seen – particularly at a time when the overall capacity of the Scottish medical workforce has been widely accepted as at best insufficient and at worst parlous[123] – see also chapter 11 and further discussion of recruitment and retention in relation to remote and rural areas below.

Nursing Issues

The burgeoning role and growth in numbers of primary care nurses seems set to continue. Apart from the traditional treatment room remit of primary care nurses, extended roles now include chronic disease management, prevention, prescribing, and telephone and face-to-face triage of acute illness. An increasingly skilled workforce of nurses is substituting for medical colleagues in new and innovative ways, including an advanced remit of nurse practitioner. The traditional role of the GP as first point of contact and gatekeeper to the NHS may be under threat but the emphasis is one of collaboration rather than competition. The evidence base underpinning enhanced roles for nurses is substantial and compelling – for example the management of chronic illness, such as the care of people with diabetes,[153, 154] depression,[155, 156] heart failure;[157] the secondary prevention of coronary heart disease;[158, 159] prescribing of medicines;[160, 161] and in-hours[140] and out-of-hours telephone triage.[152] In addition to considerations of efficacy and safety, there are also issues of cost-effectiveness – and there is some evidence that nurse practitioners are similarly cost-effective to GPs as point of first contact for acute illness.[162] Similarly, doctor substitution by nurses has been demonstrated to be acceptable to patients, for example in telephone triage,[140, 152] and in the nurse practitioner role.[162] A number of professional barriers have been identified to further development of the nurse practitioner role, including GP perceptions of threat to their status, nursing capabilities, training and scope of responsibility.[138]

As for GPs, issues of nursing workforce supply, accountability, morale and professional development were recognised in the Strategy for Nursing and Midwifery: *Caring for Scotland*, which was published in 2002.[118] This document built on other policy documents such as *Our National Health*,[32] *Nursing for Health*[117] which envisaged a greater public health role for nurses, and a *Framework for Maternity Services in Scotland*.[163, 164] All of these policy documents emphasised the importance of research,[165] evidence-based practice, development and innovation with relevance for the future of primary care.

Pharmacist Issues

Many of the issues for primary care nurses have similar resonance for pharmacists and pharmacy assistants. Again, there is a significant and growing international evidence base[166] for extended roles of clinical and community pharmacists, for example in: palliative care,[167] health promotion[168] – including smoking cessation,[169] coronary heart disease prevention,[170] depression,[171] clinical consultations,[172] drug misuse[173] and pharmacovigilance.[174] Patient satisfaction surveys also indicate that pharmacist advice is highly valued.[117, 168] There are a number of constraints which have stood in the way of further expansion of the role of community pharmacists including current UK legislative strictures, contractual matters and the lack of awareness among other health care professionals and the general public of the expertise of pharmacists.[175, 176] Another very practical barrier has been lack of appropriate premises space for personal advice.

Many of the significant contributions of clinical and community pharmacists to patient care have been unsung – as recognised in the Strategy for Pharmaceutical Care in Scotland: *The Right Medicine*,[115] published in 2002 and *Pharmacy for Health – the Way Forward*,[116] published in 2003. The exceptional potential for pharmacists in both health promotion and illness management has yet to be fully realised – with an estimated 600 000 visits to pharmacies and 190 000 GP prescriptions dispensed in Scotland daily.[115, 116] *The Right Medicine* identified a series of planned actions in a four-year programme to address barriers and to push through radical change – including: premises improvement,[177] electronic transfer of prescriptions,[131, 178] LHCC pharmacy locality groups, pharmacist prescribing, pharmaceutical needs assessment of communities and of disadvantaged individuals, workforce planning, educational development, clinical governance and harnessing research contributions.[115] Many of these are likely to have a significant impact on the delivery of primary care in Scotland.

Issues for Other Primary Care Health Professionals

In the past 20 years General Dental Practitioners (GDPs) numbers of have grown significantly along with increasing recognition of their role in the extended primary care team. In comparison, numbers of Community Dental Practitioners (CDPs) have diminished significantly. Issues of supply and demand are not only about overall workforce numbers but also about geographical distribution and the swinging balance of commitment by GDPs from NHS to private care.[179] This has resulted in restricted access to NHS primary dental care in some areas of Scotland – particularly remote locations. Primary care dentistry continues to evolve from a mainly NHS service to a mixed economy, including the potential of aggregated practices, operated by the corporate sector, and dental specialist outreach into the community.[180] In all of this, it is important that dentistry remains an integral part of the development of equitable primary care services in Scotland (see also chapter 11).[181, 182] This ambition has been reflected in the Scottish Executive's policies set out in *An Action Plan for Dental Services in Scotland*,[120] building on the earlier Oral Health Strategy,[183] with additional reports on –

workforce planning,[184] information management and technology,[185] education and training of professions complementary to dentistry[186] and clinical governance.[187]

Over the period 1980 to 2000, the number of NHS clinical psychologists expanded more than any other category of primary care health professional staff, with the exception of GP practice nurses. As for other disciplines, the evidence base for clinical psychology interventions is increasing, but appears at first sight less extensive than for some others engaged in primary care.[188-191] This reflects two issues: the need for further opportunities for research and evaluation and for a greater recognition of the contribution of clinical psychologists to primary care.[192] The importance of clinical psychology services in Scotland was set as a core element of the Framework for Mental Health Services.[87, 193] This acknowledged the commitment in *Our National Health*[32] for better services in the community for people suffering from anxiety and depression, a further emphasis on positive mental health and the future potential of LHCCs for service delivery[88, 128] – see also chapter 11 for clinical psychology workforce issues.

Provision of ophthalmic services in the community has also evolved over the last 20 years with increasing numbers of visual tests being performed annually. Extended roles have been pursued including diabetic screening[194] and direct referral to ophthalmologists has been piloted when abnormalities are encountered, by-passing the traditional GP route. One recent UK survey on low vision services provision reported that the distribution was geographically uneven, uncoordinated and required to be reviewed.[195] Because of the independent contractor status of opticians and the complexities of service provision any such review of ophthalmic services in Scotland would be challenging – however desirable.

As *Building on Success* acknowledged,[124] allied health professionals (AHPs) were also seen to play a key role in delivering effective primary care. Having grown by over 100% between 1980 and 2000, a similar order of growth in their numbers of 80% over the next 20 years was predicted by the Wanless Report in 2002.[196] AHPs include a diverse range of skills and professional expertise: art, drama and music therapists, dietitians, occupational therapists, orthoptists, orthotists and prosthetists, physiotherapists, podiatrists, radiographers, and speech and language therapists. Aside from their existing roles, *Building on Success* foresaw extensive future developments including: engagement in the development and delivery of new models of care, service redesign and clinical governance based on electronic networks.[124]

Pulling Together – Teamwork, Leadership and Quality Improvement

Comprehensive analysis of all of the significant events for individual health disciplines over the last 20 years is elusive and beyond the scope of this limited account. It is clear that there are a number of generic issues facing primary care teams including: capacity, competencies, evolving roles, skill-mix, engagement in planning as well as service delivery and the clamant need for support for professional development. In all of this, successful teamworking becomes paramount – relationships are just as important as roles, and effective networks [94, 95] are as relevant as individual proficiency. Leadership is not a professional right but rather a responsibility and as such, determined by available skills, expertise and values.[2, 197] It is possible to pull this together around the shared dynamic of quality improvement both for patient care and for professional development. This nettle was firmly grasped by successive policy documents, contractual arrangements and professional aspirations at the turn of the century.[93, 110, 113, 115–119,124, 125, 146]

The RCGP Practice Accreditation scheme has been one very tangible marker of progress for effective teamworking and quality assurance in primary care, developed under the auspices of RCGP Scotland and the Clinical Standards Board for Scotland (CSBS).[198] # By mid 2003, 364 general practices (35% of the total) had successfully completed the Practice Accreditation Scheme and 45 had attained the more challenging Quality Practice Award.##

Remote and Rural Areas – Towards Sustainable Solutions

The distinctive needs of remote and rural areas of Scotland pose significant challenges for effective health care delivery. Recognition of recruitment and retention issues for primary care is particularly acute for remote areas of Scotland and deemed to be a high priority by the SEHD. This should also be aligned with a growing evidence base demonstrating differences in prognosis

---

Continued as NHS Quality Improvement Scotland – NHSQIS the successor of CSBS in 2003

Source: MacDonald C, 2003, RCGP Scotland (personal communication)

and treatment outcomes for illnesses such as common cancers in patients living in these areas.[199, 200] The Remote and Rural Areas Resource Initiative (RARARI) was established in 2000 to help to develop and evaluate new and sustainable models of care in remote areas.[93, 104] Early progress came in the form of the commissioning of work including the Solutions Group Report,[122] which advocated PMS plus contracts,[81, 82] nurse practitioners, enhanced telemedicine links, appropriate training opportunities and the development of novel recruitment and retention packages. The broader review of the medical workforce: *Future Practice* (the Temple Report),[123] was also published in 2002 and had sustainability of services as a defining purpose. Many of its recommendations had immediacy for remote and rural practice, including: acceleration and extension of managed clinical networks,[94, 95] definition of core services with outcome standards, enhanced local public engagement and strategies for staff support linked to proposed regional planning provisions. Undoubtedly a substantial part of the solution will be educational endeavour and NHSEducation (NES) will play a pivotal role.[125, 201] 'Equity' was cited earlier as one of the key values for primary care.[7, 37] Equity issues are not only about patient imperatives but are also about development opportunities for health professionals which should not be eroded by working in remote locations.[2] Ideas for improving patient services and staff morale in remote and rural areas have not been in short supply but practical and sustainable solutions have proved more elusive. The recognition of looming crisis sharpened resolve at all levels, however, and by the end of 2002, there was a growing momentum for urgent reform.

Intermediate Care – Pursuing Integrated Services

Promoted by some as a novel solution for healthcare delivery in the millennium, the basic premise of intermediate care is not new.[121, 202] It is perhaps at its most familiar in the form of care undertaken in community hospitals, which occupy an uneasy middle ground between primary and secondary sectors.[86] Community hospitals in Scotland are valued by the communities they serve and by the professionals who work in them, but yet remain curiously under-researched.[203–206] Encouraging progress has been made, however, in establishing their role in palliative care provision[207] and clinical standards have been drafted by CSBS/NHSQIS.[208] Although traditionally seen as units with a varied combination of inpatient beds, outpatient activities and investigative facilities located in rural sites, they could also be recast as ambulatory, 'bed-less' assessment units in urban settings. In the light of LHCC and managed clinical network developments,[95, 128] the potential for new variants of community hospitals – 'community resource centres' – should be appraised for one-stop delivery of locally accessible integrated care.[205, 206] Developing intermediate care models should also consider the possibility of more advanced nursing and medical procedures being undertaken in patients' homes, with novel uses of telecare.[209–211]

Rational intermediate care developments will depend on creativity, enterprise and experiment allied to robust evaluation, and they must adapt to local needs and circumstances.[86, 121] As such, they pose a number of dilemmas as well as opportunities for generalist/specialist consensus, teamworking, resource allocation, adequate facilities, skill-mix, training and accountability.

Education, Research and Development

Many issues crowd for attention, but one of the most important has been recognition of an educational continuum instead of the former false dichotomies of undergraduate/postgraduate and unidisciplinary/multidisciplinary learning. As the roles of primary care staff evolve and additional skills and competencies are required, adequate educational and training support mechanisms should develop in tandem, as articulated in a number of policy documents and reports, including *Learning Together*.[119] In order to bring this to fruition, the combined endeavours of SEHD, NES, local NHS organisations, professional and academic bodies will need to be harnessed effectively. Relevant initiatives to date include: specific training courses for practice nurses – in chronic disease management and triage of acute illnesses and injuries; for doctors – in advanced resuscitation and life support skills[104] and NES higher professional training fellowships; for all staff – the multi-centre Scottish MSc in Primary Care.[212]

Use of primary care settings for undergraduate education increased rapidly in the nineties, particularly for medical students in the wake of the GMC report: *Tomorrow's Doctors*.[213] By the end of 2002, approximately 12% of the new medical undergraduate curriculum[Σ] was being taught by academic departments of general practice and primary care, with the support of more than 40% of all

---

[Σ] In the Medical Schools of the Universities of Aberdeen, Dundee, Edinburgh and Glasgow

general practices throughout Scotland. This represented a four-fold order of increase in primary care teaching compared to previous curricula and was enabled by access to Additional Costs of Teaching (ACT) funds[ΣΣ] for the first time in the mid 1990s. During this period, academic departments of general practice and primary care throughout the UK grew in parallel with their heightened teaching commitments and both their progress and constraints were crystallised in the report: *New Century, New Challenges.*[214, 215]

The deficit of good quality research in primary care was recognised in the mid 1980s by the Chief Scientist Office (CSO), which commissioned a report in 1987: *Research into Health Care in the Community.*[216] Initial substantive progress came in the formation of the CSO Research Practice scheme in 1996 and the early development of primary care research networks throughout Scotland. This was amplified after publication of the 1997 Department of Health Report: *R&D in Primary Care* (The Mant Report),[217] and the 1998 CSO Research Strategy Report,[218] which committed to a two-fold increase in expenditure on primary care R&D over the next four years. In 1999, the report: *Shaping the Future – A Primary Care R&D Strategy for Scotland*[219] was published and advocated the formation of a Scottish School of Primary Care (SSPC). This was established in foundation form in 2000, with joint support funding from CSO, the Primary Care Directorate in SEHD and the Scottish Council for Postgraduate Medical and Dental Education (SCPMDE), with additional assistance from the Chief Nursing Officer and the Royal Pharmaceutical Society, Scottish Department. SSPC went from foundation to fully established status in 2002, and an account of its early progress is described in the CSO 2000–01 Annual Report,[220] which also confirmed a four-fold increase in annual primary care R&D spending (£4M) since 1998.[218] The compelling arguments for continued progress in the quality and quantity of primary care R&D in Scotland were recognised consistently in contemporary SEHD nursing,[165] pharmacy,[115] dental,[125, 181] clinical psychology,[193] and AHP[124] strategies.

From Information Management and Technology to eHealth

The potential for computerised records and IM&T to underpin effective, quality assured patient care has been recognised for some time.[51, 221, 222] Although encouraging progress has occurred in some areas, much more needs to be done.[131, 178, 183, 223, 224] In the past, traditional, largely paper-based record systems have been developed separately and held at each site of care provision. In the future, successful innovation of electronic records should be patient-centred, offering accessible, secure and accurate information – in the right place and at the right time. The strengths, weaknesses and future priorities for primary care IM&T in Scotland were reviewed in 2002 for GPASS,[131] the national system used at the time by ~85% of practices. A number of urgent recommendations were made for improved functionality, ownership, priority setting, training and support. These were set in the context of the challenging quality reporting of the imminent new GP Contract,[150] the future requirements of CSBS/NHSQIS, and the stark results of a comprehensive survey undertaken by Scottish Clinical Information Management in Primary Care (SCIMP) – which found that only 3% of all general practices had achieved paperless status by early 2001.[225]

A key plank of future success was seen as encouragement of effective clinical leadership at all levels, in active partnership with technical IM&T support staff and aligned to realistic levels of infrastructural and training investment. In the early 1980s attitudinal, cultural and confidentiality barriers were predicted to be the ultimate limiting factors hindering progress, not technological constraints,[221] and this continued to hold sway some 20 years later.[131, 226]

The delivery of high quality health care, supported by effective information technology – 'eHealth' was deemed essential in *Partnership for Care*,[129] with a commitment to ongoing ministerial direction and clinical leadership. To complement this, a number of initiatives were being instigated including:[178] Scottish Clinical Information (SCI) – providing relevant technical infrastructure for shared electronic records;[227] Electronic Clinical Communication Implementation (ECCI) – providing enhanced exchange of information between primary and secondary care;[228] the Scottish Telemedicine Action Forum (STAF) – exploiting transmission of voice, pictures, images and clinical data;[229] electronic transmission of prescriptions;[230] and eCare – promoting interagency data exchange,[231] as promulgated in *A Joint Future*.[33] Likely future developments include: patient held 'smart' cards, home-based telecare and 24 hour online access to health care advice – 'eNHS24'.[129,178] In parallel, electronic networks, primarily established for transmission of patient data, should also be viewed as portals and conduits of professional 'eLearning' throughout Scotland, available to all healthcare workers – irrespective of geographical location and independent of care setting.[232]

Conclusions – Looking to the Future

In any view of the future of primary care, it is important to assimilate the lessons and experience of the past 20 years. During this period the growing international evidence base has been consistent and convincing for robust primary care as the keystone of an effective and efficient health service. Successive UK and Scottish government policies over the past 20 years have recognised this in their rhetoric, but not necessarily in their subsequent reality. While an increased proportion of NHS resources has been directed towards primary care, much of this has been consumed by the costs of medicines linked to multiple illnesses and polypharmacy in an ageing population. Upwards pressure on prescribing budgets will also continue in the form of new technologies, the implementation of evidence-based guidelines and the pursuit of quality criteria embedded in new contractual arrangements.

In tandem, the primary care workforce has increased substantially and practice nurses in particular have prospered at the expense of GPs, whose numbers have grown only marginally and insufficiently – with critical shortages in some remote and rural areas. This also reflects on enhanced roles for others including nurses, pharmacists, dental assistants, clinical psychologists and AHPs. In the future new breeds of workers will join extended teams – for example, public health practitioners, nurse technicians, paramedics, GPs and others with special clinical, educational or R&D skills. This growing amalgam of additional skills enhances and does not detract from the core generalist function of primary care. This trend will also be accentuated by new contractual arrangements – and by the aspirations of a new generation of more mobile primary care workers, requiring greater career flexibility.

In the past two decades, primary care has restructured significantly, with increasing consolidation in the provision of care – for example GP collaborative working together in out-of-hours co-operatives. As part of this trend, there has been a conceptual departure from the self-sufficiency of individual practices towards more comprehensive care services being delivered by extended primary care teams working at LHCC level or beyond. With such rationalisation comes possible tensions between comprehensiveness and continuity – requiring appropriate safeguards, including robust, shared electronic patient records. As such, there will be an increasing focus on the quality of the patient journey of care, with blurring of margins between self-care, social care, primary, intermediate and secondary care – and a new emphasis on integrated care. This appears to be the aim of Community Health Partnerships as outlined in the recent White Paper, *Partnership for Care*.[129]

Drivers for improved patient care must be considered alongside support for the expanding roles of primary care team members – equipping a high morale workforce that is fit for purpose and demonstrably so. Continuing educational and R&D innovation will play a pivotal role as will more meaningful engagement of patients in service development and delivery.[233] Challenges will continue on a number of fronts, including definition, refinement and verification of criteria and outcome indicators for quality care. In all of this, the role of primary care will be crucial for maximising health improvement and minimising health inequality.

In the next 20 years or so, it is likely that the transit of primary care away from its general practice antecedents will continue apace. As this landscape evolves and ambitions grow, it will be essential that the core generalist values of primary care continue to be recognised, revisited and refreshed.

ACKNOWLEDGEMENTS

The author would like to acknowledge specifically the following individuals and organisations for their assistance in compiling this chapter: Dr Colin Hunter; Prof TS Murray; Dr MW Taylor, NHSEducation; Mr Alasdair Munro, Mr Ross Scott, Dr Hugh Whyte, Dr Hamish Wilson, and colleagues, Scottish Executive Health Department; Mr Richard Copland, Mr Alan Jamieson, and colleagues in the Information and Statistics Division, Common Services Agency; Dr W Reith and colleagues, Royal College of General Practitioners Scotland; Mrs Pat Dawson, Royal College of Nursing Scotland; Ms Alison Strath, Royal Pharmaceutical Society (Scottish Department).

REFERENCES

1. Meads G. *Future Options for General Practice*. Oxford: Radcliffe Medical Press, 1996.

2. Ritchie LD. General Practice: Beyond the Numbers Game. *Aberdeen University Review* 1994, 191: 243–259.

3. Cushing H. *The Life of Sir William Osler*. Oxford: Oxford University Press, 1925.

4. Royal College of General Practitioners. The Educational Needs of the Future General Practitioner, *Journal of the Royal College of General Practitioners* 1969, 18: 358–360.

5. Balint M. *The Doctor, His Patient and the Illness*. London: Pitman, 1957.

6. Hart JT. *A New Kind of Doctor*. London: Merlin Press, 1988.

7. Chang WC. The Meaning and Goals of Equity in Health. *Journal of Epidemiology and Community Health* 2002, 56, 488–499.

8. Starfield B. New Paradigms for Quality in Primary Care, *British Journal of General Practice* 2001, 51: 303–309.

9. McLaren G, Bain M. Deprivation and Health in Scotland. Edinburgh: Information and Statistics Division, Common Services Agency, 1998
See also: Scottish Executive Health Department, 2002, Health in Scotland 2001: Annual Report of the Chief Medical Officer, The Stationery Office, Edinburgh.[www.scotland.gov.uk/library5/health/his01–05.asp]

10. Watt GCM. The Inverse Care Law Today. *Lancet* 2002: 360, 252–254.

11. Taylor D. *Developing Primary Care: Opportunities for the 1990s*. London: King's Institute and Nuffield Provincial Hospitals Trust, 1991.

12. Howie JGR. *Patient-Centredness and the Politics of Change*. London: Nuffield Trust, 1999.

13. Vuori H. *What is Good Primary Care?* Atun R, Lang H (eds). London: Imperial College, 1996.

14. Mihill C. *Shaping Tomorrow: Issues Facing General Practice in the New Millennium*. London: British Medical Association, 2000.

15. Scottish Intercollegiate Working Party. *Acute Medical Admissions and the Future of General Medicine*. Edinburgh: Royal College of Physicians of Edinburgh, 1998.

16. Petrie JC. Levers for Change in Medicine. *Scottish Medical Journal* 2001, 46: 35–36.

17.   Departments of Health UK. *Primary Health Care – an Agenda for Discussion*. London: HMSO, 1986.

18.   Departments of Health UK. *Promoting Better Health: The Government's Programme for Improving Primary Health Care*. London: HMSO, 1987.

19.   Departments of Health UK. *Working for Patients*. London: HMSO, 1989.

20.   Scottish Home and Health Department. *General Practice in the National Health Service: a New Contract*. Edinburgh: HMSO, 1989.

21.   Scottish Home and Health Department. *Implications for Primary Health Care Services – Scottish Working Paper* I. Edinburgh: HMSO, 1989.

22.   Scottish Home and Health Department. *Funding General Practice*. Edinburgh: HMSO, 1990.

23.   Scottish Health Service Advisory Council. *The Management of Primary Health Care Services*. Edinburgh: SHHD, 1991.

24.   NHS Management Executive. *Primary Care Development Papers*:
       Paper 1: *Towards a Strategic Framework for Primary Care*. 1994.
       Paper 2: *Supporting General Practices through the Practice Staff Scheme*. 1994.
       Paper 3: *Setting and Communicating Quality of Service Standards in General Practice*. 1994.
       Paper 4: *Primary Care Strategy: The Role of GP Practice Development Plans*. 1994.
       Paper 5: *Putting Health Promotion into Primary Care Strategies*. 1994.
       Paper 6: *Nursing in General Practice*. 1995.
       Edinburgh: SHHD, 1994–1995.

25.   NHS Management Executive. *General Practice Fundholding*. Edinburgh: SHHD, 1994.

26.   Scottish Office Department of Health. *Primary Care – the Way Ahead*. Edinburgh: SHHD, 1996.

27.   Departments of Health. *Choice and Opportunity – Primary Care: the Future – Choice and Opportunity*. London: HMSO, 1996.

28.   Scottish Office Department of Health. *Annual Report of the Chief Medical Officer: 1996 – Health in Scotland*. Edinburgh: The Stationery Office, 1997.

29.   Scottish Office Department of Health. *Primary Care: Agenda for Action*. Edinburgh:. The Stationery Office, 1997.

30.   Scottish Office Department of Health. *The Scottish Health Service: Ready for the Future*. Edinburgh: The Stationery Office, 1997.

31. Scottish Office Department of Health. *Designed to Care: Renewing the National Health Service in Scotland*. Edinburgh: The Stationery Office, 1997.

32. Scottish Executive Health Department. *Our National Health: A Plan for Action, A Plan for Change*. Edinburgh: The Stationery Office, 2000. [www.show.scot.nhs.uk/sehd/onh/onh-00.htm]

33. Joint Future Group Report. *Community Care: A Joint Future*. Edinburgh: The Stationery Office, 2000. [www.scotland.gov.uk/library3/social/rjfg-00.asp] See also Joint Future Unit Website: [www.scotland.gov.uk/health/jointfutureunit/]

34. Starfield B, Shi L. Policy Relevant Determinants of Health: An International Perspective. *Health Policy* 2002, 60: 201–218.

35. Fry J, Horder J. *Primary Healthcare in an International Context*. Oxford: Nuffield Provincial Hospitals Trust, 1995.

36. Studies cited in: Haslam D. 'Schools and Hospitals' for 'Education and Health'. *British Medical Journal* 2003, 326: 234–235.

37. Shi L, Starfield B, Kennedy B, Kawachi I. Income Inequality, Primary Care and Health Indicators. *Journal of Family Practice* 1999, 48: 275–284.

38. Gulliford MC. Availability of Primary Care Doctors and Population Health in England: is there an Association? *Journal of Public Health Medicine* 2002, 24: 252–254.

39. Scottish Executive. *Public Attitudes to the NHS in Scotland*. Edinburgh: Scottish Executive, 2001. [www.scotland.gov.uk/cru/kdo1/purple/]
See also: Scottish Household Surveys. [www.scotland.gov.uk/shs/]

40. Royal College of General Practitioners (Scotland). Scottish General Practitioners Committee. *Valuing Scottish General Practice*. Edinburgh: Royal College of General Practitioners, 2000.

41. Rivett G. *From Cradle to Grave – Fifty Years of the NHS*. London: King's Fund, 1988.

42. General Medical Services Committee, BMA. Report of the New Charter Working Group. London: BMA, 1979.

43. Royal College of General Practitioners. *Towards Quality in General Practice*. London: RCGP, 1985.

44. Jarman B. Underprivileged Areas: Validation and Distribution of Risk Scores, *British Medical Journal* 1984, 289: 1587–1592. See also: Carstairs V, Morris R. *Deprivation and Health in Scotland*. Aberdeen: Aberdeen University Press, 1991.

45.   Department of Health and Social Security. *Neighbourhood Nursing: a Focus for Care*. Chair: Cumberlege J. London: HMSO, 1986.

46.   Bowling A, Stilwell B. *The Nurse in Family Practice*. London: Scutari Press, 1989.

47.   Jarman B, Cumberlege J. Developing Primary Health Care. *British Medical Journal* 1987, 294: 1005–1008.

48.   Charter for General Practice. (Editorial) *British Medical Journal* 1965, 1, 669.

49.   Scottish Home and Health Department. *Indicative Prescribing Budgets*. Edinburgh: SHHD, 1990.

50.   Scottish Home and Health Department. *Introducing Scottish Prescribing Analysis (SPA)*. Edinburgh:SHHD, 1990.

51.   Taylor MW, Ritchie LD, Taylor RJ et al. General Practice Computing in Scotland, *British Medical Journal* 1990, 300: 170–172.

52.   General Medical Services Committee. *Building Your Own Future*. London: BMA, 1991.

53.   Howie JGR, Heaney DJ, Maxwell M, Porter AM, Hopton JL, Light CJ. The Chief Scientist Reports: The Scottish General Practice Fundholding Project – Outline of an Evaluation. *Health Bulletin* 1992, 50: 316–328.

54.   Maxwell M, Heaney DJ, Howie JGR, Noble S. General Practice Fundholding: Observations on Prescribing Patterns and Costs Using the Defined Daily Dose Method. *British Medical Journal* 1993, 307: 1190–1194.

55.   Howie JGR, Heaney DJ, Maxwell M. Evaluating Care of Patients Reporting Pain in Fundholding Practices. *British Medical Journal* 1994, 309: 705–710.

56.   Howie JGR, Heaney DJ, Maxwell M. *General Practice Fundholding: Shadow Project – an Evaluation*. Edinburgh: University of Edinburgh, Department of General Practice, 1995.

57.   Howie JGR, Heaney DJ, Maxwell M. Care of Patients with Selected Health Problems in Fundholding Practices in Scotland in 1990 and 1992: Needs, Process and Outcomes, *British Journal of General Practice* 1995, 45: 121–126.

58.   Howie JGR, Heaney DJ, Maxwell. *Measuring Quality In General Practice – Pilot Study of Needs, Process and Outcome Measures*. Occasional Paper 75. London: Royal College of General Practitioners, 1997.

59.   Information and Statistics Division. *Scottish Health Statistics 1999*. Table L 1.6. Edinburgh: ISD, 2000. [www.show.scot.nhs.uk/isd]

60.   Whynes DK, Heron T, Avery AJ. Prescribing Cost Savings by GP Fundholders: Long-term or Short-term? *Health Economics* 1997, 6: 209–211.

61.   Smith RD, Wilton P. General Practice Fundholding: Progress to Date. *British Journal of General Practice* 1998, 48: 1253–1257.

62.   Glennerster H. Competition and Quality in Health Care: the UK Experience, *International Journal for Quality in Health Care* 1998, 10: 403–410.

63.   Corney RH. Changes in Patient Satisfaction and Experience in Primary and Secondary Care: the Effect of General Practice Fundholding. *British Journal of General Practice* 1999, 49: 27–30.

64.   Koperski M, Rodnick JE. Recent Developments in Primary Care in the United Kingdom: from Competition to Community-orientated Primary Care. *Journal of Family Practice 1999*, 48: 140–145.

65.   Ritchie LD, Bisset AF, Russell D, Leslie V, Thomson I. Primary and Preschool Immunisation in Grampian: Progress and the 1990 Contract. *British Medical Journal* 1992, 304: 816–819.

66.   Rudiman R, Gilbert FJ, Ritchie LD. 1995, Comparison of Uptake of Breast Screening, Cervical Screening and Childhood Immunisation, *British Medical Journal* 1995, 310: 229.

67.   Scottish Office Health Department. Hutton D. GP Out of Hours Services Working Group. Chairman: D Hutton) Edinburgh: SOHD, 1998. [www.scotland.gov.uk/library/documents-wl/gpooh-01.htm]

68.   Secretary of State for Health. *The National Health Service: A Service with ambitions.* London: HMSO, 1996.

69.   Secretary of State for Health. *Primary Care: Delivering the Future.* London: HMSO, 1996.

70.   NHS Management Executive. *Primary Care – the Way Ahead: Response to Consultation Exercise.* Edinburgh: SHHD, 1996.

71.   Royal College of General Practitioners. *The Nature of General Medical Practice.* London: RCGP, 1996.

72.   General Medical Services Committee. *Core Services: Taking the Initiative.* London: BMA, 1996.

73.   Fugelli P, Heath I. The Nature of General Practice. *British Medical Journal* 1996, 312: 456–457.

74.   Leese B, Bosanquet N. Changes in General Practice and its Effects on Service Provision in
      Areas with Different Socioeconomic Characteristics. *British Medical Journal* 1995,
      311: 546–550.

75.   NHS Management Executive Directorate of Primary Care. NHS MEL(1997)19, MEL
      (1997)49, Personal Medical Services Pilots. Edinburgh: SOHD, 1997.

76.   Scottish Executive Health Department. *Personal Medical Services Pilots*. Edinburgh: SEHD,
      2000. [www.scotland.gov.uk/library3/health/pmsp]

77.   Directorate of Primary Care Health Department. NHS MEL(1999)60. Personal Medical
      Services: Second Round. Edinburgh: SEHD, 1999.
      [http://www.show.scot.nhs.uk/sehd/mels/1999]

78.   Scottish Executive Health Department. Review by Scottish Ministers of Personal Services
      Medical Services Pilots under the Primary Care Act 1997. Edinburgh: SEHD, 2000.
      [www.scotland.gov.uk/library3/health/pmsp]

79.   Directorate of Service Policy and Planning. Personal Medical Services (PMS) Evaluation –
      University of Southampton Final Report. Edinburgh: SEHD, 2002.

80.   PMS National Evaluation Team. National Evaluation of First Wave NHS Personal
      Medical Services Pilots – Summaries of Findings from Four Research Projects. 2002.
      [http://www.doh.gov.uk/pricare/pmsfirstwaveeval02.htm]

81.   Lewis R, Gillam S. Personal Medical Services. *British Medical Journal* 2002,
      325: 1126–1127.

82.   Directorate of Services Policy and Planning. PW103703. *Personal Medical Services*.
      Edinburgh: SEHD, 2002.

83.   Departments of Health UK . *The Patient's Charter*. London: HMSO, 1991.

84.   Secretary of State for Health. *The New NHS*. London: HMSO, 1997.

85.   Scottish Office Health Department Management Executive. Ritchie LD. *Community
      Hospitals: Purpose and Potential – Discussion Paper*. Edinburgh: NHSiS, 1994.

86.   Ritchie LD. *Community Hospitals in Scotland: Promoting Progress*. Aberdeen: University of
      Aberdeen, Department of General Practice and Primary Care, 1996.

87.   Scottish Office Health Department. *Framework for Mental Health Services in Scotland*.
      Edinburgh: SOHD 1997.

88.   Woods K, McCollam A, McLean J, MacCallum E. *Delivering Integrated Mental Health Care in
      Scotland's Primary Care Trusts*. Ayr: Institute of Healthcare Management, 2001.

89. General Practitioners Committee of the BMA. Annual Report. London: BMA, 1999.

90. Royal College of General Practitioners Scottish Council. *Promoting Good Practice: Responding to Clinical Governance.* Chairman: CM Hunter. Edinburgh: RCGP, 1998.

91. Royal College of General Practitioners Scottish Council. *Practical Guidance on the Implementation of Clinical Governance in Primary Care in Scotland.* Chairman: CM Hunter. Edinburgh: RCGP, 1999.

92. Hunter CM, Campbell M. Personal Communication, 2002. SPICE–PC: the Scottish Programme for Improving Clinical Effectiveness in Primary Care.
Note: SPICE-PC is overseen by the Clinical Effectiveness Steering Group (CEPSTEG). [www.ceppc.org/spice]

93. Scottish Office Department of Health. *Acute Services Review.* Chairman: DC Carter. Edinburgh: The Stationery Office, 1998.

94. Scottish Office Department of Health. NHS MEL(1999)10, *Introduction of Managed Clinical Networks within the NHS in Scotland.* Edinburgh: SOHD, 1999.

95. Scottish Executive Health Department. NHS HDL (2002) 69. *Promoting the Development of Managed Clinical Networks in Scotland.* Edinburgh: SEHD 2002.

96. Campbell NC, Thain J, Deans HG, Ritchie LD, Rawles JM. Secondary Prevention in Coronary Heart Disease: Baseline Survey of Provision in General Practice. *British Medical Journal* 1998, 316: 1430–1433.

97. Campbell NC, Grimshaw JM, Ritchie LD, Rawles JM. Cardiac Rehabilitation in Scotland: is Current Provision Satisfactory? *Journal of Public Health Medicine* 1996, 30: 478–480.

98. Scottish Office Department of Health. NHS MEL (1998) 34. *Promoting Thrombolysis in Scotland.* Edinburgh: SODoH, 1998.

99. Rawles J, Ritchie LD. Thrombolysis in Peripheral Practices in Scotland: Another Rule of Halves. *Health Bulletin* 1999, 57: 9–15.

100. Rawles J, Sinclair C, Jennings K, Ritchie LD, Waugh N. 1998, Call to Needle Times after Acute Myocardial Infarction in Urban and Rural Areas of Scotland: an Observational Study. *British Medical Journal* 1998, 317: 576–578.

101. Scottish Executive Health Department, NHS Scotland. *Coronary Heart Disease/Stroke Task Force Report.* Chairman: AR Lorimer. Edinburgh: The Stationery Office, 2001.

102. Report of the Dumfries and Galloway Cardiac Services Managed Clinical Network Project, 2002. Lead Clinician: C Baker. [www.show.scot.nhs.uk/mcn]

103. Scottish Executive Health Department, NHS Scotland. *Coronary Heart Disease and Stroke Strategy for Scotland*. Chairman: N Boon. Edinburgh: The Stationery Office, 2002. [www.scotland.gov.uk/library5/health/chds]

104. Remote and Rural Areas Resource Initiative (RARARI).*About RARARI- Progress Report*. Fort William: RARARI, 2000. [http//:www.rarari.org.uk]

105. Scottish Office Department of Health. *Towards a Healthier Scotland*. Edinburgh: The Stationery Office, 1999.

106. Scottish Office Department of Health. *Working Together for a Healthier Scotland*. Edinburgh: The Stationery Office, 1998.

107. Scottish Needs Assessment Programme. *Needs Assessment In Primary Care: a Rough Guide*. Chairman: J Cavanagh. SNAP, Edinburgh: SNAP, 1998.

108. Gillam S, Murray S. *Needs Assessment in General Practice*. Occasional Paper. London: RCGP, 1996.

109. Hopton JL, Dlugolecka M. Need and Demand for Primary Healthcare: a Comparative Survey Approach. *British Medical Journal* 1995, 310: 1369–1373.

110. Scottish Executive Health Department. *Review of the Public Health Function in Scotland*. Chairman: DC Carter. CSEHD, Edinburgh: CSEHD, 1999. [www.scotland.gov.uk/library2/doc09/rphf]

111. Scottish Executive Health Department. *Fair Shares for All – the Report of the National Review of Resource Allocation for the NHS in Scotland*. (Arbuthnott Report) Edinburgh: The Stationery Office, 1999.

112. Scottish Executive Health Department. *Fair Shares for All – Final Report*. Edinburgh: The Stationery Office, 2000.

113. Scottish Executive Health Department. Report from the Primary Care Modernisation Group. *Making the Connections, Developing Best Practice into Common Practice*. Chairman: F McKenzie. Edinburgh: The Stationery Office, 2002. [www.show.scot.nhs.uk/sehd/publications/mcbp-01.htm]

114. Scottish Executive Health Department. *Nurse Prescribing – Extension of Nurse Prescribing in NHSScotland. A Guide for Implementation*. NHS HDL(2002)56, SEHD, Edinburgh: SEHD, 2002.[www.show.scot.nhs/sehd/mels/HDL2002_56.pdf] See also: [www.show.scot.nhs.uk/sehd/nurseprescribing/progress.htm]

115. Scottish Executive Health Department. *The Right Medicine: A Strategy for Pharmaceutical Care in Scotland*. Edinburgh: The Stationery Office, 2002.

116. Public Health Institute for Scotland. *Pharmacy for Health: The Way Forward for Pharmaceutical Public Health in Scotland*. Glasgow: PHIS, 2003.

117. Scottish Executive Health Department. *Nursing for Health: A Review of the Contribution of Nurses, Midwives and Health Visitors to Improving the Public's Health in Scotland*. Chairman: A Jarvie. Edinburgh: The Stationery Office, 2001.

118. Scottish Executive Health Department. *Caring for Scotland: The Strategy for Nursing and Midwifery in Scotland*. Edinburgh: The Stationery Office, 2002.

119. Scottish Executive Health Department. *Learning Together – A Strategy for Education, Training and Lifelong Learning for All Staff in the NHS*. Edinburgh: The Stationery Office, 1999.

120. Scottish Executive Health Department. *An Action Plan for Dental Services in Scotland*. Edinburgh: SEHD, 2000. [www.scotland.gov.uk/library3/health/apds]

121. Hunter CM, Ritchie LD. *Intermediate Care: A Discussion Paper*. Edinburgh: RCGP Scotland, 2001.

122. Remote and Rural Areas Resource Initiative. *Solutions for the Provision of Health Care in Remote and Rural Areas*. Chairman: D Murray. Fort William: RARARI, 2002. [www.rarari.org.uk]

123. Scottish Executive Health Department. *Future Practice: A Review of the Scottish Medical Workforce*. (Temple Report) The Stationery Office, Edinburgh: The Stationery Office, 2002. (plus Response of the Scottish Executive, July 2002).

124. Scottish Executive Health Department. *Building on Success: Future Directions for the Allied Health Professions in Scotland*. Edinburgh: The Stationery Office, 2002.

125. NHS Education for Scotland. *Education and Training for the Dental Team in Remote and Rural Regions of Scotland*: Report of a Working Group. Chairman: JS Rennie. Edinburgh: NES, 2003.

126. Scottish Executive Health Department. *Towards a Safer Healthier Workplace* – Occupational Health and Safety Services for the Staff of the NHS in Scotland. Edinburgh: The Stationery Office, 1999.

127. NHS24. *Vision for NHS24*. [www.nhs24.com]. (Initial roll-out began in Grampian in May 2002, Greater Glasgow in November 2002, with planned cover of whole of Scotland by end 2004).

128. Scottish Executive Health Department. *LHCC Development: the Next Steps*. Edinburgh: SEHD, 2001. [www.show.scot.nhs.uk/lhcc]

129. Scottish Executive Health Department. *NHS Scotland, 2003, Partnership for Care.* Edinburgh: The Stationery Office, 2003.
[www.show.scot.nhs.uk/sehd.publications/PartnershipforCare.hwp.pdf]

130. See: [www.show.scot.nhs.uk/isd/heart_disease/cmr/handbook/].

131. Information and Statistics Division. *Primary Care IM&T in Scotland: Promoting Progress, Securing Success.* Report of the GPASS Review Group. Chairman: LDRitchie.Edinburgh: ISD, 2002. [www.show.scot.nhs.uk/gpasslg/GPASSReview]

132. Milne RM, Taylor MW, Taylor RJ. Audit of Populations in General Practice: the Creation of a National Resource for the Study of Morbidity in General Practice, *Journal of Epidemiology and Community Health* 1998, 52: Suppl 1, 20S–24S.

133. Aylin P, Majeed FA, Cook DG. Home Visiting by General Practitioners in England and Wales. *British Medical Journal* 1996, 313: 207–210.

134. Salisbury C, Trivella M, Bruster S. Demand for Out of Hours Care from General Practitioners in England and Scotland: Observational Study Based on Routinely Recorded Data. *British Medical Journal* 2000, 320: 618–621.

135. McKinley RK, Stevenson K, Adams S, Manku-Scott TK. Meeting Patient Expectations of Care: the Major Determinant of Satisfaction with Out-of-Hours Medical Care? *Family Practice* 2002, 19: 333–338.

136. Shipman C, Payne F, Hooper R, Dale J. Patients Satisfaction with Out-of–Hours Services: How do GP cooperatives compare with deputizing and practice based arrangements? *Journal of Public Health Medicine* 2000, 22: 149–154.

137. Scott A, Watson MS, Ross S. Eliciting Preferences of the Community for Out of Hours Care Provided by General Practitioners: a Stated Preference Discrete Choice Experiment. *Social Science and Medicine* 2003, 56: 803–814.

138. Wilson A, Pearson D, Hassey A. Barriers to Developing the Nurse Practitioner Role in Primary Care – the GP Perspective. *Family Practice* 2002, 19: 641–6.

139. Richards DA, Meakins J, Tawfik J, Godfrey L, Duttin E, Richardson G, Russell D. Nurse Telephone Triage for Same Day Appointments in General Practice: Multiple Interrupted Time Series Trial of Effect on Workload and Costs. *British Medical Journal* 2002, 325: 1214–1217.

140. Jones K, Gilbert P, Little J, Wilkinson K. Nurse Triage for House Call Requests in a Tyneside General Practice: Patient's Views and Effect on Doctor Workload. *British Journal of General Practice* 1998, 48: 1303–1306.

141. Scottish Executive Health Department. *Adding Life to Years: Report of the Expert Group on HealthCare of Older People.* Chairman: EM Armstrong. Edinburgh: The Stationery Office, 2002.. [www.show.scot.nhs.uk/sehd/publications/alty]

142. Scottish General Practitioners Committee. *The Reality Behind the Rhetoric: A Survey of the Views of GPs in Scotland on Morale, Service Provision and Priorities for Improving Primary Care.* Chairman: K Harden. Edinburgh: BMA Scotland, 2001.

143. Sibbald, B, Bojke C, Gravelle H. National Survey of Job Satisfaction and Retirement Intentions among General Practitioners in England. *British Medical Journal* 2003, 326: 22–24.

144. Jewell D. Are We Downhearted? (Editorial) *British Journal of General Practice* 2003, 53: 92–93.

145. Lambert TW, Evans J, Goldacre MJ. Recruitment of UK-trained Doctors into General Practice: Findings from National Cohort Studies, *British Journal of General Practice* 2002, 52: 364–372.

146. Scottish Executive Health Department and Department of Health. *Unfinished Business – Proposals for Reform of the Senior House Officer Grade.* Chairman: L Donaldson. Edinburgh: The Stationery Office, 2002.

147. General Medical Council. *Good Medical Practice.* London: GMC, 2001.

148. General Practitioners Committee of the British Medical Association, Royal College of General Practitioners. *Good Medical Practice for General Practitioners.* London: RCGP, 2002.

149. Scottish Executive Health Department. *Report of The Short Life Working Group on Identifying and Preventing Under Performance Amongst General Medical Practitioners.* Chairman: H Whyte. Edinburgh: SEHD, 2001. [www.scotland.gov.uk/library3/health/pbtc-00.asp]

150. General Practitioners Committee and the NHS Confederation. *Investing in General Practice: New GMS Contract 2003.* London: BMA, 2003.
See also: General Practitioners Committee. *Your Contract, Your Future.* London: BMA, 2002. [www.bma.org.uk/]

151. Scottish General Practitioners Committee. *Annual Report 2002.* London: BMA, 2002. [www.bma.org.uk/ap.nsf/Content/sgpc+ann+rep+02]

152. Lattimer V, George S, Thompson F, Thomas E, Mullee M, Turnbull J, Smith H, Moore M, Bond H, Glasper A. Safety and Effectiveness of Nurse Telephone Consultation in Out of Hours Primary Care: Randomised Controlled Trial. *British Medical Journal* 1998, 317: 1054–1059.

153. Vrijhoef H, Diediriks C, Spreeuwenberg C. The Nurse Specialist as Main Care-Provider for Patients with Type 2 Diabetes in A Primary Care setting: Effects on Patient Outcomes. *International Journal of Nursing Studies* 2002, 39: 441–451.

154. Renders DM, Valk GD, Griffin SJ, Wagner EH, Eijk Van JT, Assendelft WJ. Interventions to Improve the Management of Diabetes in Primary Care Outpatient and Community Settings: A Systematic Review. *Diabetes Care* 2001, 24: 1821–1833.

155. Kation W, Von Korff M, Line E, Simon G. Rethinking Practitioner Roles in Chronic Illness: the Specialist, Primary Care Physician and the Practice Nurse. *General Hospital Psychiatry* 2001, 23: 138–144.

156. Gilbody S, Whitty P. Improving the Recognition and Management of Depression in Primary Care. *Effective Health Care* 2002, 7: 1–11.

157. Blue L, Lang E, McMurray JJ, Davie JP, McDonagh TA, Murdoch DR *et al*. Randomised Controlled Trial of Specialist Nurse Intervention in Heart Failure. *British Medical Journal* 2001, 323: 715–718.

158. Campbell NC, Ritchie LD, Thains J, Deans HG, Rawles JM, Squair JL. Secondary Prevention in Coronary Heart Disease: a Randomised Trial of Nurse Led Clinics in Primary Care. *Heart* 1998, 80: 447–482.

159. Murchie P, Campbell N, Ritchie LD, Simpson JA, Thain A. Secondary Prevention Clinics for Coronary Heart Disease: Four Year Follow-up of a Randomised Controlled Trial. *British Medical Journal* 2003, 326: 84–86.

160. Brooks N, Otway C, Rashid C, Kilty E, Maggs C. The Patient's View: the Benefits and Limitations of Nurse Prescribing. *British Journal of Community Nursing* 2001, 6: 342–348.

161. Rodden C. Nurse Prescribing: Views on Autonomy and Independence. *British Journal of Community Nursing* 2001, 6: 350–355.

162. Venning P, Durie A, Roland M, Roberts C, Leese B. Randomised Controlled Trial Comparing Cost Effectiveness of General Practitioners and Nurse Practitioners in Primary Care Settings. *British Medical Journal* 2000, 320: 1048–1053.

163. Scottish Executive Health Department. *A Framework for Maternity Service in Scotland*. Edinburgh: The Stationery Office, 2001.

164. Scottish Executive Health Department. *Implementing a Framework for Maternity Services in Scotland*. Edinburgh: SEHD, 2002. [www.scotland.gov.uk/library5/health/ifms]

165. Scottish Executive Health Department. *Choices and Challenges: The Strategy for Research and Development in Nursing and Midwifery in Scotland*. Edinburgh: The Stationery Office, 2002. [www.scotland.gov.uk/library5/health/cac]

166. Carter BL, Helling DK. Ambulatory Care Pharmacy Services: Has the Agenda Changed? *Annals of Pharmacotherapy* 2000, 34: 772–787.

167. Needham DS, Wong IC, Campion PD. Evaluation of the Effectiveness of UK Community Pharmacists' Interventions in Community Palliative Care. *Palliative Medicine* 2002, 16: 219–225.

168. Anderson C. Health Promotion in Community Pharmacy: the UK Situation. *Patient Education and Counseling* 2000, 39: 285–291.

169. Sinclair HK, Bond CM, Lennox AS, Silcock J, Winfield AJ. Knowledge of and Attitudes to Smoking Cessation: the Effect of Stage of Change Training for Community Pharmacy Staff. *Health Bulletin* 1998, 56: 526–539.

170. Geber J, Parra D, Beckey NP, Korman L. Optimising Drug Therapy in Patients with Cardiovascular Disease: the Impact of Pharmacist Managed Pharmacotherapy Clinics in a Primary Care Setting. *Pharmacotherapy* 2002, 22: 738–747.

171. Finley PR, Rens HR, Pont JT, Gess SL, Louie C, Bull SA, Bero LA. Impact of a Collaborative Pharmacy Practice Model on the Treatment of Depression in Primary Care. *American Journal of Health-Systems Pharmacy* 2002, 59: 1518–1526.

172. Chen J, Britten N. 'Strong Medicine': an Analysis of Pharmacist Consultations in Primary Care. *Family Practice* 2000, 17: 480–483.

173. Matheson C, Bond CM, Pitcairn J Community Pharmacy Services for Drug Misusers in Scotland: What Difference does Five Years Make? *Addiction* 2002, 97: 1405–1412.

174. Layton D, Sinclair HK, Bond CM, Hannaford PC, Shakir SA. Pharmacovigilance of Over-the-Counter Products based in Community Pharmacy: Methodological Issues from Pilot Work Conducted in Hampshire and Grampian. *Pharmacoepidemiology and Drug Safety* 2002, 11: 503–513.

175. Rutter PR, Hunt AJ, Jones IF. Exploring the Gap: Community Pharmacists' Perceptions of their Current Role Compared with their Aspirations. *International Journal of Pharmacy Practice* 2000, 8: 204–208.

176. Edmunds J, Calnan MW. The Reprofessionalisation of Community Pharmacy? An Exploration of Attitudes to Extended Roles for Community Pharmacists amongst Pharmacists and General Practitioners in the United Kingdom. *Social Science and Medicine* 2001, 53: 943–955.

177. Scottish Executive Health Department Primary Care Unit. 2002. NHS Circular: PCA (P) (2002)1, Phase 2 of Scheme to Support the Creation of Areas in Community Pharmacies for the Provision of Personal Advice.

178.   NHSScotland. *National Strategic Programme for Information Management and Technology*. Edinburgh: SEHD, 2002. [www.show.scot.nhs.uk/imt/Nationalstrat.htm]

179.   Russell EM, Leggate M, Hamilton R. Dentists in General and Community Practice: a Scottish Survey. *British Dental Journal* 2002, 193: 333–337.

180.   Mason D. General Dental Practice – Challenges and Opportunities: A Personal View. *British Dental Journal* 1995, 179: 350–354.

181.   Burke FJ, Pendlebury ME. 2001, Academics for Dental Primary Care. *British Dental Journal* 2001, 191: 64–65.

182.   Haughney MG, Devennie JC, MacPherson LM, Mason DK. Integration of Primary Care Dental and Medical Services: A Three Year Study. *British Dental Journal* 1998, 185: 343–347.

183.   Scottish Office Health Department. *Oral Health Strategy for Scotland*. Edinburgh: The Stationery Office, 1995 . [www.scotland.gov.uk/library/documents/oral01.htm]

184.   Scottish Executive Health Department. *Workforce Planning for Dentistry in Scotland: A Strategic Review: Interim Report*. Edinburgh: SEHD, 2000. [www.scotland.gov.uk/library3/health/sacd-00.asp]

185.   Scottish Executive Health Department. *Dentistry in the New Millennium: An Information and Technology Strategy for Dentistry in Scotland*. Edinburgh: SEHD, 2001. [www.scotland.gov.uk/library3/misc/dinm-00.asp]

186.   Scottish Executive Health Department. *Dentistry in the New Millennium: Education and Training of the Professionals Complementary to Dentistry in Scotland*. Edinburgh: SEHD, 2002. [www.scotland.gov.uk/library5/health/dinm-00.asp]

187.   Scottish Executive Health Department. *National Dental Advisory Committee: Clinical Governance in Dental Primary Care*. Edinburgh: SEHD, 2001. [www.scotland.gov.uk/library3/misc/cgpc-00.asp]

188.   Tata P, Eagle A, Green J. Does Providing More Accessible Primary Care Psychology Services Lower the Clinical Threshold for Referrals? *British Journal of General Practice* 1996, 46: 469–472.

189.   Huey DA, Britton PG. A Portrait of Clinical Psychology. *Journal of Interprofessional Care* 2002, 16: 69–78.

190.   Wood JM, Garb HN, Lilienfield SO, Nezworski MT. Clinical Assessment. *Annual Review of Psychology* 2002, 53: 519–543.

191. Simpson S. The Provision of a Telepsychology Service to Shetland: Client and Therapist Satisfaction and the Ability to Develop a Therapeutic Alliance. *Journal of Telemedicine and Telecare* 2001, 7, Suppl 1: 34–36.

192. Department of Health. *Treatment Choice in Psychological Therapies and Counselling: an Evidence Based Clinical Practice Guideline.* London: DOH, 2001. [www.doh.gov.uk/mentalhealth/treatmentguidelines/treatment.pdf]

193. Scottish Executive Health Department Community Care Division. NHS HDL(2001)75. Edinburgh: SEHD, 2001. [www.show.scot.nhs.uk/sehd/mels/HDL2001_75.htm]

194. Hammond CJ, Shackleton J, Flanagan DW, Herrtage J, Wade J. Comparison Between an Ophthalmic Optician and an Ophthalmologist in Screening for Diabetic Retinopathy. *Eye* 1996, 10: 107–112.

195. Culham LE, Ryan B, Jackson AJ, Hill AR, Jones B, Miles C, Young JA, Bruce C, Bird AC. Low Vision Services for Visual Rehabilitation in the United Kingdom. *British Journal of Ophthalmology* 2002, 86: 743–747.

196. HM Treasury. *Securing Our Future Health: Taking a Long Term View.* Final Report. (The Wanless Report) London: HM Treasury, 2002. [www.hm-treasury.gov.uk/consultations_and_legislation/wanless/

197. Pendleton D, King J. Values and Leadership. *British Medical Journal* 2002, 325: 1352–1355.

198. Clinical Standards Board for Scotland and RCGP Scotland. *Quality Assurance in Primary Care: RCGP Practice Accreditation Progress Report.* Edinburgh: CSBS, 2002. [see also: www.ceppc.org/spice].

199. Campbell NC, Elliott AM, Sharp L, Ritchie LD, Cassidy J, Little J. Rural and Urban Differences in Stage at Diagnosis of Colorectal and Lung Cancer. *British Journal of Cancer* 2001, 84: 910–914.

200. Campbell NC, Elliott AM, Sharp L, Ritchie LD, Cassidy J, Little J. Impact of Deprivation and Rural Residence on Treatment of Colorectal and Lung Cancer. *British Journal of Cancer* 2002, 87: 585–590.

201. Scottish Council for Postgraduate Medical and Dental Education. *Seeking Solutions: Education and Training for Remote and Rural Health Professionals.* Report of a Multidisciplinary Conference. Edinburgh: SCPMDE, 2000.

202. Steiner A. *Intermediate Care: a Conceptual Framework and Review of the Literature.* London: King's Fund, 1997.

203. Grant JA. Community Hospitals: *A Study in Resource Use, Decision Making and Patient Outcome.* MD Thesis. Glasgow: University of Glasgow, 2002.

204. Royal College of General Practitioners and Associations of General Practitioner
      Community Hospitals. *Community Hospitals – Preparing for the Future*. Chairman: ND Jarvie.
      Occasional Paper 43. London: RCGP, 1990.

205. Ritchie LD, Robinson K. Community Hospitals: New Wine in Old Bottles? *British Journal
      of General Practice* 1998, 48: 1039–1040.

206. Scottish Association of Community Hospitals (SACH). *Intermediate and Integrated Care*.
      Report of Conference 2001.Chairman: HD Greig. Brechin: SACH, 2002.

207. Centre for Health and Social Research (CHSR). Commissioned by the Scottish
      Association of Community Hospitals. *The Provision of Palliative Care in Community Hospitals in
      Scotland*. Edinburgh: CHSR, 2002.

208. Clinical Standards Board for Scotland. *Community Hospitals – Draft Clinical Standards*.
      Chairman: A Short. Edinburgh: CSBS, 2002.

209. Jester R, Hicks C. Using Cost-Effectiveness Analysis to Compare Hospital at Home and
      Inpatient Interventions, Parts 1 and 2. *Journal of Clinical Nursing* 2003, 12: 13–27.

210. Wilson A, Wynn A, Parker H. Patient and Carer Satisfaction with 'Hospital at Home':
      Quantitative and Qualitative Results from a Randomised Controlled Trial. *British Journal of
      General Practice* 2003, 52: 9–13.

211. Shepperd S, Iliffe S. Hospital at Home Versus Inpatient Hospital Care. *Cochrane Database of
      Systematic Reviews* 2001, 3: CD000356.

212. Scottish MSc in Primary Care: See Scottish School of Primary Care Website:
      [www.sspc.uk.com]

213. General Medical Council. *Tomorrow's Doctors*. London: GMC, 1993. (under revision
      2002–2003)

214. Society for Academic Primary Care (SAPC). *New Century, New Challenges: A Report from the
      Heads of Departments of General Practice and Primary Care in the Medical Schools of the United
      Kingdom*. Chairman: C Dowrick. London: SAPC, 2002.

215. Morrison J, Watt G. New Century, New Challenges for Community Based Medical
      Education. *Medical Education* 2003, 37: 2–3.

216. Chief Scientist Office, Scottish Home and Health Department. *Report of the Working Group
      on Research into Health Care in the Community*. Chairman: JGR Howie. Edinburgh: SHHD,
      1987.

217. Department of Health. *R & D in Primary Care*. Chairman: D Mant. London: DOH, 1997.

218. Chief Scientist Office, Scottish Office Department of Health. *Research Strategy for the National Health Service in Scotland*. Edinburgh: SODOH, 1998. [www.show.scot.nhs.uk/cso/publications/Research.Strategy.doc]

219. Scottish Forum for Academic General Practice. *Shaping the Future: A Primary Care Research and Development Strategy for Scotland*. Edinburgh: RCGP Scotland, 1999.

220. Chief Scientist Office, Scottish Executive Health Department. *Annual Report 2000–01*.Edinburgh: SEHD, 2001. [www.show.scot.nhs.uk/cso/publications/] See also SSPC Website for updates on progress: [www.sspc.uk.com]

221. Ritchie LD. Computers in General Practice: A Review of the Current Situation. *Health Bulletin* 1982, 40: 248–254.

222. Ritchie LD. *Computers in Primary Care*. London: Heinemann Medical, 1986.

223. Mitchell M, Sullivan FM. A Descriptive Feast but an Evaluative Famine: Systematic Review of Published Articles on Primary Care Computing during 1980–97. *British Medical Journal* 2001, 322: 279–282.

224. Majeed A. Ten Ways to Improve Information Technology in the NHS. *British Medical Journal* 2003, 326: 2002–206.

225. Morris L, Campbell M, MacDonald C. *SCIMP Survey of Computer Use in General Practice*. Edinburgh: RCGP Scotland, 2002. [www.ceppc.org/scimp].

226. Confidentiality and Security Advisory Group for Scotland. *Protecting Patient Confidentiality: FinalReport*.Edinburgh: SEHD, 2003. [www.show.scot.nhs.uk/sehd/publications/ppcr/ppcr-00.htm]

227. See Websites: [www.show.scot.nhs.uk/sci]; [www.diabetes.scot.nhs.uk]

228. See Website: [www.show.scot.nhs.uk/ecci]

229. See Website: [www.show.scot.nhs.uk/telemedicine]

230. See Website: [www.show.scot.nhs.uk/imt/programmes/programme5.htm]

231. See Website: [www.show.scot.nhs.uk/ecare]

232. See Website: [www.elib.scot.nhs/uk]

233. Scottish Executive Health Department. *Patient Focus and Public Involvement*. Edinburgh: SEHD, 2001.

9. Scotland's Acute Hospital Services

David Carter

Acute hospital services are a vital component in the provision of healthcare and an area of continuing major change. This chapter examines trends in the delivery of acute care in Scotland over the past 20 years. It focuses particularly on events since the publication of *Designed to Care – Renewing the National Health Service in Scotland*[1] in 1997 and the Acute Services Review in 1998.[2]

The historically higher level of funding of health care in Scotland than the rest of the United Kingdom (see chapter 1) has sustained a larger acute hospital sector. This means that whatever indicator of supply is used, Scotland has greater provision than its UK counterparts. Using 1995–96 data as an example, standardised mortality rates in Scotland are generally higher than elsewhere in the UK while life expectancy is lower and NHS expenditure is greater (Table 9.1).[3] Scotland possesses more inpatient beds per head than other parts of the UK, has a greater number of hospital doctors per head and has proportionately fewer people on waiting lists for inpatient or day case care.

Nonetheless, the pressures on acute hospital services have been and remain intense. Changing levels of demand, technological advances, and growing expectations have raised questions about the adequacy of service models developed from the 1960s and 1970s, an era which encouraged a substantial investment in Scotland's district general hospitals over the following decades.

TABLE 9.1 Indicators of health need set against basic indicators of service provision in England, Scotland, Wales and Northern Ireland in 1995–96 (Dixon et al 1999)

	England	Scotland	Wales	N. Ireland
Standardised mortality ratio				
Male	97	118	103	109
Female	98	119	101	106
Life expectancy (years)				
Male	74	71.9	73.6	72.7
Female	79.3	77.4	78.4	78.3
Total NHS expenditure[*]	683 (73%)	855 (70%)	803 (62%)	717 (64%)
Hospital beds/1000 population	4.3	8.0	5.5	6.1
Hospital doctors/1000 population	0.9	1.2	1.0	1.1

[*]Refers to expenditure per capita. Figures in parentheses show percentage of NHS expenditure devoted to hospital and community health services.

In 2000, the total net expenditure on the NHS in Scotland was £5.244M,[4] roughly four times greater than expenditure in 1981. Of this, some £3.436M was spent as revenue and £0.91M as capital on hospital and community health services; 85% of this money was expended on hospital services. These figures do not include expenditure on central health services (such as the Common Services Agency), the Scottish Ambulance Service, Scottish Council for Postgraduate Medical and Dental Education, State Hospital and Clinical Standards Board for Scotland, among others (Table 9.2).

TABLE 9.2 Net costs of the NHS in Scotland: a comparison between expenditure in 1981 and 2000. Data from Scottish Health Statistics 2000; expenditure shown in £'000s and years refer to year ending 31 March).

	1981	2000
Health board administration	48 883	44 132
Hospital / community health services		
Revenue	910 303	3 436 144
Capital	61 888	91 205
Family practitioner services	227 036	1 214 392
Central health services	43 252	165 212
Scottish Ambulance Service		92 496
Scottish Council for Postgraduate Medical and Dental Education		131 819
State Hospital	4 867	19 736
Other costs	18 953	48 557
Central Government administration	5 238	12 322
Total Cost	**1 329 420**	**5 256 755**

Acute hospitals, beds and activity trends

The changes in the health system in Scotland over the past 20 years are described in detail in chapter 1. Major policy shifts in the past 20 years have resulted in profound changes in the organisation of acute services, culminating in the most recent policy document published in 2000, *Our National Health. A plan for action, a plan for change.*[5]

Acute Hospitals

The past 20 years have seen a great reduction in the number of hospitals dispensing acute services in Scotland. Taking Edinburgh as an example, acute medical and surgical care has been withdrawn progressively from smaller urban hospitals (such as the Bruntsfield, Deaconess, Leith, Northern General, Eastern

General, City and Princess Margaret Rose Hospitals) and concentrated in the Royal Infirmary and the Western General Hospital. This rationalisation of the NHS Estate has been driven by multiple and inter-related factors including costs of upkeep and modernisation, need for new building, sustainability of services, need to centralise high-technology expensive specialist services, provision of emergency services and manpower considerations (not least of which is the need to sustain rotas in the face of increasing pressure posed by the European Working Time Directive).

As shown in Table 9.2, capital spending in respect of hospital and community services in Scotland has remained low. In 1981, it represented 6.8% of the total expenditure on these services; since 1996 the figure has declined from 6.9% to a low of 2.5% and 2.7% in 1999 and 2000 respectively. Of course these data do not reflect the costs of the current NHS Hospital Building Programme with its six new facilities and significant extensions to Glasgow Royal Infirmary and the Western General Hospital, Edinburgh (Table 9.3). The total estimated cost of this programme is £485M of which £357 has been raised through the Private Finance Initiative (PFI), £106M from public funds and £22M from capital receipts.

TABLE 9.3 NHS Scotland Hospital Building Programme (SOURCE Health in Scotland 2000, Report of the Chief Medical Officer, Stationery Office).

Project	Value	Planned opening date
New Royal Infirmary, Edinburgh	£180M (PFI)	Spring 2002 – 03
Wishaw General Hospital	£100M (PFI)	June 2001
Hairmyres Hospital	£68M (PFI)	April 2001
East Ayrshire Community Hospital	£9M (PFI)	August 2000
Glasgow Royal Infirmary (extension)	£52M (publicly funded)	Late 2001
Western General Hospital, Edinburgh (extension)	£47M (publicly funded)	September 2001
Southern Isles Community Hospital	£7M (publicly funded)	April 2001
Aberdeen Childrens Hospital	£22M (publicly funded)	2003

The extent and possible extension of private involvement in the NHS remains controversial. The proportion of total health spend that is private has been about 15% in the UK, low by comparison with a European average of around 24%.[6] PFI is a mechanism by which the private sector builds and maintains NHS hospitals and runs ancillary services. The economic case against PFI has been strongly articulated with particular reference to the anxiety that the high costs of capital could translate into adverse effects on service provision, bed capacity and workforce.[7-10] The initiative has also been consistently opposed by the British Medical Association (BMA) which regards it as an unaffordable long-term strategy for increasing capital investment in the NHS. That said, the BMA has been willing to consider alternative means of extending private involvement in the NHS and the possibilities offered by Public Private Partnerships (PPPs).[11] The stated aims of PPPs are to modernise the NHS, improve patient care, and increase the quality and efficiency of services through exploring new ways of working. The NHS already has a working relationship with the private sector. The majority of GPs, for example, work as independent contractors, many hospital consultants work in the private sector, and ancillary services are often provided privately. Future partnerships could include diagnostic and treatment centres, dedicated elective surgery units, management of NHS Trusts and the provision of capacity and expertise for intermediate care.

In Scotland, the private sector has generally had even less involvement with the NHS than in England. Significantly, one of the largest private facilities offering an extensive range of surgical care, the HCI Hospital at Clydebank, has just been acquired in 2002 by the NHS in Scotland at a cost of £37.5M from the Abu Dhabi Investment Company. This hospital is being developed as a national waiting times centre for patients requiring complex cardiac surgery, major orthopaedic operations, plastic surgery and cardiac investigations such as coronary angiography. The centre will not simply serve the population of Glasgow; it is available for use by the NHS throughout Scotland and may well continue to offer services to other parts of the United Kingdom on an appropriate contractual basis.

Beds

In keeping with the general trend throughout the UK, the number of available staffed beds of every type in Scottish hospitals has shown a progressive decline since 1980/81, falling from 59 571 to 34 696 in 1999/2000.[4] The number of acute hospital beds fell from 19 537 to 14 692 over the same period. Within this total the decline in number of acute surgical beds has been sharper and more sustained (from 10 817 to 6471) than that of acute medical beds (7662 to 6870). Indeed in the past few years the number of acute medical beds has risen slightly from a nadir of 6018 beds in 1996/97. Inpatient throughput (average number of cases per bed) has risen from 39.2 in 1990/91 to 52.6 in 1999/00, while mean stay per inpatient episode in acute specialties has fallen from 22.9 days in 1980/81 to 5.3 days in 1999/00. These trends reflect continuing improvements in medical, surgical and anaesthetic care, with increased use of minimally invasive surgery, interventional radiology, interventional endoscopy, and day patient care.

Whereas the number of acute medical and surgical beds in Scotland fell by only 2.2% between 1999 and 2000, the decrease in non-acute specialties has been much more marked. The number of psychiatric beds, for example, fell by 6.1%, learning disability beds by 14.4% and geriatric medicine beds by 5.4% over the same period. Over the last 20 years the fall in the number of psychiatric and learning disability beds has been profound (from 16 953 to 8145, and from 7092 to 2223 respectively).[4]

The fall in the number of hospital beds is not a uniquely Scottish phenomenon. Over the past 20 years the average number of acute beds per thousand population in OECD countries has fallen from just over 5.5 to just under 4. In England the trend has been similar but the fall began from a lower starting point (just over 5 to just over 3 per 1000). The recent National Beds Inquiry [12] undertaken by the Department of Health reports a fall of just over 2% per annum since 1980 in beds available for acute, general and maternity care, despite a rise in acute and general admissions of 3.5% and a bed occupancy rate that has increased to around 83%. The picture that emerges is one of an NHS struggling to cope and in urgent need of different approaches to care management. The rising number of medical and surgical emergency admissions, increasing proportion of elderly patients and delayed discharge (because of lack of access to rehabilitation, intermediate care, home care and other social services interventions) account in large part for the stresses and strains currently imposed on acute hospital beds.

The National Beds Inquiry reported that two-thirds of hospital beds were occupied by people aged 65 years and over, and its literature review estimated that around 20% of bed usage by older patients was probably inappropriate had alternative facilities been available. In Scotland, the July 2001 Census showed that there were 2954 patients ready for discharge; 87.6% of the patients were aged 65 years and over and 68% of them were outwith the six week discharge planning period.[13] The top five reasons for delay were awaiting start/completion of post-hospital social care assessment (21%), non-availability of public funding for nursing home place (17%), awaiting place in non-NHS funded nursing home (13%), awaiting bed in other NHS hospital/specialty/facility (7%) and patient exercising statutory right of choice (6%).

Activity trends

Activity in the acute sector of the NHS in Scotland has risen continually since 1981 to plateau in 1999–2000 (Figure 9.1). Inpatient episodes have increased modestly while day patient episodes have risen almost threefold.

Figure 9.1 Annual number of inpatient episodes and discharges and outpatient episodes in acute specialties in NHS Scotland 1981–2000 (SOURCE ISD Scotland)

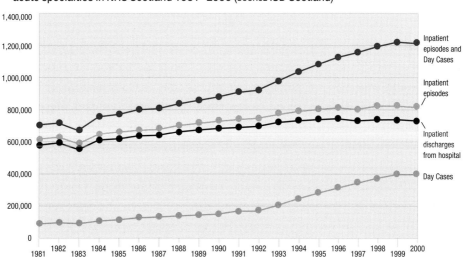

Year ending 31 March

Perhaps the most dramatic trend has been the progressive reduction in elective inpatient activity against a backdrop of rising emergency activity (Figure 9.2). Emergency admissions now account for 67% of all inpatient admissions to acute specialties.[1]

Figure 9.2   Trends in inpatient and day case activity in acute specialties in NHS Scotland 1981–2000 (SOURCE ISD Scotland – SMR1 & SMR 01)

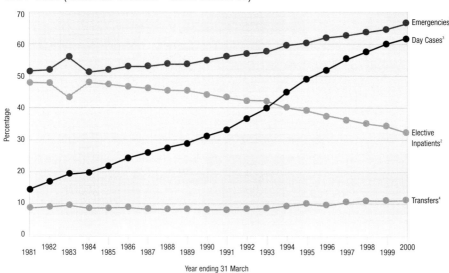

In 1981 day patient activity accounted for only 14.6% of acute sector activity; it now accounts for 62.6% of all elective inpatient/day case admissions in acute specialties.[4] The advantages of day surgery have been identified and advocated in two key reports in Scotland; the 1992 report *Day Surgery in Scottish Hospitals* (Scottish Office Audit Unit) [14] and the 1997 report, *Better by the Day? – Day Surgery in Scotland* (Accounts Commission).[15] Current targets relate to 19 day case procedures and are based on the targets proposed by the Audit Commission. Average performance of Trusts now exceeds the 1997 targets in 10 operations but fails in all but one instance (inguinal hernia in adults) to achieve the revised targets set recently by the Health Department. This 'failure' should not be misconstrued in that targets are deliberately intended to be stretching but ultimately achievable in the constant drive for improved efficiency. Variation between Trusts remains striking.

The increasing productivity of the acute sector has struggled to keep pace with demands placed on the service. Bed crises, traditionally associated with pressures on general medical beds as a result of respiratory-related illnesses in winter, are now more common at other times of the year. Multiple admissions of very elderly people for unrelated episodes of care are also a significant factor. As a consequence of these forces, waiting lists for elective admission remain problematic and resistant to sustained improvement. In 1990 the total hospital waiting list[*] stood at 79 866 and in 2001 at 81 968. Determined efforts in 2002 brought the figure down to 71 962, but if history repeats itself this will not be sustained. Some improvement in waiting times has been achieved, however, particularly for patients waiting unreasonably long times. The Patient's Charter (see chapter 1) set guarantees for maximum waiting times and successive governments have devoted considerable effort and money to ensuring that no-one waits for more than one year for any inpatient admission (a target achieved in recent times). Less impressive has been the fact that in 2002 one in 10 patients had to wait for more than six months to see a consultant. Public concern has pushed waiting times to the top of the political agenda and has resulted in periodic accusations that undue emphasis on these times is distorting clinical priorities by displacing more serious and urgent cases from operating lists. In a broader context, the reduction in waiting times inevitably draws resources from other needs in both the acute sector and elsewhere in the NHS.

It is worth emphasising that when presented in a different manner, Scotland's waiting list data can tell a more encouraging story. In 2002, 70% of outpatients were seen within 13 weeks, and almost 80% of inpatients were admitted within three months, the median being 34 days. Recent initiatives by the Scottish Executive to implement booked outpatient appointments are designed to build on this record. Improving communication between primary and secondary care services should help further to reduce the concerns of patients at an anxious time in their lives.

The Acute Services Review

The Acute Services Review was undertaken in 1997–98 to look critically at the delivery of acute services in an NHS operating within a framework of

---

[*] www.show.scot.nhs.uk/isd/acute-activity

partnership rather than the constraints of the internal market. It was a major exercise undertaken by a Steering Group chaired by the Chief Medical Officer and supported by seven Sub-Groups established to consider the following aspects of the acute sector;

- Management of renal disease

- Management of cardiac disease

- Management of neurological/neurosurgical disease

- Management of peripheral vascular disease

- Treatment services for children

- Diagnostic and support services

- Quality assurance and accreditation

The areas were chosen not because they were deemed to have particular priority or because they were perceived to be in crisis. In particular, the four disease areas were selected because they offered opportunities to use specific issues to develop principles and service models that could be applicable to the acute sector as a whole. Each Sub-Group and the Steering Group were asked to consider evidence on clinical effectiveness and outcomes; patient convenience; medical technologies; trends in demand; relationships between services and between the acute sector and primary and community care; training needs of the clinical workforce; and research and development activity. All eight Groups were multidisciplinary, involved both clinicians and management, and all had lay representation. A series of open meetings allowed full engagement with the wider professional community and the public, and written submissions were welcomed at every stage.

From the outset, the Review was concerned with equity of access, quality of services, quality of outcomes (and in particular the relationship between service volume and outcome), optimal use of resources, networking, emergency pressures, service design and responsiveness, and clinical effectiveness. Throughout its course, the Review was alert to workforce issues, notably service pressures, training needs, continuing professional development and job satisfaction. It was recognised that implementation of the Review's recommendations would take time and that there could be no quick fix. Some of the issues considered by the Acute Services Review are examined in further detail in the sections that follow.

Quality and performance of acute services in Scotland
(see also chapter 10)

Scotland has taken a leading role in various aspects of the 'clinical quality agenda' including the use of clinical audit, development of clinical outcome indicators, and the formulation of evidence-based guidelines by the Scottish Intercollegiate Guideline Network (SIGN). It has been well served by the availability of excellent clinical activity and outcome data, and linkage between various registries has provided comprehensive information about health and health care. This has enabled analysis of both the strengths and weaknesses of health care in Scotland, and has fuelled the increasing public appetite for information about health services.

Clinical audit has been a particularly prominent feature of acute sector activity in Scotland. Surgical audit in Lothian, for example, has been in existence for over 50 years and was a major factor in the early development of specialist vascular surgery and urology in Edinburgh. Scotland's Clinical Resource and Audit Group (CRAG) has played a lead role by fostering local and national multiprofessional audit [for example, Scottish Audit of Surgical Mortality (SASM), Renal Registry, Scottish Trauma Audit Group], publishing Clinical Outcome Indicator reports and sponsoring and supporting SIGN. As a national extension of surgical audit, SASM has monitored all deaths after surgery and provided critical peer review by consultant anaesthetists and surgeons of each death. In addition to focusing attention on lessons to be learned, this audit has highlighted resource issues such as the need for critical care beds, and is viewed as a useful tool in the continuing drive for quality.

Nine Clinical Outcome Indicator reports between 1993 and 2002 have presented data at Health Board or Trust level and some indicators have been reviewed more than once (see also chapter 10). Topics examined at Health Board level include rates of teenage pregnancy, suicide, hospitalisation for childhood asthma and survival from various cancers. Topics examined at Trust level include rates of 30-day mortality after emergency admission with hip fracture, myocardial infarction and stroke, re-operation after transurethral prostatectomy, and emergency re-admission rates after operations such as appendicectomy, hysterectomy and hip replacement. Data are standardised for age and sex, and where appropriate, by Carstairs deprivation category. Confidence intervals are provided and trends over time are now being set out. The need for careful and cautious interpretation is stressed repeatedly; the indicators are intended to highlight issues that might require further scrutiny and not to provide a basis for inferences about the quality of care and construction of league tables.

The clinical outcome indicator reports have been well received and dealt with responsibly by the media who have generally avoided the use of lurid headlines and inappropriate allusion to 'death tables'. Some have found it hard, however, to resist the temptation to see the indicators as league tables and as a platform for naming and shaming. A postal questionnaire conducted by the Scottish Executive in 1997 indicated that the indicators were of some practical value to health professionals and in some instances had helped to change practice if not behaviour.[16] Independent review found that indicators had helped to raise awareness of quality issues among Trust staff and may have alerted providers to some issues requiring further investigation.[17] Indicators had been used to support applications for further funding and service development. Disappointingly, they were rarely used directly to stimulate continuous quality improvement or share best practice between organisations.

The work of the Acute Services Review on clinical quality assurance and accreditation was widely welcomed by public and professionals alike and led directly to the creation of the Clinical Standards Board for Scotland (see chapter 10). It will be interesting to monitor the impact of this initiative on quality improvement as its work moves from a developmental into a fully operational stage.

The volume-outcome debate

A key challenge for the Acute Services Review was to develop an appropriate balance between the benefits of concentrating specialist services and resources and the provision of good quality local services. At the time (1997–98), many of the published claims for a positive relationship between the volume of activity in a given service and the quality of outcome obtained were not supported by robust evidence. Analysis such as that undertaken by the York NHS Centre for Reviews and Dissemination, for example,[18] was beginning to show objective evidence for a relationship between volume-outcome relationship in specific areas such as the treatment of cardiac disease and some aspects of surgery for vascular disease and cancer.

The Acute Services Review concluded that:

- The critical mass needed to achieve the benefits that might flow from increased volume of activity can come through managed clinical networks (MCNs – see below) rather than enforced centralisation/concentration of services.

- Evidence-based practice, accreditation and clinical quality assurance will be more important factors in improving outcomes than simply increasing the volume of activity.

- Significant pressures within the NHS can be balanced across a range of organisations and structures that compromise neither the development of centres of excellence nor local provision.

These conclusions have underpinned the development of MCNs in Scotland in the drive for high quality services that make optimal use of available resources. They are not invalidated by the hardening evidence base that outcome is indeed related to volume after specific surgical and other interventions.[19, 20] As the Acute Services Review clearly recognised, however, centralisation of services will be both unavoidable and desirable for some highly specialised services such as liver transplantation (see below) or open heart surgery in children.

The case for concentration and National Services

The National Services Division (NSD) of the Common Services Agency was created in 1993 to commission and fund a range of services where a national rather than regional perspective was required. The range of services commissioned by NSD has changed with time but it currently includes such components as the prevention of drug misuse and its treatment, HIV/AIDS services, and heart and liver transplantation. Although top slicing of funds for designated national services may have seemed at odds with the basic tenets of an internally competitive NHS, NSD survived the internal market era and its continuation was assured in *Designed to Care*.[2] In 2000 a total of £39.2 million was expended by NSD.

Liver transplantation provides a good illustration of a highly specialised service where the annual case load/demand is too small (some 50 transplants in Scottish adults a year) for the work to be undertaken by multiple units. After an expert working group had concluded that Scotland needed a liver transplantation unit, Edinburgh Royal Infirmary was selected in competition as the national site. Approximately £2M per annum was top-sliced to NSD from the NHS budget to establish a sustainable robust service and avoid the difficulties of trying to run such a service within an internal market. In such a market, not every Health Board (and particularly the small Island Boards) might have felt it necessary to strike a deal annually with the national unit just in case one or more of its inhabitants required a transplant. While the case for a national adult transplantation unit was agreed, it was felt (correctly) that the case load for paediatric liver transplantation was too small to justify the establishment of a Scottish centre. Children requiring transplantation continue to be referred to specialist children's units in England. This is important: it is not sensible to try to provide every specialist service within Scotland and the limitations imposed by a population size of 5.1 million.

Open heart surgery in children offers an example of a different type of problem. Scotland has been well served over the years by two centres offering this type of surgery (Edinburgh and Glasgow) but surgery was undertaken latterly by only one consultant in Edinburgh and two in Glasgow. While both services appeared to achieve acceptable outcomes, concerns about case-load and the sustainability of relatively small volume services led to consideration of the need to create one such centre serving all of Scotland. In the event, this type of surgery has been concentrated in Glasgow. Such decisions are difficult and can never be universally popular. Great care must be taken to consider all implications; for example, would removal of one specialised service, in this case cardiac surgery, imperil the viability of the paediatric intensive care unit (ICU) in Edinburgh? The ability to take a Scotland-wide perspective is immensely helpful and parallel decisions about Edinburgh's role in paediatric neurosurgery and the transfer of critically ill and injured children have offset any concerns about ICU case-load and sustainability.

Access to acute hospitals in Scotland

The majority of Scots inhabit the Central belt or East Coast in reasonable proximity to major urban centres and large teaching hospitals. The recent Review of the Scottish Workforce,[21] chaired by Professor John Temple, suggested that 89% of the population live within 30 minutes drive time of the 35 hospitals classified as accepting acute admissions (Table 9.4), and that 84% live within 30 minutes drive time of the 22 hospitals classified as having an Accident and Emergency Unit. Reassuring though these statistics may seem with regard to access, it must be borne in mind that some of these are small hospitals serving remote areas and that a significant number of the Scottish population do not have ready access to acute hospital care. These statistics also fail to reflect the fact that specialists such as neurosurgeons, medical oncologists and paediatric surgeons are based only within large urban centres or larger district hospitals.

TABLE 9.4 Proximity to acute hospital care as expressed by drive times to hospitals accepting acute admissions and those with accident and emergency units. (Data from Future Practice: A review of the Scottish Medical Workforce. Scottish Executive 2002)

Drivetime	No. of population living within drive time of hospital accepting acute admissions*	No. of population living within drive time of hospital with accident and emergency department**
< 30 minutes	4 365 249	4 102 637
30–60 minutes	375 188	414 481
60–90 minutes	75 690	173 389
90–120 minutes	17 297	36 956
>120 minutes	53 582	159 543

*Hospitals accepting acute admissions were defined as those with consultant physicians or surgeons based on site, excluding day and community hospitals. Hospitals providing care of the elderly, maternity services, psychiatric care and paediatric care were excluded unless they were also thought to undertake general medicine or general surgery. The six 'remote and rural' hospitals at Oban, Fort William, Wick, Stornoway, Kirkwall and Lerwick were included.

** Hospitals with a major Accident and Emergency Unit were defined as those with full-time consultant staff in Accident and Emergency Medicine, accepting that some units may have combined cover and that cover in some units may also be provided by consultants from other specialties.

A constant problem is the need to balance local access with the provision of services of acceptably high quality that are appropriate for the location concerned, sustainable and cost-effective. While the public understandably wish to have services within easy reach, they also appreciate that not every household can be served by a nearby hospital offering the full range of specialist services. The public also understand that to have local access to a service of inferior quality is not in their best interests.

To take a hypothetical example, the people of the small northern town of Wick almost certainly understand that if their child is injured in a road traffic accident there will not be a neurosurgeon, let alone a paediatric neurosurgeon, standing by on the staff of their local hospital. If their son had the misfortune to develop testicular cancer, these same parents would have little difficulty understanding the desirability of transfer to a distant specialist centre, offering as it would, an excellent prospect of regaining normal life expectancy. At the same time, they might have profound difficulty understanding why either of them would need to be referred to a distant centre for hernia repair or cholecystectomy or treatment of a simple fracture.

Sustainability of Services

The fact that a significant proportion of the Scottish population are dispersed in remote and rural areas makes it particularly difficult to provide every inhabitant with a sustainable local consultant-delivered acute service. Surgery provides a good example of the difficulties involved. Traditionally, some remote areas (for example, the island of Skye) have been served by a single consultant surgeon who lived in the community. While such single-handed surgeons may well have given long and devoted service, the arrangement is no longer sustainable or indeed, acceptable. Its problems include the impossibility of sustaining round-the-clock services throughout the year, having a surgeon serve as a generalist while at the same time attempting to provide specialist care, the need to maintain surgical skills on a relatively small surgical caseload, professional isolation and the difficulty of continuing professional development. While some of these problems can be overcome or at least ameliorated, those that remain are usually so great that alternative solutions to single-handed working have to be found.

Simply increasing the number of consultants based in a small community may create or compound as many problems as it solves. To have two consultant surgeons living and working on Skye, for example, might lessen (but not necessarily to an acceptable degree) the amount of time spent on call, but would halve an already small workload with detriment to the maintenance of clinical and operative skills. It is also naive to view surgical (or any other specialist) services as simply dependent on the availability of appropriate consultant skills. Much depends on maintaining a skilled nursing staff, providing safe anaesthesia, and if surgery of any complexity is being undertaken, availability of high-dependency/intensive care.

Although this section has used surgery as its prime example, similar considerations apply to other specialties. There is a growing realisation that remote communities may be better served by dropping all pretence of maintaining a round-the-clock consultant service delivered by one individual who lives locally. For a community such as Skye, more can be achieved by regarding the island as part of a wider area being served by a sustainable service of acceptable quality. In the example being used here, the single-handed surgeon on Skye is replaced by adding a third consultant to the staff of the Belford Hospital in Fort William. Services in the Belford Hospital become immediately more sustainable. Elective surgery is still carried out on Skye by having one of the three consultants travel to Skye to conduct regular outpatient and operating sessions. Given that these consultants are working together to serve a larger population, they find it easier to retain surgical and clinical skills and avoid professional isolation. Virtually all the elective surgery undertaken on Skye in earlier years continues to be carried out there. The only elective surgery not performed on Skye involves more complex surgery (for example, anterior resection of the rectum) where transfer to a larger centre such as Inverness is, and always has been, merited because of the potential need for specialist care and high dependency/intensive care.

It is very difficult to reassure people who live in remote areas and who may be anxious about the proposed loss of 'our own surgeon'. There is no way of avoiding the fact that a small number of patients and their relatives will be inconvenienced by the need for travel in this new model where the needs of the Skye population are subsumed into those of the regional population. The availability of emergency transportation by land or air is a major consideration as there will be occasions when a critically ill or injured individual has to be transferred urgently to an appropriate centre. Skye at least has a bridge to the mainland although some of its people live more than two hours drive from the nearest large district general hospital at Inverness. In the case of some island communities, drive time is irrelevant and it must not be forgotten that our three island Health Boards each serve an archipelago rather than one island.

The Acute Services Review[2] fully recognised the particular needs of remote and rural communities and the tyranny of distance. It argued for the continued role of community hospitals, flagged concern about recruitment and retention of healthcare professionals, and made a strong case for regional services with improved outreach as a means of providing sustainable services for remote communities. Arguably, its most imaginative recommendation was to press for the creation of a Resource Centre that would oversee, co-ordinate and underpin training needs and the support of professionals working in the Highlands and Islands. In the event, the Scottish Executive responded by creating a Remote and Rural Areas Resource Initiative (RARARI) that would further the development of healthcare for all remote and rural parts of Scotland. The Initiative is in receipt of £2M annually over a three-year period starting in 2000.

Affordability and cost-effectiveness have not been advanced to this point in the argument about sustainable quality services. This is not to say they are unimportant as resources for healthcare are finite. Money spent on maintaining services that are inappropriate or inappropriately configured, is money that could surely be spent more wisely elsewhere. The main argument on sustainability, however, hinges on the question of quality. Local access will always be highly desirable but must never be provided at the expense of quality. Sustainability requires a critical mass of individuals who are appropriately skilled, sufficient in number to provide round-the-clock services and able to deal with a case-load that allows them to maintain skills and continue their professional development. These problems have already been alluded to in the example of surgical services for Skye but they are not confined to remote and rural communities. Existing and forecast shortages in the workforce, the increasing desire of professionals to work flexibly and the need to implement the European Working Time Directive for doctors in training all have profound implications for service sustainability (see chapter 11).

Scotland's District General Hospitals

As mentioned earlier, the Acute Services Review argued for retention of community hospitals. What about the case for retention of District General Hospitals (DGHs) in Scotland? At the start of the Review, colleagues in some smaller DGHs were apprehensive that it would recommend that they cease to offer specialist services if they failed to achieve an arbitrary case load or did not provide a fully comprehensive service. Breast cancer provides a good case in point. Should the Borders General Hospital cease to treat breast cancer patients because it undertakes less than say 75 mastectomy operations a year and cannot administer radiotherapy? Should all patients from the Borders be diverted immediately to the specialist Breast Unit in Edinburgh where they can receive the full spectrum of treatment from highly specialised staff? The answer of course is no. Provided the staff of the Borders General Hospital can demonstrate that they are using evidence-based guidelines, achieve acceptable outcomes (demands now placed on all hospitals by the Clinical Standards Board) and have a sustainable service, they should continue to provide local treatment for patients in their area. This is not to say that a linear accelerator now needs to be built in Melrose. Patients requiring radiotherapy should still travel to Edinburgh but they may not need to do so if they require chemotherapy. Much depends on effective linkage between professionals in Edinburgh and Melrose, a linkage ideally achieved by creation of a managed clinical network (see below).

Retention of a network of district general hospitals does not mean that every hospital should attempt to offer every specialist service or develop highly specialised services that are usually the preserve of large University hospitals. In many regions, it is not sensible or feasible to have specialised services duplicated (and often unsustainable) in hospitals that may be close in terms of both distance and travelling time. In attempting to rationalise services in their region, health boards have frequently encountered opposition from patients and practitioners alike who may perceive any bid to close a service in 'their hospital' as a major threat. Much effort is still being expended, for example, on the rationalisation of acute services in Glasgow, Forth Valley, Tayside and Fife. Ambulatory care deserves special mention in this context in that prompt access to efficient day patient services would in most peoples' minds compensate for loss of a particular service in a given neighbourhood hospital. As outlined in the Acute Services Review, the model Ambulatory Care Centre could capitalise on modern technology to provide a one-stop service to investigation and treatment. Minimally invasive surgery, interventional radiology and interventional endoscopy lend themselves to ambulatory care and would be major components (although not by any means the only components) of the services on offer.

Service delivery and managed clinical networks

Extended access to improved and seamless services was given great impetus by *Designed to Care* and the Designed Healthcare Initiative established in 1997. The 50 or so projects that followed were intended to redesign services from a patient's perspective and use a 'whole systems approach' to make optimal use of professional skills, challenge traditional ways of working, reduce waiting times, and generally improve responsiveness and quality of care. Examples of service redesign highlighted in *Health in Scotland 2000* [22] include initiatives in Lothian (one-stop breast clinic), and Glasgow (one-stop colorectal clinic; dedicated stroke unit with one-stop clinic for patients with transient ischaemic attacks), and improved access to mental health services, child health services and services for older people in Borders, Dumfries and Galloway, and Ayrshire and Arran respectively.

The concept of managed clinical networks (MCNs) was developed as part of the Acute Services Review as an alternative to conventional hub and spoke models in which patients are channelled centripetally to centralised specialist services. Existing networks for the care of diabetes (Tayside) and cancer surgery (Highlands and Islands) were of seminal importance in developing the MCN concept. The work of the Vascular Sub-Group in developing the model of an Integrated Regional Vascular Service (IRVS) was also particularly important, setting out as it did the core criteria for such a network. A minimum population base of 500 000 was identified as necessary for this particular type of vascular network to take account of audit of clinical activity, staffing requirements, rota needs of a consultant-led emergency service, clinical throughput needed to meet training standards, and critical mass to warrant appointment of specialist senior staff. It was envisaged that each IRVS would be formed by integration of adjacent existing vascular services, with emergency and 'high technology' care being undertaken in a single centre. At the same time, local access would be enhanced by a network of local clinics offering day surgery, venous surgery, post-acute care and rehabilitation.

The concept of MCNs was well received after publication of the Acute Services Review and has subsequently been admired outwith Scotland.[23] Core principles guiding their development have been set out clearly in the Management Executive Letter MEL (1999).[10] Managed clinical networks are defined as linked groups of health professionals and organisations from primary, secondary and tertiary care, working in a co-ordinated manner, unconstrained by existing professional and health board boundaries, and ensuring equitable provision of high quality clinically effective services throughout Scotland. Flexibility and pragmatism were seen as vital in network development. Networks, for example, might be specialty-based or disease-based. They might cover local care, care in a health board region, or care that was supra-regional or national. The general principles of accountability and clinical governance were to apply to MCNs in the same way that they applied to the rest of the NHS.

Managed clinical networks are now in development in a number of disease areas and regions. The diabetes network in Tayside (DARTS) continues to develop and new initiatives are underway in areas that include intensive care of critically ill and injured children, stroke, vascular services, management of cleft lip and palate, coronary heart disease, end-stage renal failure and home parenteral nutrition. Perhaps the most striking new development is in the field of cancer where earlier work to develop MCNs in palliative care (HDL(2000)10) is now being extended to cancer care in general (see chapter 5). HDL(2001)71 sets out the expectation that by 2002 networks should be in place for the management of all cancers. Particular emphasis is given to the early creation of networks for the management of lung and colorectal cancer.

Managed clinical networks remain an exciting prospect but enthusiasm has to be tempered by the realisation that traditional attitudes to management, funding flows and service delivery by clinicians may need to alter when developing networks that cross Trust and Health Board boundaries. The concept of a lead clinician (or manager) has central importance and this individual must be empowered by management and the health professionals concerned if the network is to be driven forward. Clinicians concerned must owe allegiance to their network rather than to a single institution/hospital as has tended to happen in the past. The strong support and authority of the Scottish Executive Health Department will continue to be crucial and links to the Clinical Standards Board for Scotland and its successor are seen as particularly helpful. Managed clinical networks must make a positive difference if they are to be retained and extended. The prospect of consistent quality improvement, benefit to patients, improved training opportunities and enhanced job satisfaction for professionals make a prize worth struggling for.

Future considerations

Because Scotland has traditionally enjoyed greater funding and manpower than England in respect of acute services it is arguably better placed to move forward into the 21st century and the continuing drive for service quality. This contention, however, must be offset by Scotland's greater burden of disease, its higher levels of deprivation and the problems posed by population dispersal in remote and rural areas. As in all civilised countries, the performance of healthcare systems is subject to ever-increasing scrutiny, public expectation and unwillingness to accept anything less than ideal outcomes. Although real increases in Government funding will go some way to improve health and health care, including the provision of acute services, it would be naïve to assume that great pressures will not remain. Health care is liable to become more rather than less costly with the advent of expensive new technologies and treatments, and the benefits of improved population health will take time to become manifest.

This means that pressure on the acute sector is liable to remain intense with pressure on acute hospitals, acute beds and staff. There can be no doubting the beneficial transition that is now taking place in terms of hospital building but pressure, and in particular emergency pressure, seems certain to continue. The emphasis on sustainable quality of clinical services has been a most welcome recent development. Further innovation is needed to capitalise on the concepts developed by initiatives such as the Acute Services Review, and service design and delivery will need to continue to evolve to benefit patients and professionals alike.

REFERENCES

1.   *Designed to Care. Renewing the Health Service in Scotland.* Edinburgh:Scottish Office Department of Health, 1997.

2.   *Acute Services Review Report.* Edinburgh:Scottish Office Department of Health, 1998.

3.   Dixon J, Inglis S, Klein R. Is the English NHS underfunded? *British Medical Journal* 1999, 318: 522–6.

4.   *Scottish Health Statistics.* Edinburgh: Information and Statistics Division. National Health Service in Scotland, 2000.

5.   4. *Our National Health. A plan for action, a plan for change.* Edinburgh: Scottish Executive Health Department, 2000.

6.   Organisation for Economic Cooperation and Development. *OECD health data 99: a comparative analysis of 29 countries.* Paris: OECD. CREDES, 1999.

7.   Gaffney D, Pollock A. *Can the NHS afford the private finance initiative?* London: BMA, 1997.

8.   Health Policy and Economic Research Unit. *The private finance initiative: briefing and update.* London: BMA, 1999.

9.   Gaffney D, Pollock A, Price D, Shaoul J. The private finance initiative: PFI in the NHS – is there an economic case? *British Medical Journal* 1999, 319: 116–119.

10. Gaffney D, Pollock A, Price D, Shaoul J. The private finance initiative: The politics of the private finance initiative and the new NHS. *British Medical Journal* 1999, 319: 249–53.

11. Health Policy and Economic Research Unit. *Extending private involvement in the NHS.* London: BMA, 2001.

12. *Shaping the Future NHS.* Long Term Planning for Hospitals and Related Services. Consultation document on the findings of the National Beds Inquiry. London: Department of Health, 2000.

13. *Patients Ready for Discharge in NHS Scotland* – figures from 15 July 2001 census. Edinburgh: ISD Scotland, September 2001.

14. *Day Surgery in Scottish Hospitals.* Edinburgh: Scottish Office Audit Unit, 1992.

15. *Better by the Day?* Day surgery in Scotland. Edinburgh:Accounts Commission, 1997.

16. Kendrick S, Cline D, Finlayson A. Clinical outcome indicators in Scotland: lessons and prospects. In Davies H, Malek M, Nielson A, Tavolaki M (eds.) *Managing quality and controlling costs.* Aldershot: Ashgate Publishing, 1999.

17. Mannion R, Goddard M. Impact of published clinical outcome data: case studies in NHS Hospital Trusts. *British Medical Journal* 2001, 323:260–3.

18. *Concentration and choice in Provision of Hospital Services.* York: NHS Centre for Reviews and Dissemination, 1997.

19. Halm EA, Lee C, Chassin MR. How is volume related to quality in health care? A systematic review of the research literature. *Interpreting the Volume – Outcome Relationship in the Context of Health Care Quality.* Washington DC: Institute of Medicine, 2000.

20.   Birkmeyer JD, Siewere AE, Finlayson EVA *et al.* Hospital volume and surgical mortality in
      the United States. *New England Journal of Medicine* 2002, 346:1128–37.

21.   *Future Practice* A Review of the Scottish Medical Workforce. Edinburgh:Scottish Executive
      Health Department, 2002.

22.   *Health in Scotland.* Report of the Chief Medical Officer. Edinburgh: The Scottish Executive,
      2001.

23.   Edwards N. Clinical networks. *British Medical Journal* 2002, 324: 63.

10. Quality Health Care in Scotland

David Steel

Introduction

'Good quality heath care delivered consistently and to a high standard must be a key objective of the NHS in Scotland. It is a shared responsibility of everyone working in the NHS, and covers all aspects of health care including the effectiveness of clinical practice, the environment in which it is delivered, and responsiveness to the needs of patients.' [1]

This statement might have been made at any time in the history of the National Health Service. That it appeared at the beginning of the first substantive chapter of a White Paper in 1997 is a clear signal of the changes that have occurred in recent years and that are the subject of this chapter: the health care quality agenda has become more explicit, more corporate, and more all-embracing.

The statement also provides a menu for the coverage of the chapter. The focus is on steps taken to improve and to monitor the quality of clinical care and treatment – often described as clinical effectiveness – but it will also include non-clinical factors that have an impact upon the care provided to patients and, of increasing importance, the involvement of patients and, where appropriate, carers in decisions about their care and treatment.

The last 15 years have seen a steady accretion in the components of what is known as 'the clinical effectiveness cycle'. Building upon a longstanding research base, first clinical audit, next clinical guidelines, and later standards-based quality assurance and health technology assessment, have been added. The challenge now is to bring all these elements together into a co-ordinated strategy designed to improve the quality of clinical care. In parallel over the same period, there have been moves to extend patient involvement, increasingly on clinical issues, and more recently to integrate this with the rest of the agenda.

These trends have been largely unaffected by the changes in government that occurred during this period. While the current quality agenda looks very different in comparison with the mid-1980s, there has also been a remarkable continuity in approach. One important aspect of this continuity has been the maintenance of a distinctive Scottish approach, which is a further theme of the chapter. Whereas many of the changes have occurred in response to UK-wide factors, the solutions adopted have had a strong Scottish character with the result that there are now marked cross-border differences in both institutions and culture.

Clinical Audit

The Scottish approach to clinical effectiveness has been built upon a long tradition of excellence and innovation in medicine and in health care generally. The reputation of Scotland's medical schools and its medical colleges is truly international. Closely linked is the tradition of research and development in which the Chief Scientist Office, which celebrated its 25th anniversary in 1998, is one key component. There is also a widely envied record of national data collection led since 1974 by the Information and Statistics Division (ISD) of the Common Services Agency. Even the practice of audit is well-established, surgical audit having been operating in Lothian for more than 50 years.

A step change, however, started to occur in the mid-1980s. Prompted by the introduction of general management (after publication of the Griffiths Report in 1985)[2] and a stronger focus on planning and on efficiency and effectiveness, two initiatives were taken in Scotland. First, in 1985 a Scottish Health Management Efficiency Group (SCOTMEG) was established, initially as an alternative and subsequently as a complement to competitive tendering, to make recommendations and spread good practice in relation to a variety of services. Its focus was mainly non-clinical but its work over the next 10 years became increasingly clinical.[3]

Secondly, in 1987 a Clinical Resource Use Group (CRUG) was formed out of an earlier Transfer of Resources Group that existed to identify good clinical practice from a clinical and economic standpoint so as to encourage the transfer of resources from acute services into the long-stay sector.[4] CRUG was chaired by the Chief Medical Officer and its membership was overwhelming medical, including representatives of the BMA, although it was later widened to include a nurse and a general manager; its remit was to identify and disseminate examples of effective use of resources in the clinical field.

The first major milestone came in 1989 with the publication of the Thatcher Government's White Paper *Working for Patients*.[5] One of its main themes was the need to ensure that 'the money available to hospitals buys the best possible care for patients'.[6] To this end, within two years all hospital doctors were to participate in medical audit, and equivalent steps were encouraged in primary care. Audit – the systematic, critical analysis of the quality of medical care – was seen as essentially a professional matter for peer review, but one in which government and management had a supportive role. In Scotland it was decided that CRUG should be translated into a Clinical Resource and Audit Group (CRAG). As its title suggests, it retained the remit of its predecessor but also assumed responsibility for determining a national audit strategy, for sponsoring audit practice at national level, and for support and oversight of local audit activity.

Over the next 13 years, CRAG was to play a central role not only in relation to audit but also to wider developments in clinical effectiveness. It proved to be one of the lasting and most highly regarded legacies of *Working for Patients* which survived the dismantling of the internal market and was disbanded only in 2002 when its work was subsumed into a new organisation designed to strengthen the co-ordination it had sought to provide.

CRAG started by promoting unidisciplinary medical, nursing, dental and pharmaceutical audit. Quite quickly, however, the emphasis turned to multidisciplinary clinical audit and in 1993 four separate committees were combined into a single Clinical Audit Sub-Committee which produced two years later a 'Strategic Framework for Clinical Audit in Scotland' designed to consolidate earlier guidance and to complement Health Boards' local audit strategies.[7] At national level, a National Projects Committee (NPC) was established to stimulate and manage a programme of national audits. In 1998 NPC was superseded by a Clinical Effectiveness Programmes Sub-Group, with a remit wider than clinical audit and the aim of funding linked work through the development of a series of clinical effectiveness programmes.[8] The Clinical Audit Sub-Committee was also replaced with an Implementation Sub-Group to support NHSScotland in taking forward the clinical effectiveness agenda and to encourage implementation of its products.

Through these various groups, CRAG has supported a major programme of national audits including initiatives such as the Scottish Audit of Surgical Mortality and the Scottish Renal Registry; and it has developed programmes in relation to the national clinical priorities of cancer, coronary heart disease and for specific areas of activity such as reproductive health and primary care. Initially, a significant proportion of CRAG's funding was allocated to Health Boards for local audit but since 1994/95 these funds have been included in Boards' general allocations. CRAG continued to take a close interest in the use of this money: providing guidance [9]; and conducting regular meetings with Health Board area clinical audit committees to review progress.

Clinical Guidelines

CRAG was also instrumental in the establishment of the Scottish Intercollegiate Guidelines Network (SIGN). In 1993 it published a report *Clinical Guidelines*, highlighting the need for guidelines on clinically effective practice that were based upon scientific evidence rather than received wisdom. This prompted the Academy of Royal Colleges and Faculties in Scotland to set up SIGN to develop multidisciplinary, evidence-based clinical guidelines for NHSScotland. SIGN is a network of doctors and other healthcare professionals that is dependent upon the commitment of the individuals who work to develop each guideline; and it is involving patients in the development of its guidelines. By 2002 it had grown into an internationally renowned organisation, with over 60 guidelines to its name. [10]

Clinical Outcome Indicators

SIGN provides a good example of the Scottish approach to clinical effectiveness: collaboration between the healthcare professions and government; multidisciplinary (but almost always medically led); and rigorous in its methodology but at the same time largely informal in the way it has operated. The same characteristics enabled Scotland to pioneer the publication of clinical outcome indicators as part of the drive to use information to improve the quality of care. In its very early days, CRAG had explored the possibility of using the high quality national data sets available in ISD to produce a range of clinical indicators. [11] A first set of indicators was produced in 1993. The following year the bold decision was taken to publish such information; and subsequently nine reports have been published containing over 45 indicators, broken down on a named Board, Trust or hospital basis.[12] That this was possible reflects the quality of the data, the benefits of record linkage between hospital records collated by ISD and the death records of the Registrar General for Scotland, and the maturity of relationships within the NHS community in Scotland.

Patient's Charter and Framework for Action

All the initiatives outlined so far were professionally led. In tandem, however, there were a range of parallel developments taking place in relation to other aspects of quality.

First, as part of the introduction of general management, there was growing interest in various schemes designed to improve standards of care such as King's Fund Organisational Audit and ISO 9000.

Secondly, as part of the Citizen's Charter initiative, the Scottish Office produced in 1991 a Patient's Charter setting out what people should expect from the NHS.[13] Its focus was on waiting times and on issues such as patient information and feedback, but it also introduced the idea of setting national standards for health care services. It was accompanied by a complementary document *Framework for Action* aimed at those working in the NHS.[14] It began to link the various agendas, bringing together the patient focus of the Charter, multidisciplinary work on clinical audit, and the initiatives being taken by nurses and allied health professionals to develop standards and statements of good practice. One of its accompanying documents set out approaches to and key principles in both setting standards and quality assurance[15]; and one of the initiatives it announced was the commissioning of CRAG and SCOTMEG to work together to identify and promote good practice and to develop standards for four patient groups/services: people with mental illness, older people, maternity services and accident and emergency services.

Mid-point Stocktake

By the mid-1990s many of the building blocks were in place. Much had been achieved but its quality was variable and its coverage patchy, shortcomings that reflected the innovative stage of development. Four specific challenges were apparent.

First, the agenda was being driven by enthusiasts pursuing their own particular interests. This had enabled rapid progress in some areas but it was insufficiently linked to the priorities of the NHS. The need for a stronger strategic focus in this and other areas prompted the development in the 1990s of annual Priorities and Planning Guidance including what became known as the common core work programme.[16] Initially, this was allied to the internal market; subsequently it underpinned the development of Board health improvement programmes and Trust implementation plans. To reinforce these developments, a Clinical Effectiveness Strategy Group was created in 1998, comprising representatives of all the key organisations, under the chairmanship of the Chief Medical Officer, to provide a forum for discussion of priorities and to improve co-ordination of activity.[17]

Secondly, progress on clinical effectiveness had not been matched in the field of cost-effectiveness. As part of the internal market, a Scottish Health Purchasing Information Centre provided a number of valuable reports but its work had been insufficiently integrated with complementary developments. As a result there was growing unease among managers that the advice and guidance becoming available on clinical practice failed to take account of its affordability and cost-effectiveness.

Thirdly, there was the challenge of involving patients and the public in this agenda. The NHS was subject to the same kind of pressures affecting all public services as individuals expected to become involved in decisions about the services they receive. A start had been made, for example with the publication of clinical outcome indicators and with the establishment by SIGN of a patient information and participation group, but these developments were at a very early stage and had only a marginal impact upon the programme as a whole.

Fourthly, and most important, was the challenge of implementation. A great deal of effort had been invested in clinical effectiveness, but what impact was it having? Was it leading to changes in clinical practice and to improvements in the quality of care and treatment provided to patients; and were these changes occurring consistently across NHSScotland?

Quality Assurance

Concerns such as these prompted the then Chief Medical Officer, Sir David Carter, to include in the Acute Services Review that he established a sub-group, chaired by Professor Sir Robert Shields, to consider whether a system of quality assurance and accreditation was needed for clinical services. Although its report was published in 1998, the decision to establish the review predated the change of government in 1997 and many of the changes introduced by the new administration had been heralded in a White Paper produced by outgoing Ministers in February 1997.[18]

The Acute Services Review recommended the development of a national system of assuring the quality of clinical services in Scotland.[19] It was to build not only on the work of CRAG and SIGN but also on quality assurance schemes already in existence such as those for the breast and cervical screening programmes and Clinical Pathology Accreditation (UK) for laboratories, and on the work of the Scottish Health Advisory Service, established in 1970 to inspect services for older people and for those with mental illness or learning or physical disability. It too was to be professionally led, with multidisciplinary groups responsible for developing standards and peer review as the means of assessing performance against the standards, but patients and the public were to be involved in all its processes and its reports were to be published.

On acceptance of these recommendations by Ministers, a Clinical Standards Board for Scotland (CSBS) was established in April 1999. Its remit was to develop and run a national system of quality assurance of clinical services designed to promote public confidence that the services provided by NHSScotland are safe and meet nationally agreed standards and to support NHSScotland in delivering the highest possible standards of care.[20]

Initially, CSBS focused on the national clinical priorities of cancer, coronary heart disease and mental health, publishing six sets of standards and conducting over 100 review visits before the production of six national overviews and over 100 local reports in late 2001/early 2002. Simultaneously, it developed a set of generic clinical governance standards, conducting a baseline review across Scotland during 2001/2002.[21] It also endorsed practice accreditation as the way forward for quality assurance in primary care, supporting the roll-out across

Scotland of the Royal College of General Practitioners' Practice Accreditation Scheme. Further sets of condition-specific standards have been issued and a phased programme of reviews has been put in place.

Designed to Care

Although the Acute Services Review had not been concluded, its recommendations regarding quality assurance were trailed in the incoming administration's White Paper *Designed to Care*, published in December 1997.[22] It also announced two further initiatives: first, a Nursing and Midwifery Practice Development Unit (NMPDU) to encourage networking and the sharing of good practice in nursing and midwifery; and second, a Scottish Health Technology Assessment Centre to evaluate and provide advice to the NHS on the clinical and cost effectiveness of new and existing health technologies, including medicines, devices, clinical procedures and health care settings. After consultation, a Health Technology Board for Scotland (HTBS) was established with this remit in April 2000.

HTBS has developed a process for undertaking each year a number of health technology assessments – comprehensive, systematic evaluations of the assumptions for, and consequences of, the application of health technology – which include close consultation with NHSScotland, patients, the public and other interested parties (including where appropriate the pharmaceutical industry).[23] These lead to the publication of a report summarising the evidence relating to the clinical and cost effectiveness of the health technology and providing advice on value for money. In addition, HTBS has provided a Scottish commentary and guides for patients and carers on the advice on new drugs issued by its counterpart in England and Wales, the National Institute for Clinical Excellence.

Clinical Governance

HTBS filled one of the gaps in a comprehensive national framework for quality improvement in NHSScotland; and the role of CSBS is to check that the tools that are now available to NHSScotland are being used to improve the quality of care and treatment being provided. At local level too steps have been taken to ensure that this is happening. *Designed to Care* announced the introduction of clinical governance, defined as 'corporate accountability for clinical performance', and this was given legislative force by the Health Act 1999 that imposed upon the board of each NHS body in Scotland a statutory duty to monitor and improve the quality of the healthcare it provides.[24] This duty in effect made clinical effectiveness **mandatory,** in the sense that it was no longer a voluntary or optional activity but a requirement on every part of the NHS and everyone who works in it; **mainstream,** in that it was to be a core activity for organisations and individuals; and **managed**, by being targeted on the priorities of the NHS, planned and resourced.

Each NHS Trust and Island NHS Board was to establish a Clinical Governance Committee, chaired by a non-executive Trustee, to monitor implementation of clinical governance, akin to the role played in financial and corporate governance matters by the Audit Committee.[25] At national level the CSBS' generic standards in effect became clinical governance standards and were to be subject to annual review, the first national and local reports being published in April 2002.[26]

Our National Health

The developments of 1999/2000 represented a further milestone in the history of clinical effectiveness in Scotland. While they retained many of the characteristics of earlier initiatives, there was also a significant shift in emphasis. The importance of professional ownership was still emphasised but it was now coupled with a much more explicit and proactive role for managers and with increasing political interest in its results. This was confirmed in the Scottish Executive's first Health Plan, *Our National Health*, published in December 2000.[27] It laid great emphasis on the setting and monitoring of national clinical standards for NHSScotland, and extended the remit of CSBS to include service standards on food, cleanliness, infection control and other matters. It also announced the development of a new performance and accountability framework with clinical quality as one of its core elements and into which CSBS reports would be a major input; and the intention to strengthen significantly patient and public involvement in all aspects of healthcare.

NHS Quality Improvement Scotland

Shortly after devolution, the Scottish Executive commissioned a report on Scotland's leading edge work on clinical quality. This recorded the range of initiatives that had been taken and the significant progress that was being made.[28] The number of different groups involved, however, was felt to be creating problems in terms of dissipation of energy and effort and overlapping responsibilities. *Our National Health*, therefore, announced that the Chief Medical Officer, Dr Mac Armstrong, would undertake a review to achieve better integration and co-ordination of those national organisations and professional bodies with an interest in clinical quality. As a first step, a mapping exercise was undertaken to identify relationships among the organisations and any gaps or overlaps. This confirmed that, despite considerable informal collaborative effort, there was a lack of cohesion in this field. NHSScotland was confused by multiple priorities and felt overburdened by an increasing number of review visits from different organisations with overlapping information requirements.

This assessment, and a round of discussions led by Dr Armstrong led to the production of a consultation paper in March 2002 recommending the establishment of a new special health board, NHS Quality Improvement Scotland.[29] Bringing together CRAG, CSBS, HTBS, SHAS and NMPDU, it was to be responsible for developing and delivering a co-ordinated strategy for improving clinical effectiveness and the quality of patient care. After formal consultation, the Executive announced in August 2002 its intention to proceed with the establishment of the new Board, to come into existence in January 2003.[30] In addition to continuing the functions of the merging organisations, the Board will have significant additional responsibilities including supporting the introduction of clinical governance locally, undertaking investigations into serious clinical service failures at the request of the Minister for Health and Community Care or on its own initiative, and linking with the English-based National Patient Safety Agency. The Board will also take over CRAG's role in commissioning guidelines from SIGN.

Distinctive Features of the Scottish Approach

Most of the developments outlined in this chapter have their equivalents in other parts of the UK. Scotland, however, is generally regarded as being ahead of its neighbours and to have pursued a distinctive approach.

The main difference lies in the extent of clinical leadership and clinical ownership of the initiatives that have been taken. North and south of the border the roles of successive CMOs have been crucial; but in Scotland they have been accorded greater freedom to shape and deliver the agenda. CRAG has been chaired by four CMOs during the 13 years of its existence, each of whom has used it as a major vehicle for delivering a clinical agenda which to a large extent he has moulded. Similarly, the creation of CSBS was the result of a CMO chaired initiative, the Acute Services Review. Within this context, great stress has been laid upon winning and sustaining clinical ownership of the developments that have occurred. Political and managerial support has of course been required but the emphasis, at least initially, has been on securing clinical 'buy-in'.

This approach has been facilitated by the relatively small size of Scotland. This encourages a real sense of family or community within the NHS, reinforced by shared training and work experience; and it has produced a relatively small cadre of leaders – in the NHS, in the civil service and in Scotland's universities. A further factor helping to strengthen the sense of community has been the strong public sector ethos and the relative insignificance of the private health care sector.

These factors have made it easier to undertake initiatives and have influenced their character significantly. Two examples illustrate this very clearly. First, the decision in 1993 to publish the clinical outcome indicators rather than to restrict circulation to medical networks, was taken with the active support not only of the Colleges but also of the BMA (somewhat to the alarm of their colleagues elsewhere in the UK). Second, although CSBS and HTBS have equivalents in England – the Commission for Health Improvement and the National Institute for Clinical Excellence – there are major differences in the way in which they operate. Both CHI and CSBS are chaired by distinguished doctors; but CSBS has been allowed to develop an approach that is much more in tune with health care professionals. In particular, its standards-based approach and its condition-specific reviews have received enthusiastic endorsement. CSBS has also been allowed to develop without direct political intervention. Ministers have been supportive of its work but they have not put CSBS under overt pressure to deliver immediate results and, very significantly, they have eschewed the language of 'naming and shaming' or the use of league tables. In contrast, CHI has attracted intense political interest at the highest levels in England and its clinical governance reviews have been developed in tandem with Ministerially directed 'star ratings'.

A similar difference in emphasis is apparent in the case of HTBS and its English counterpart, NICE. NICE's agenda is much more politically driven and it has been less able to develop a methodology that is acceptable to both the NHS and to the pharmaceutical industry.

This is an area therefore in which useful comparisons can be drawn. Governments north and south of the border have similar aims – reassuring the public and improving the quality of health care – and have put in place mechanisms that have many common features. However there have also been significant differences in approach and context, not only since 1998 but also in the changes that are being introduced in 2002/03 to strengthen the scope and powers of the bodies responsible for inspecting and monitoring quality.[31]

Challenges Ahead

In many respects, Scotland's record in clinical effectiveness is impressive. NHS Quality Improvement Scotland has solid foundations upon which to build but the scale and challenge of its agenda should not be underestimated.

There are good reasons why the development of an overarching strategy for clinical quality has eluded its predecessors: in part historical, reflecting the stage in development of these activities, but also the inherent difficulty of the task. Such a strategy will also present challenges to everyone affected by it. Government, managers and clinicians will be bound publicly by the priorities it sets and their freedom of manoeuvre will thus be circumscribed. And the public will find the NHS less amenable to pressure.

Equally, bringing together a diverse range of bodies, each of which has developed an organisational culture appropriate to its specific task, will require careful handling if the strengths of each is not to be lost in a mix that is characterised by the lowest common denominator of all; and the task of integration is to be achieved at the same time as new functions such as patient safety and the conduct of investigations into serious clinical failures are to be added. Moreover, while the merging of organisations will reduce some duplication of effort, other boundaries remain, for example with the standards and associated visits connected with professional education and training, and with parallel developments that are occurring in connection with complementary services provided by local authorities and the private sector.

While these tasks are being addressed, there are various major challenges that affect all the new Board's activities. First, although Scotland's information systems compare favourably with others, there are still major gaps in the ability to monitor clinical effectiveness and the quality of care on a consistent basis across the NHS. There is a real challenge to define what data are needed – for the delivery of clinical practice itself as well as for monitoring – and to put in place systems that will capture these data consistently and cost-effectively across Scotland, if not further afield, so as to allow appropriate comparative assessments to be made.

One aspect of this challenge is to ensure that the whole patient journey of care is captured. Despite the advances of recent years, clinical practice is usually divided into episodes of care. Seamless care with linked data across journeys of care and records that move with patients has been an objective for many years but all too frequently is still no more than an aspiration.

Next, although an encouraging start has been made with patient and public involvement, it is no more than a start.[32] Greater clarity is required about the role of lay people in the clinical quality agenda so that appropriate recruitment and support mechanisms can be put in place to enable them to deliver it. There is also a need to determine how patient and public views can be deployed both in setting standards and reviewing performance alongside increasingly scientific clinical evidence.

Better information will allow the performance of the NHS to be assessed more effectively. But it is only a means to other ends. It will demonstrate much more clearly the quality of clinical care over time, in different parts of Scotland, and between Scotland and other similar countries. Already the issues of 'postcode prescribing' and 'the lottery of care' are generating a considerable amount of political debate. The tools that have been developed and are in prospect will enable politicians and managers to target resources much more effectively than previously to address gaps in service provision and areas where standards fall short of what is required. This has major implications for them and for patients and the public by making explicit choices that in the past have generally been avoided.

For those who run the NHS, it is likely to result in greater central direction of resource allocation as additional money is targeted on particular problems that have been identified. For individual patients, it will allow informed decisions to be made whether and where to obtain treatment; and for communities it will encourage and strengthen campaigning to secure equity with standards being achieved elsewhere. For the NHS to cope with pressures such as these, requires an ability to manage expectations and a mature response on the part of the media that have not generally been apparent in the first 50 years of its existence.

Finally, although the NHS still spends much less on quality assurance and related processes than most other organisations of its size and complexity, it is nonetheless essential that these activities are themselves subject to rigorous evaluation to demonstrate that money being spent this way rather than on direct patient care is producing measurable benefits for patients. Moreover, the political stakes have risen significantly as a result of the substantial increases in NHS funding in recent years. Ministers attach great importance to these processes as means both of ensuring that the NHS delivers promised improvements in patient care, and of demonstrating that the principles on which the NHS has been based since 1948 remain valid for the 21st century.

Note: This chapter was written in mid-2002.

REFERENCES

1.   *Designed to Care: Renewing the National Health Service in Scotland.* Cm 3811. London: HMSO, 1997, page 4.

2.   *NHS Management Inquiry.* London: DHSS, 1983.

3.   *The SCOTMEG Portfolio 1985–1995: A Compendium Report.* Edinburgh: SCOTMEG, 1996.

4.   *The History and Development of CRAG.* CRAG website: www.show.scot.nhs.uk/crag

5.   *Working for Patients.* Cm 555. London : HMSO, 1989.

6.   op.cit. p39.

7.   *Strategic Framework for Clinical Audit in Scotland.* Edinburgh: CRAG, 1995.

8.   *Review of CRAG.* Edinburgh: CRAG, 1998.

9.   For example – the Thomson Report: *The Interface between Clinical Audit and Management.* Edinburgh: CRAG, 1993 and *Goals for Clinical Effectiveness*, issued by CRAG from 1996–1999.

10.   SIGN's methodology is outlined in *SIGN 50: A Guideline Developers' Handbook.* Edinburgh: SIGN, 2001 (updated 2002).

11.   *Clinical Outcome Measures.* Edinburgh: CRAG, 1992.

12.   The most recent report is *Clinical Outcome Indicators.* Edinburgh: CRAG, 2002, which includes a summary of all the indicators published.

13.   *The Patient's Charter: A Charter for Health.* Edinburgh: Scottish Office, 1991.

14.   *Framework for Action.* Edinburgh: Scottish Office, 1991.

15.   *Framework for Action Improving Health Care: A Guide.* Edinburgh: Scottish Office, 1992.

16.   *Clinical Effectiveness. Common Core Work Programme.* MEL (1995) 84 and MEL (1997) 26. Edinburgh: Scottish Office, 1995 and 1997.

17.   *Review of CRAG.* Edinburgh: CRAG, 1998.

18.   *The Scottish Health Service: Ready for the Future.* Cm 3551. London: HMSO, 1997.

19.   *Acute Services Review Report.* Edinburgh: HMSO, 1998, chapter 8.

20.   CSBS' methodology and its record in its first three years are outlined in its *Annual Report 2001/02.* Edinburgh: CSBS, 2002.

21.   *Improving Clinical Care in Scotland – Generic Clinical Governance Standards: National Overview.* Edinburgh: CSBS, 2000.

22.   *Designed to Care: Renewing the National Health Service in Scotland.* Cm 3811. London: HMSO, 1997.

23.   HTBS' methodology and its record in its first two years are outlined in its *Annual Report 2001/02.* Glasgow: HTBS, 2002.

24.   *Health Act 1999*, section 51.

25.   *Clinical Governance.* MEL (1998) 75 and MEL (2000) 29. Edinburgh: Scottish Office/Executive, 1998 and 2000.

26.   *Improving Clinical Care in Scotland – Generic Clinical Governance Standards: National Overview.* Edinburgh: CSBS, 2002.

27.   *Our National Health: A Plan for Action, A Plan for Change.* Edinburgh: Scottish Executive, 2000.

28.   *A Focus on Quality: Improving Health Care in Scotland.* Edinburgh: Scottish Executive, 2000.

29.   *A Quality and Standards Board for Health in Scotland:* Consultation Paper. Edinburgh: Scottish Executive, 2002.

30.   *Quality and Standards Board for Health in Scotland: Response to the Consultation Process.* Edinburgh: Scottish Executive, 2002.

31.   In England and Wales, a new body – the Commission for Healthcare Audit and Inspection – is to be established incorporating CHI, the value for money work of the Audit Commission, and the private sector inspectorate role of the National Care Standards Commission.

32.   *Patient Focus and Public Involvement.* Edinburgh: Scottish Executive, 2001.

11. The Scottish Health Service Workforce

Graham Buckley

Introduction

Scotland has a long and distinctive tradition within the United Kingdom in its arrangements for educational provision and management. An important consequence has been the role of Scotland as a supplier of trained professionals to the rest of the United Kingdom. For medicine and dentistry, an illustration of this distinctive history, was the Scottish Council for Postgraduate Medical Education (SCPME). It was established in 1970 as a non-statutory body following the Royal Commission on Medical Education (the Todd Report). In addition to serving as a forum, it had responsibility for regional postgraduate education committees (each led by a Postgraduate Medical Dean or Director), and used working groups to address specific educational issues. In 1972 SCPME assumed responsibility for postgraduate dental education (becoming SCPMDE). After review in 1991 by an Advisory Group chaired by the then Chief Medical Officer for Scotland, Sir Kenneth Calman, SCPMDE was strengthened so that it could carry out executive as well as advisory functions. Accordingly, it became a Special Health Board in 1993 with responsibility for the entire budget for all doctors and dentists in training (in contrast to the situation in England where only 50 % of the funding was so transferred). In 1998 SCPMDE's financial responsibilities were extended to the funding of general practice vocational training components, and in 1999 its remit was extended to the training of clinical psychologists.

Although quinquennial review in 2000/2001 gave strong endorsement to SCPMDE as a well managed, efficiently run and cohesive organisation, a new Special Health Board, NHS Education for Scotland, was brought into being on 1 April 2002. The objective was to extend the management of postgraduate/ post-qualification training and education by combining SCPMDE with the National Board for Nursing, Midwifery and Health Visiting, and the Post Qualification Education Board for Pharmacists. This new Board has the ambitious task of promoting the education, training, and continuing development of all NHSScotland staff. There is no equivalent body in the rest of the United Kingdom.

Scope of this chapter

This overview of the healthcare workforce in Scotland will focus on staff employed within NHSScotland in five main professional groups – Dentistry, Clinical Psychology, Medicine, Nursing, and Midwifery. Nursing and Midwifery will be covered under one heading since they have traditionally been considered together in workforce analysis. Many other professional groupings are of course also involved in delivering services – notably the Allied Health Professions and the large number of support workers. Health care professionals working in Social Work Departments and in the independent sector also make significant contributions but detailed information on these groups is difficult to capture in a uniform and systematic way.

For all the health professions NHSScotland is the main employer. Through the annual Information Services Division (ISD) census of employed staff and targeted enquiries, it is possible to discern the general trends and specific workforce pressures that impact on health care provision. Comparing and contrasting the changes occurring in the four professional groups chosen for analysis over the past decade will highlight the interaction between policies, labour markets, demography, and regulation in shaping the composition of the NHSScotland workforce.

Basic statistics

The headline figures for the NHSScotland workforce are set out in Table 11.1. They indicate an apparent stability in the composition and size of the workforce. Increases in medicine and in the allied health professions have been offset by reductions in ancillary workers because of contracting out of domestic services. Examination of particular groups of staff in more detail reveals that there have been significant shifts within professions. There was, for example, a doubling of the number of nurses working within general medical practices in the 1990s. In medicine all of the increase over this decade occurred in hospital practice. The number of general medical practitioners remained constant with the figure for whole time equivalents probably falling. The word probably is important. The interpretation of workforce data requires the detailed knowledge of practitioners within each professional group to provide the appropriate understanding of context and complexity. The four professional groups analysed have been chosen because there has been recent work published with practitioner participation in the review of workforce data.

In spite of these caveats, the overall figures do show remarkable stability in the NHSScotland workforce. At one level this is not surprising since health services are labour-intensive with over 70% of health care spending devoted to salaries. Constraints on total health spending are consequently experienced as constraints on workforce expansion. Similarly, although there have been many aspirations expressed about service re-design, involving changes in skillmix and in professional roles, regulatory and employment constraints make the UK health service one of the more conservative of the developed countries with respect to this kind of innovation. The major changes that have occurred in the work of nurses working in general medical practice reinforce this basic message as they operate outside the employment framework of other NHS nurses.

TABLE 11.1 National trends

Scotland	1990		1995		2000	
	Headcount	*WTE*	*Headcount*	*WTE*	*Headcount*	*WTE*
All staff	135 751	111 993	138 002	114 110	136 167	113 144
Medical	10 908	9 852	1 175	10 597	12 777	11 557
Dental	2 321	2 156	2 486	2 355	2 687	2 539
Nursing & Midwifery	63 144	52 284	63 273	52 416	61 464	51 228
Scientific & Professional	1 216	1 159	1 565	1 462	1 907	1 718
Allied Health Professions	5 694	4 733	7 171	5 919	8 560	7 014

SOURCE: ISD Scotland

Dentistry

Dentistry has been selected as the first case study because it provides a well-defined, relatively simple, and largely uni-professional context to explore issues of importance and relevance to the rest of the complex healthcare system in Scotland. The focus of analysis is on the 2500 dentists working in Scotland, recognising that they are supported by a range of staff in the professions complementary to dentistry (PCD): dental hygienists, dental therapists, dental nurses, and dental technicians. Information is not routinely gathered for these professional groups or for the receptionists and practice managers but it is estimated that there are around 5000 such staff in Scotland working in over 1000 different practice and hospital locations.

An increasing workforce?

Figure 11.1 illustrates the steady rise in the number of dentists working in Scotland over the past decade: CDS refers to dentists in the community dental service and GDS includes all the dentists working as general dental practitioners. Almost all of this increase has occurred in general dental practice (337) reflecting the fact that three-quarters of all dentists work in this sector. The steady increase in the number of dentists contracted to the NHS in Scotland has occurred during a period of major fluctuations in the supply of Scottish dental graduates, policy shifts in the details of pension and remuneration packages, major changes in the oral health of the population, and increasing demand for dental services.

Figure 11.1 Trend in the number of NHS Scotland dentists

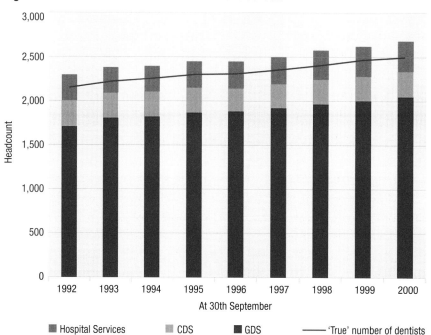

The total financial NHS resource devoted to dental services was tightly constrained during the 1990s. One consequence of this has been major growth in the amount of non-NHS dental care. The true extent of this provision is difficult to quantify but at one level it can be gauged from the fact that the proportion of dentists providing more than a 75% commitment to the NHS fell from 70% to 50% over the decade.

During the 1990s the percentage of female general dental practitioners rose from 26% to 33%. This trend is likely to continue as the percentage of women graduating from the Dental Schools in Scotland has risen to 60% of the total output compared with the UK figure of 50%. Numerous studies have shown that many female dentists choose to work on a less than full-time basis. The impact of this feminisation of the dental workforce is examined further later in this section.

Consequently, although the headcount for general dental practitioners rose by 20%, the combination of an increase in non-NHS work and more part-time working suggests that whole-time equivalence for general dental practice in the NHS in Scotland has at best remained static during a period of sustained increase in demand.

Reviews of the dental workforce carried out on a United Kingdom basis in the 1980s indicated a likely surplus of dental graduates and led to reductions in student intake of 10% which resulted in the closure of three dental schools. One of these was the University of Edinburgh Dental School. From a peak of 159 Scottish dental graduates in 1987, output from the Scottish dental schools fell to 66 in 1994 rising to 125 in 1999. These reductions were based on false assumptions about fluoridation of the water supply and improved oral health. Part of an analysis of recruitment and retention of dentists for NHSScotland from 1993-2000 is shown in Table 11.2. The relatively low percentage contribution of recent Scottish graduates to the total is of interest. It reveals why the reductions in output from the dental schools did not immediately impact significantly on the workforce. Potential shortfalls can in the short term be compensated for by recruitment from within an active UK market and by attracting more returners back into work. Table 11.3 focuses on general dental practitioners and also shows wide variation in the contribution to total recruitment by the different categories of joiners. The information on leavers below the age of 55 years illustrates the dynamic nature of the dental workforce with an average net outflow of 60 per year. This dynamism and net outflow is of considerable interest. Scotland has traditionally been a net exporter of trained health care professionals. This has been particularly true for dentists and has led to a sense of security and comfort regarding recruitment within senior management in the health service. Has the cushion of excess supply now gone? The next section looks at the factors impacting on the need and demand for dentists in Scotland and current evidence to support future workforce modelling.

TABLE 11.2 Scottish Dental Workforce – Leavers and Joiners: Summary 1993 – 2000

	Annual number			
	Average	*Minimum*	*Maximum*	*%*
Leavers from NHS Scotland	**152**	**135**	**158**	**100%**
Aged <55	121	107	129	79%
Aged 55+	31	26	39	21%
Joiners to NHS Scotland	**195**	**177**	**210**	**100%**
Returner	60	46	73	31%
Scottish recent graduate[*]	79	13	117	40%
Other UK graduate[*]	10	4	15	5%
Overseas joiner	15	10	18	7%
Other joiner UK qualified	16	9	27	8%
Other joiner – unknown	16	2	89	8%

[*] Graduated in previous three years

TABLE 11.3 Summary of leavers and joiners from/to General Dental PractitionerWorkforce in Scotland 1994 – 2000

| | Annual number | | | |
	Average	Minimum	Maximum	%
Leavers	**94**	**73**	**110**	**100%**
Left NHSScotland <55	61	53	68	65%
Left NHSScotland 55+	20	11	26	21%
Left to other sector	13	7	17	14%
Joiners	**126**	**100**	**142**	**100%**
Joiner from VT	58	53	63	44%
Joiner from other sector	10	6	15	11%
Returners	41	26	48	34%
New – UK	12	6	18	13%
New – Overseas	4	1	7	5%

TABLE 11.4 Factors influencing the supply and demand for dental services

Demand Factors	Estimated Effect on Demand
Trend of increased demand for all health services	Increased demand
Increasing proportion of the elderly in the population	Increased demand
Increasing number of individuals who have natural teeth	Increased demand
Increase average of retained natural teeth	Increased demand
Increasing number of more complex treatments available	Increased demand
Increasing public expectations of dental treatments/services	Increased demand
Increasing proportion of children with untreated decay	Increased demand
Reduction in oral disease	Reduced demand
Technological	Increase/Reduction

TABLE 11.4 (continued)

Supply Factors	Estimated Effect on Supply
Predicted decline in numbers of registered dentists	Reduction in supply
Increased early retirements	Reduction in supply
Increased part-time working	Reduction in supply
Increased proportion of women in dental workforce	Reduction in supply
Reduction of UK dental graduates	Reduction in supply
Loss of dental workforce to other countries	Reduction in supply
Increase in non-NHS working	Reduction in supply
Working time directives, conditions of service, eg. maternity leave	Reduction in supply
Dissatisfaction with working conditions	Reduction in supply
Lack of PCDs	Reduction in supply
Reduction in number of hygienists being trained	Reduction in supply
Lack of funding for PCD training	Reduction in supply

Increasing demand

Within the broad context of workforce development for the whole of dental services, it is possible to identify the factors influencing the need for dentists over the next 10 to 20 years: (Table 11.4). The most significant is the increase in demand for dental services. This flows from an increase in the number of adults in the population who still have teeth and the linked increase in public awareness of what Scottish dentists can provide. It seems incredible that in 1972 only 56% of the adult population had any teeth and over the age of 65 years only 14% had any teeth remaining. A national survey carried out in 1998 showed that major changes have occurred. There are now one million more people in Scotland who require regular dental treatment than there were in 1972. In spite of the undoubted improvements in oral health, evidence of unmet need for dental care in Scotland is strong. The only evidence-based factor with the potential to reduce significantly the demand for dental services through prevention of disease is water fluoridation. A clearer example of the direct relationship between politics, health care policy and workforce planning would be hard to find.

In the 1990s the closure of the University of Edinburgh Dental School, an increase in early retirements, more part-time work, and more non-NHS working combined to reduce the availability of dentists to NHSScotland. The increase in part-time working is linked to the increasing number of women in dentistry. Women make up two-thirds of the total increase in the number of dentists in Scotland between 1990 and 2000. The ratio of females to males at entry to dental school is now 6:4. More women dentists than men work part-time and many take career breaks when they have young children. The feminisation of the dental workforce is linked to an apparent decrease in overall geographical mobility of dentists. This phenomenon is not solely a result of the gender change in the composition of the workforce and is observed in other professional groups. Problems in the recruitment of dentists mount with increasing distance from main urban centres.

Although almost all direct dental care is provided by dentists, significant hands-on services are delivered by dental hygienists. It is estimated that about 360 hygienists are working in Scotland. Until recently, there has been no central planning or funding for their two-year training course. There has been a similar lack of central planning for the training of dental therapists. Consequently, there has been a decline of 30% over the past five years in the output of trained hygienists and there are only a handful of dental therapists in Scotland. Reduction in supply and poor career structures mean that these groups are not yet playing the role they could in improving oral health. Dentists are still carrying out tasks that should be undertaken by hygienists and therapists.

There is similar lack of planning in the training and recruitment of dental nurses. Local and ad hoc arrangements have led to concerns about the levels of competence of this staff group. This is important in itself but also impacts on the efficiency and effectiveness of dentists.

In combination, the above factors raise questions about the ability of Scotland to provide high standards of dental care for the whole of its population. Incorporating these factors and historical trends in the dental workforce into a modelling exercise to predict future numbers of dentists suggests that Scotland has reached a turning point. From the expensive but comfortable position of being a provider of qualified dentists to the rest of the UK, NHSScotland is now struggling to meet the demand for dental care. If reliance on attracting dentists from outside Scotland is to be avoided, measures are needed to improve retention of Scottish graduates in Scotland and increase the number of returners after career breaks. Simply increasing the number of dental students will not necessarily solve the problem. Increasing the number of postgraduate vocational training opportunities in Scotland is likely to be more effective as current evidence shows that almost 80% of the dentists completing postgraduate vocational training or general professional training (GPT) remain in the NHSScotland workforce. There is also evidence that many of these dentists wish to remain close to their training practices. This can have a beneficial effect on the even distribution of dentists around Scotland through appointing rural dentists as trainers. Scotland has led the UK in implementing GPT. A relatively modest increase in the number of places could be the best way of ensuring adequate numbers of dentists in Scotland in the future. The short duration of GPT at two years provides a mechanism for fine tuning supply without undue delay in response to changes in demand. Long lead times in training make effective responses to shifts in demand almost impossible.

This exploration of workforce issues in dentistry has highlighted the following issues which will be examined further in relation to the other professions:

- Scotland recruiting within an active UK labour market

- Increasing and changing patterns of demand for services

- Feminisation of the workforce

- Increasing significance of the private sector

- Public policy impacting directly on health

- The need for improved workforce planning

- Evidence base for policy developments.

Clinical Psychology

Clinical and other applied psychologists constitute a maturing profession. This is in contrast to dentistry in the sense that there is a secure public understanding of the work undertaken by dentists. Almost everyone comes into contact with dentists at some stage in their lives. Although there are continuing technical developments in dentistry, the range of interventions provided by dentists and the context in which they work are familiar to us. Psychologists contribute to all aspects of health care but, as yet, in small numbers. They assess, formulate, intervene, and advise in helping patients who have psychological problems using a bio-psycho-social model of health. However, as yet, there is no simple shared view amongst the public, health service managers, or other clinicians about the future role of psychologists in NHSScotland.

Supply and Demand

Clinical psychologists make up more the 95% of the total number of applied psychologists in the NHS. Formal postgraduate training in clinical psychology started in Scotland in the 1960s in the Universities of Edinburgh and Glasgow with an intake of two or three diploma 'probationers' to each of the two-year courses. Although there has been a significant increase in the numbers in training from such slender beginnings, Scotland has not kept pace with England and Wales in the rate of expansion (Table 11.5).

TABLE 11.5 Training for Clinical Psychology

	England and Wales	Scotland
1996	262	27
1997	281	33
1998	313	33
1999	346	32
2000	381	32
2001	402	32

The demand for trained psychologists outstrips supply. Detailed evidence gathered in 1998 suggested a minimum of 44 (13%) posts had been vacant in Scotland for more than three months. This service demand for psychologists is being driven by patient demand. Of the six 'closed' waiting lists identified by the Scottish Executive in 2001, three were for psychology services. This increase in demand reflects growing recognition and awareness of the psychological dimensions of health and evidence of the benefits of psychological interventions. This evidence is strong across the whole spectrum of health care including the treatment of people with cancer and those affected by chronic illnesses such as diabetes. At present over three-quarters of qualified clinical psychologists work in the traditional areas of adult mental health (including direct referrals from primary care), learning disabilities, and the care of children. The contributions of psychologists in other areas of care are at such a low level as to make the service vulnerable. In 2001, for example, there were only 2.2 whole-time equivalent qualified psychologists in the whole of NHSScotland specialising in the care of people with cancer.

A raft of policy statements and Scottish Executive Health Department initiatives, ranging from *Our National Health* to the *Framework for Mental Health*, all point to the need for more capacity for psychological interventions in promoting the health and wellbeing of patients across the lifespan. The 'Joint Future' agenda emphasises the wide range of settings where these health care interventions need to be delivered.

All health professionals have a part to play in contributing to the psychological health of patients. The role of trained psychologists includes direct work with patients who have complex psychological disorders and the support of colleagues in other health professions who also provide psychological services. The balance between providing direct patient care and advising other practitioners varies with the context, the area of care and, paradoxically, with level of demand. The immediate pressure of long waiting lists often means that psychologists find it difficult to free up the time needed to work creatively with others in establishing a more strategic approach to service provision and re-design.

Workforce Planning

The current position for clinical psychology can be viewed as a failure in workforce planning. Belated recognition of service needs for their services has now resulted in a commitment to double training numbers over the next three years with a view to doubling the qualified psychologist workforce by 2010.

Why has this serious under-supply of one professional group occurred in Scotland? Similar shortages were recognised earlier in England. There the expansion in training numbers began in 1996 and has been maintained as the output has not yet matched service needs. The reason for inactivity in Scotland appears to have been the difficulty experienced by a small professional group in influencing policy decisions. Qualified clinical psychologists constitute less than 0.4% of the NHSScotland workforce. For the postgraduate course in clinical psychology decisions on training numbers take place within the Health Department of the Scottish Executive. Devolution has made a significant difference in this decision-making process. Debate within the Scottish Parliament highlighting significant gaps in the provision of psychological services has provided a new counterbalance in the competition for new resources. Health Boards and the big battalions of the nurses and doctors in their submissions to the Health Department have not until now given a high priority to the psychological dimensions of health.

Career Structure

Shortages in the supply of psychologists in the 1990s have had a distorting effect on career structures and in the distribution of staff. Undergraduates are actively advised against considering a career in clinical psychology because of barriers to training. Nonetheless, the availability of large numbers of Scottish graduates with good first degrees in psychology, who are motivated to work in the field of health care, makes it easy to recruit unqualified staff to poorly paid positions as Assistant Psychologists. Typically, they work at this level for at least two years while applying for clinical training. Indeed time served as an Assistant is virtually a pre-requisite for entry to postgraduate training. Individuals in this phase lasting one or two years have no guarantee of career progression. Assistant Psychologists are vulnerable to exploitation and this route of entry to the profession is having a significant effect on the way a career in the NHS is being perceived by undergraduates. This could contribute to the fact that 90% of the intake to postgraduate training are women.

Shortages in the supply of qualified clinical psychologists have resulted in the rapid promotion of relatively junior and inexperienced staff, so truncating the planned career structure of A and B grades. A second impact has been the exaggerated effect in clinical psychology of more general geographical recruitment patterns. Qualified psychologists can pick and choose from a large pool of vacant posts and choose to remain close to their training base in either Edinburgh or Glasgow.

Other centres that have managed to establish a critical number of psychologists are holding their own in recruiting staff but the picture elsewhere is poor. The consequent patchy nature of service provision across Scotland is fuelling demands to create training opportunities away from the Central Belt.

Regulation and Competence

The form of postgraduate training for Clinical Psychology is unusual in that the trainees are both NHS employees and full-time students who are required to undertake research as a core element of the course. Research awareness and understanding of research methods are required by other professions. It is the nature of the research participation during the three-year course in Clinical Psychology that is being questioned. This raises an issue of central importance in workforce development in the NHS: who defines the competence and fitness for purpose of practitioners at entry to the service? As for other professions, Universities determine fitness for award subject to the inspection and approval of professional bodies, in this case The British Psychological Society. The NHS until now has been a passive recipient of graduates, largely because of the difficulty it has had in articulating the competencies required to deliver a service. There are signs that this is changing with the setting of occupational standards across a wide range of clinical services. One body being set up to do this, Skills for Health, is doing so on a UK basis. As NHSScotland develops its own approach to service delivery, will it be possible to have uniform occupational definitions and standards for the whole of the UK? The question of how these will inform the competencies defined by professional regulatory bodies has yet to be resolved.

Additional workforce issues highlighted in this brief analysis of Clinical Psychology are:

- Big P and little p politics in determining numbers in training

- Challenging interface between NHS as commissioners of training and Universities as providers

- Shortages in supply distorting career structures

- Major inequities in provision of services

Medicine

The publication in July 2002 of *Future Practice*, a review of the medical workforce in Scotland commissioned by the Scottish Executive, is timely. This review by Professor John Temple, at the invitation of the Minister for Health, examines the demand and supply of doctors in Scotland in a systematic and wide-ranging fashion. The implications for the future configuration of health services in Scotland are profound. This section will highlight the key findings and recommendations contained in the review report and where appropriate provide a critique. In many ways the workforce patterns in medicine mirror those described for dentistry. The complex professional interrelationships required to deliver comprehensive medical care, however, pose even more formidable challenges. Shortening waiting times for operations, for example, requires adequate numbers of anaesthetists, theatre personnel, and well staffed surgical wards as well as sufficient surgeons. In addition and, in contrast to most dentists and psychologists, doctors function mainly within settings that provide services with 24 hour and 7 day access. Permitted maximum working hours are consequently of major significance in determining the size and distribution of the medical workforce.

International Comparisons

Table 11.6 makes comparisons between the medical workforce figures for Scotland, England, UK and Europe. They show that in UK terms Scotland is relatively well served by doctors. The average figure for European countries needs to be interpreted with caution because of fundamental differences in health care systems and in the definition of 'active' doctors. The table also reveals the considerable contribution that Scotland has made in providing qualified doctors to the rest of the UK. This tradition extends back to the eighteenth century and has had a major cultural and scientific impact on British medicine.

Since the inception of the NHS in 1948, the UK has depended on overseas qualified doctors to maintain its health services. The House of Commons Health Committee reported on the NHS Workforce in England in 2000. It questioned both the strategic and ethical basis of attracting large numbers of overseas qualified doctors and the risk for exploitation of these doctors in the UK. The Committee recommended a step increase in the number of medical students in England.

TABLE 11.6 Medical Workforce : Comparative Parameters

	Scotland	England	UK	Europe
Population:				
Population (2000)	5 115 000	49 997 000	59 756 000	
Population projection to 2020	-1%	+ 8%		
Density Persons per sq km	65	383	246	
Life Expectation at birth – male*	72.6	75.1	74.8	EU Average 74.6
Life Expectation at birth – female*	78.1	80	79.8	EU Average 80.9
Expenditure on health:				
NHS Expenditure per capita (1998/9)	£904	£740	£766	
Public health expenditure as % of GDP:	6.7%	n/a	5.7%	EU Average 6.5%
Medical Workforce:				
Nos doctors (1999) NHS	12 253	92 537	114 059	
Nos doctors per 1000 population (1997)	2.4	1.9	1.9	Many EU countries: around 3.0
Intake to medical schools: 1997:				
Actual intake medical schools	811 **	3 872	5 062	
Intake/100,000 (2000 population)	15.9	7.7	8.5	
2005:				
Expected intake medical schools	811 ***	6 006	7 248	
Intake/1000,000 (2000 population)	15.9	12.0	12.12 *	

* Life expectancy figures are for the period 1997 – 99;

** Excludes the intake to St Andrews University which has been included within the intake to English clinical medical schools;

*** Planned target intake is 772. Actual intake may be higher than the planned intake.

Career Structure

In spite of being a net exporter of doctors, Scotland also depends on doctors who qualified in other countries (Figure 11.2). Many overseas doctors wish to come to this country to train and a significant number remain to contribute to the NHS in career posts. Immigration rules were changed in 2001. Until then it was not possible for overseas qualified doctors to train for General Practice unless they had the right to permanent residence in the UK. The group employed as staff grade doctors give some cause for concern. The career structure in medicine is unusual in retaining qualified doctors within training grades for up to 12 years and in having in effect only two professionally approved career grades: Consultant and Principal in General Practice. Doctors in other career grades of clinical assistant or staff grade are perceived within the profession to be of low status or even worse as failures. A survey of doctors in the staff grade in Scotland in 1997 showed that it is largely made up of male

Figure 11.2   NHS Scotland Medical Staff: Percentage by Country of Qualification

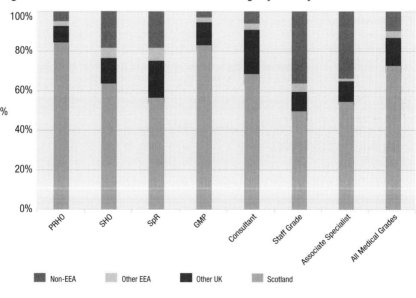

SOURCE: Future Practice. Figures for the year 2000

PRHO = Pre-registration House Officers
SHO = Senior House Officers
SpR = Specialist Registrars
GMP = General Medical Practitioners

overseas qualified doctors who would like to progress to a consultant post and female UK qualified doctors who like their working conditions but would like to have more respect from medical colleagues.

The career structure in medicine is also unusual in that more than half the total hospital medical workforce are doctors in the training grades of Pre-registration House Officer, Senior House Officer, and Specialist Registrar. The average length of this training is 10 years. During this time the training and service demands on the doctors are difficult to keep in balance. The combination of the grades of Registrar and Senior Registrar into that of Specialist Registrar in 1996 was intended to shorten the duration of training. This has not happened but the supervision and planning of training has improved. Training for general practice requires a minimum of four years after qualification. After a serious dip in recruitment in the early 1990s to less than 200 per annum, the output from vocational training for general practice has risen back to 280 per annum. This pattern paralleled the picture in England.

Enough Doctors?

Even when the increase in intake to medical schools in England is fully implemented in 2005, Scotland without any increase will still be producing more doctors pro-rata than England. Will Scotland have enough doctors in 2010 and 2020? *Future practice* does not provide a definitive answer. Instead it examines the factors influencing the demand for doctors, their likely working patterns, and their recruitment and retention.

The crucial factor in increasing the demand for doctors and the one that will drive service re-design and re-configuration is a change in working hours. Medical staff have tried to provide a 24 hour service with a workforce designed for a conventional working day. First line evening, night, and weekend medical cover in hospital has been provided by the least experienced doctors working anything up to 100 hours per week. The intensity and technical demands of modern acute medical practice make this unacceptable but it is the legal force of the European Working Time Directive that will drive significant change over the next five years. Shift working akin to the working arrangements for nurses will become the norm for doctors in all grades in the acute specialties as the move to a 48 hour working week is implemented. Experience in countries elsewhere in the European Union who have already implemented the Directive indicates that the minimum number of doctors required to cover a 24 hours 7 day service is five with seven as the preferred number. All of these doctors require to be competent to work without supervision otherwise the total complement of doctors to run the service is higher. The implications of these basic facts are very serious for the provision of health care in Scotland. Many more doctors will be required. Acute hospital services that currently function with less than seven senior medical staff will either have to recruit more doctors, combine with other units, or redesign the provision of care so that generalists or non-medical staff can provide first line care. As experience in trying to create a new approach to maternity services in Scotland has shown, none of these options will be easy to adopt. It may be assumed that these problems will be confined to the small and remote hospitals but this is not the case. Almost all departments within the district general hospitals in Scotland function at present with less than seven senior medical staff.

Reforms in General Practice

General practice has already tackled the issue of working hours through a radical change in the nature of service provision at night and weekends. In 1990 local and ad hoc duty rotas covering up to three or four practices were the norm for out-of-hours services. Many practices in the urban centres also used commercial deputising services. In 1998, agreement between Government and the profession created the financial and organisational infrastructure to create co-operatives of general practitioners covering wide geographical areas and populations of up to one million. This shift in working patterns has been a success. General practitioners within the areas served by co-operatives have a predictable working week and receive mutual support from each other in handling difficult urgent medical problems. Public acceptance of the new arrangements has been positive. Most people see the benefits of being seen at night by doctors who are not exhausted and who have good immediate backup from a support team. Recruitment of doctors to work in practices not covered by co-operatives is poor. These practices are geographically isolated and the problems of attracting staff to work in remote and rural locations has been exacerbated in general practice because of the increasing contrast in out-of-hours commitments of doctors working in the urban and rural parts of Scotland. Co-operatives in general practice can function because of the inter-changeability of one doctor from another within their medical workforce.

Specialisation

The latter half of the twentieth century can be viewed in medical practice as a period of increasing specialisation. This has been a world-wide phenomenon but, as outlined above, it creates special problems in Scotland because of the uneven distribution of the population. The Acute Services Review undertaken in 1998 proposed the creation of managed clinical networks and intermediate care as ways of tackling this problem.

Remote and rural practice also raises a constitutional issue in the context of devolution. No training programmes approved by UK statutory bodies fully equip doctors to work in primary or secondary care in remote areas. Regulation of the professions is a reserved matter for the Westminster Parliament. This weakens the ability of the Scottish Parliament to decide the way in which it will determine the design and delivery of health services to the whole of the population it serves. The Scottish Council for Postgraduate Medical and Dental Education and now NHS Education for Scotland have provided training opportunities in general practice and in general surgery to help equip doctors who do wish to work in these locations but are hampered in doing so by UK professional regulatory framework.

Reinventing generalism in acute hospital medicine may be one solution. General Medicine is an approved specialty but there are no Specialist Registrars in Scotland who emerge with this as their only accreditation. Instead they acquire dual certification in General Medicine and a sub-specialty such as: Gastroenterology, Respiratory Medicine, or Cardiology. As these dually certificated consultants progress in their careers, their daytime work tends to become exclusively devoted to their sub-specialty. Assuming responsibility at night for the whole range of acute medical problems presenting to hospital becomes increasingly difficult for these doctors. The response from within the medical profession is to seek to create a new specialty of Acute Medicine. This could be a sensible step if service developments and configurations provide predictable career opportunities that would encourage doctors to train for this type of work.

Workforce Planning

At present workforce planning in medicine in Scotland consists of annual requests to NHS Trusts for information on expected vacancies for consultants in each specialty for the next five years. These figures are used to guide the intake into Specialist Registrar training programmes. There are major weaknesses in this arrangement. The average length of training for Specialist Registrars is six years. This is too long for a rapid response to qualitative and quantitative changes in demand for trained staff. Although the implicit policy in Scotland has been to overproduce trained doctors, lack of linkage between output from training programmes and recruitment into consultant posts undermines the value of this strong supply position. Data collected during 2001 suggests that up to 50% of doctors leave Scotland immediately after completing their specialist training, most to work in England.

Retention of general practitioners is less easy to define. Overall there are difficulties in recruitment to Principal posts in general practice. Young doctors are able to pick where and how they wish to work. They are choosing to spend several years in short-term posts before committing themselves to long-term financial and service responsibilities as a partner in a general practice. Accurate figures are difficult to assemble but it is estimated that there are currently about 800 qualified general practitioners who are working as locums in general practice in Scotland. The figures from ISD in Table 11.7 indicate that it may take more than five years from completion of vocational training for general practice for doctors to be appointed as Principals. Only half of the output from the training programmes eventually take up permanent posts in general practice in NHSScotland. The rest are almost equally divided between those who choose to work in hospital or community based specialties in Scotland and those who leave to work in either general practice or in hospital in the rest of the United Kingdom.

TABLE 11.7 Destination of Scottish GP Registrars after training

Destination/ Number years after training	1	3	5	10
GP Principal – Scotland	13%	28%	48%	53%
GP Principal – England/Wales	1%	4%	8%	11%
Hospital Specialties – Scotland	27%	13%	13%	14%
Community/Public Health – Scotland	1%	3%	4%	5%
Non GP Specialties – England/Wales	3%	3%	5%	6%
Unknown	55%	38%	22%	10%

Future Practice recommends more active management of the labour market in medicine and the need for national and regional mechanisms to co-ordinate the supply, demand and distribution of doctors. At present, Scotland can be accused of squandering its advantageous position with regard to the supply of doctors and is consequently suffering shortages in a number of specialties, notably Radiology.

This section has highlighted the following:

- Tensions emerging between UK and Scotland in regulation and planning of medical workforce.

- Special need in Scotland to achieve effective balance between generalist and specialist provision of care by medical workforce.

- Strong supply of doctors not matched by effective retention, resulting in shortages in key areas.

- Increasing vulnerability of recruitment to rural and remote parts of Scotland related to widening gap in working conditions between doctors working in these areas and in urban centres.

Nursing and Midwifery

Although traditionally bracketed together in workforce analysis, nursing and midwifery differ in their history, recruitment patterns and professional ethos. During the 1990s the average age at completion of nurse education rose from 26 in 1992 to over 30 in 2000. In contrast the age of midwives at qualification has remained relatively steady at 27 years. This latter figure has remained stable in spite of the fact that a significant number of midwives first train as nurses. However, direct entry to midwifery education has now risen to 75% and the two professions now appear to be recruiting from rather different populations.

Major changes in the education, composition, and workforce planning of the nursing profession took place in the 1990s. Most of these changes mirrored those taking place in the rest of the UK. One difference has been the lack of reliance in Scotland on the recruitment of overseas qualified nurses. In England it is estimated that there are 22 000 nurse vacancies and overseas recruitment campaigns are taking place to meet this workforce crisis.

Project 2000 dominated the 1990s for both nurses and midwives. Until 1992 students in these professions were NHS employees and were regarded as part of the workforce. Under Project 2000 responsibility for education progressively transferred from the Colleges of Nursing and Midwifery to Higher Education Institutions. By 1996 contracts with seven universities in Scotland had been agreed with the Scottish Executive to provide the three-year courses in nursing or midwifery leading to a diploma and registration with United Kingdom Central Council for Nursing and Midwifery and Health Visiting (UKCC). Students on these courses receive bursaries as full-time students rather than employees. In addition 10% of students undertake four-year degree courses funded through the general Scottish Higher Education Funding Council allocation to Universities. Nurses who wish to become midwives require to complete an 18-month course. There is also a range of one to two-year courses for graduates and enrolled nurses to enable them to become registered nurses with the UKCC (replaced in 2002 by the Nursing and Midwifery Council (NMC)). It is anticipated that 80% of students entering nurse and midwife courses from September 2001 onwards will exit with a Scottish ordinary degree, together with NMC registration.

Table 11.8 shows the number of students in each category in Scotland in 2000/01 and table 11.9 the overall trend for the latter part of the 1990s.

TABLE 11.8 Number Commenced Approved Courses 2000 / 01

3 year course	Shortened course for graduates	Integrated degree course	Conversion courses for registered first level nurses	Conversion courses for registered second level nurses	Total
2604	171	261	83	379	3498

TABLE 11.9 Year end Training Population Summary 1997 – 2001 (effective date 31 March)

	1997	1998	1999	2000	2001
Nursing	6747	7059	7383	7600	8028
Midwifery	595	584	594	606	604

How have these changes in the education profile of nurses and midwives impacted on the workforce in these professions in Scotland?

The first important piece of evidence is that recruitment into nursing and midwifery training remains buoyant. Table 11.10 shows the output from education programmes for the past five years. What these figures do not show is the high dropout rate from nurse education. The average attrition from the three-year diploma courses over the past 10 years has been between 20% and 30%. In October 2000 the Royal College of Nursing carried out a postal survey of 2000 student nurses. This revealed the following reasons for leaving the course:

● Financial hardship 58%

● Dissatisfaction with course 52%

● Dissatisfaction with clinical placements 30%

TABLE 11.10 Completions of Training for 3-year Diploma Courses 1996/7 – 2000/1

Course of Study	Year of completion				
	1996/7	1997/8	1998/9	1999/0	2000/1
Part 12 (Adult Nursing)	1067	965	1070	1156	1084
Part 13 (Mental Health Nursing)	297	269	268	279	248
Part 14 (Learning Disability Nursing)	66	60	42	45	38
Part 15 (Children's Nursing)	87	90	90	102	111
Total	**1517**	**1384**	**1470**	**1582**	**1481**

Similar responses were given to a Unison survey which also revealed that 95% of students took on extra work to supplement their bursaries. The rules on bursaries are a factor in the rise in the average age of nursing student in that a higher rate is paid to students over the age of 26 years on entry to the course.

TABLE 11.11 Destinations of Qualifiers from 3 year Diploma Courses

	1996	1997	1998	1999	2000
Leaving Scotland	140	65	82	138	117
Scottish Independent Health Care	173	103	33	78	108
NHSScotland	1002	684	560	938	720
Seeking Employment as Nurse	207	42	42	107	52
Not Pursuing Nursing Career	43	20	16	13	6
Not Known	394	568	415	508	480
Other	2	17	23	21	24
Total Number of New Qualifiers	**1961**	**1499**	**1171**	**1803**	**1507**

Table 11.11 shows that only 50% of nurses are known to enter NHSScotland on registration. The data set is clearly incomplete but many nurses enter the independent sector and up to 10% leave Scotland. Vacancy rates over the past five years (Table 11.12) can be interpreted to reflect a good recruitment position for NHSScotland. The demand forecast by NHS employers for nurses over the next four years (Figure 11.3) shows a dramatic shift between 2000/1 and 2001/2. Previous confidence in the supply position in Scotland in nursing may not continue. Examining the profile of vacancies in Table 11.12 shows the current pressure points in recruitment. Care of the elderly, mental health, community (including district nursing and health visiting) feature prominently in total vacancies but only learning disability and theatre nursing appear to have long-term vacancies. In contrast to England the use of bank and agency nurses to fill long-term vacancies is limited. A survey by the Accounts Commission in 2000 estimated an annual spend on bank and agency nursing in Scotland in 1997/98 of £25m. Cover for unplanned absences is the most common reported reason for employing an average of 500 such nurses each day in the NHS in Scotland. Marked variations between Trusts suggest differences in management practices.

TABLE 11. 12 National Trend of All Vacancies for Nurse and Midwifes

	1996	1997	1998	1999	2000	2001
Nurses	3.8%	3.8%	3.7%	3.1%	2.7%	3.7%
Midwives	1.9%	1.3%	1.3%	2.1%	1.1%	1.3%
Total Qualified Staff	**3.7%**	**3.6%**	**3.5%**	**3.1%**	**2.6%**	**3.6%**

Figure 11.3   Forecast of NHS Employers' Demand for Nursing and Midwifery in 2000 and 2001

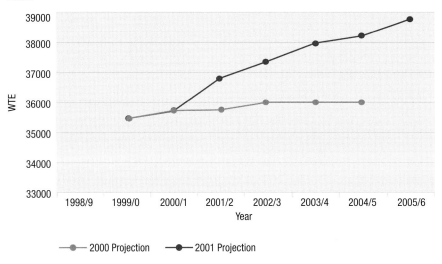

There is an interesting contrast between different sections of the nursing and midwifery professions in part-time working. Almost half the total number of midwives and half the nurses in adult general and in paediatrics work part-time. Less than 20% of nurses in adult mental health and learning disability work part-time. The average contracted hours of part-time staff is 23 hours. These figures have remained stable for the past 10 years, except in midwifery which has seen an increase in part-time working.

In summary, the nursing and midwifery workforce in Scotland in comparison to the rest of the UK is in a healthy state. Increasing demands from the service may test the recruitment capacity of what is now the key target group : women in their mid 20s.

Nursing is by far the largest staff group in the NHS and in absolute terms makes up a significant part of the overall workforce in Scotland. This means that overall demographic shifts in the population will impact on nursing. The Wanless report highlighted this issue for Scotland. A decreasing birth rate and a rise in the percentage of the population who are aged over 75 years is anticipated over the next 20 years. This will increase the demand for nurses in both the NHS and independent sector. At the same time there will be a decrease in the number of potential recruits with many other career options available to young people. The immediate challenge is to make the education or preparation for nursing and midwifery more attractive so that the present attrition rates come into line with other vocational courses. The next area to tackle in a systematic way will be the career structure within both nursing and midwifery. At present career advancement in these professions largely equates to increasing managerial responsibility. Professional leadership through a clinical academic career pathway is beginning to become established through the creation of nurse consultant posts and clinical professorships but as yet there is little overt structure or coherence about this dimension to career development. Many nurses and midwives fund their own higher education with little or no guarantee that this will lead to the opportunity to apply the new skills that they acquire. The publication of *Learning Together* by the Scottish Executive in 1999 was of particular importance for nursing. It signalled the requirement for NHS Trusts and Boards to produce Local Learning Plans to give coherence to the continuing professional development of their staff. As the largest and most diverse group of staff in the NHS nurses are a group with many career opportunities outside the NHS. They will be the touchstone to test whether NHSScotland can compete successfully with other sectors in recruiting and retaining skilled workers and so provide high standards of health care.

The Future

This chapter has looked at the workforce of NHSScotland by concentrating first on two of the smaller professional groups in dentistry and clinical psychology. It has also concentrated on training issues. This has been done as a way of cutting through the complexities encountered in the larger staff groups such as nursing and medicine. Complexity linked to specialist practice is a core problem in the delivery of modern health care. There are 26 separate training pathways in Internal Medicine alone, 12 in Surgery, and there is a multiplicity of Specialist Nursing Qualifications. The trend to specialisation in all sections of the workforce poses special problems in Scotland because of the uneven distribution of its population.

The case studies reveal the reality of a UK market for doctors and dentists, with less mobility for clinical psychologists and nurses. Compared with England the output from pre-registration courses is at a high level for almost all the health professions. Clinical Psychology is an obvious exception as are some of the Allied Health Professions. The reasons for this are the lack of priority given to the smaller professions in allocating funding for their training and the rapidly increasing service demand for qualified staff in these professions. For most of the other professions and staff groups, workforce problems when they occur relate to poor retention and recruitment at a local level. This mainly relates to adverse geographical factors. In a Scottish and UK workforce market health professionals prefer to work in or close to major urban centres.

The report of the Scottish Integrated Workforce Planning Group published in 2000 recommended that patient needs translated into service developments should drive workforce planning in qualitative and quantitative terms. In spite of devolution this has not yet happened. Supply is largely based on historical norms and training programmes conform to the standards and patterns set by UK regulatory bodies. This is in spite of the increasingly distinctive nature of NHSScotland. The plans, announced by the Scottish Executive Health Department, to bring workforce planning and development to the centre of its activities are welcome.

Although the basic statistics on the workforce are reassuring, the demography of Scotland presents a major challenge for the future. Recruitment into NHSScotland will be from a shrinking pool of young adults while demand for services increases with an ageing population. From being a net exporter of trained staff, Scotland may need to be more effective in marketing itself to attract high calibre staff from the rest of the UK and from other countries.

SOURCES

1. *Acute Services Review Report.* Edinburgh: Scottish Office, 1998.

2. Clinical Workforce Planning Group. *Psychology Planning.* Draft Report. Edinburgh: SCPMDE, 2002.

3. Clinical Psychology Workforce Planning Group. *NHS Education for Scotland.* Report. Edinburgh: SCPMDE, 2002.

4. *Facing the Future.* Report of the Convention on Recruitment and Retention in Nursing and Midwifery. Edinburgh: Scottish Executive, 2001.

5. *Future Practice.* A Review of the Scottish Medical Workforce. Edinburgh: Scottish Executive, 2002.

6. Medical Workforce Standing Advisory Committee. *Planning the Medical Workforce.* Second Report. London: Department of Health, 1995.

7. *Securing our future health: taking a long-term view.* The Wanless Report. London : HM Treasury, 2002.

8. *Skillmix Review and Forward Look.* Glasgow: The Royal College of Physicians and Surgeons of Glasgow, 2002.

9. Workforce Planning for Dentistry in Scotland. *A Strategic Review.* Interim Report and Recommendations. Edinburgh: Scottish Executive, 2000.

10. Workforce Planning for Dentistry in Scotland. *Characteristics and Supply Dynamics of the Dental Workforce in Scotland and Projecting Future Supply.* Edinburgh: SCPMDE/ISD Scotland, 2001.

12. The Future for Scotland's Health and Health Services

Kevin Woods and David Carter

In this final chapter we take a look into the future for Scotland's health and its health care services. It is something of a perilous exercise, as the view ahead is clouded by great uncertainties. As the previous chapters have shown, so much has changed over the past 15 years, and often in unexpected ways, that it would be foolhardy to pretend that a chapter such as this can be, in the end, anything other than speculative. On the other hand, there are trends discernible now which will influence the next few years. There have also been a number of measured attempts to identify possible 'futures' or 'scenarios'. The Wanless Review[1] of future funding needs of the health services in the UK, and the Nuffield Trust's *Policy Futures Project* [2] are two recent examples of such studies concerned with health. None of these studies has a specifically Scottish focus, though an attempt has been made to describe *The Possible Scot,*[3] an aspirational study of potential improvements in our national health status.

Does this suggest that the capacity for longer term planning may be a weakness in Scotland's health care sector? The pressures of the moment may make the creation of such a capacity appear to be a luxury that cannot be afforded, but the cost of not doing so may be greater in the future. Without such a perspective how can our political leaders hope to see beyond the next election, and how can the people of Scotland be engaged in the necessary public debate about the priorities for investment and the need for change?

Policy futures

The Nuffield Trust's Report *Policy Futures for UK Health* [2] offers a framework for thinking about these matters. It began by adopting 2015 as its planning horizon, and commissioned technical papers to scan the health policy environment, before subjecting them to wide review and debate. Analyses of trends in disease, society, environment, governance, economics, and industry, generated a series of key issues for policy-makers up to 2015. In summary, these are:

- Rising public expectations

- The ageing population

- Assessing new technologies

- Information and communication technology and information management

- Workforce education and training

- System performance and quality.

Three key conclusions emerged from this analysis, and they are undoubtedly relevant to the Scottish situation. First, health improvement needs a longer term perspective than governments sometimes give it, requiring sustained support across all of their activities, and, in a world of growing globalisation, acknowledgement of the need for international collaboration. The current concern with the health consequences of bio-terrorism and SARS are a chilling illustration of the last point. The hard to quantify threat of Variant CJD, the upward trend in HIV and other bloodborne infections, as well as the return of more traditional diseases, such as tuberculosis, in new virulent forms, demand the attention of many government departments and agencies. Reduction of social and other inequalities in health is likely to be achieved by a mixture of health-based initiatives, fiscal policy and economic performance. This will require skilled inter-government co-ordination and collaboration, involving political leaders at local, Scottish, UK, European, and global levels. In a shrinking world, the health problems of Scotland are neither unique nor will the solutions to them be found entirely within our borders. The challenge is to see our problems in the context of an increasingly inter-connected world.

Secondly, the Nuffield Trust Report raised the awkward question of how to manage public expectations of our health care system and pay for them. The ingenuity of our scientists and technologists in creating new therapeutic opportunities, and our experience of service delivery outside the health care sector, are among the factors that drive public expectations. The 'baby boomers' of postwar Scotland, who have lived all their lives with the NHS are likely to be less tolerant of the care on offer to them in their older age than were their parents, and their children may well question why in a world of round the clock services it remains difficult to access health care when and where they want. The explosion in the availability of information is already changing the doctor-patient relationship, as people arrive in surgeries concerned that the care they receive should be in accordance with the latest research findings posted on a reputable (or not) website. The acceleration in the generation of new knowledge, founded on the largest ever capacity for medically related research makes it increasingly difficult for professionals to remain up-to-date other than by becoming increasingly specialised. These are irresistible forces, but of course they are not new, nor is the principal dilemma that they pose, how to pay for them?

The history of the NHS and the experience of all developed nations is that the capacity to do more technically and the aspirations of the population run ahead of the economy's ability to accommodate them all. This is a particularly pressing problem in the NHS which attempts to be a comprehensive service, universally available throughout the country, and publicly funded from taxation. In reality, it has never achieved this, though it comes close; co-payments are long-established in the form of prescription charges; some forms of care have become largely the preserve of the individual and the private sector – dentistry and optometry being the best examples – and it is comparatively easy to find examples of what has come to be known as the 'postcode lottery' of care where, new technologies (usually drugs), are available to some but not others.

Wanless Review of NHS Funding

The political pressures that flow from this reality led the current UK Government to take a long-term look (until 2022) at the funding needs of the country's health services, undertaken on behalf of the Chancellor of the Exchequer by Derek Wanless, until recently the Chief Executive of the Natwest Bank.[1] In passing, it is worth noting that the UK Treasury alone commissioned this study, though in keeping with tradition, consultations with devolved administrations did take place. Observing that the cost drivers in each part of the UK were similar, the report sought to quantify the impact on costs of quality improvements, rising expectations, ageing, technology, changing health needs, pay and prices, and productivity. It avoided the obvious difficulty of finding 'the' answer amid the uncertainty of a 20-year forward projection by developing three alternative scenarios.

The first, described as *Solid Progress* envisaged a health service world where life expectancy improves, and the population is more engaged in their own health; the NHS becomes a more responsive service, with high levels of technology, and more efficient use of resources. The second scenario, *Slow Uptake,* is a more pessimistic view in which health status improves slowly at best, and the health service is relatively unresponsive, making limited use of new technology and with only small gains in productivity. Most optimistic is the third scenario, *Fully Engaged,* where public involvement in health drives substantial gains in life expectancy, and population health status improves significantly. A health service making extensive use of new technology is much more responsive and the efficiency of resource use improves substantially. Of course, the one thing we know with some certainty is that the future will be somewhat different from the scenarios developed by Wanless, but at least they offer a helpful conceptual framework for thinking about these matters.

The least expensive scenario is the third, with an estimated price tag for the UK of £154 billion, and most expensive is the second, with an estimated cost of £184 billion. Meeting these bills requires an average annual real terms increase in NHS resources of between 4.2% and 5.1% over the 20 year period, and because of the need to catch up caused by past 'underfunding,' the earlier years require higher growth levels (between 7.1% and 7.3%). In his budget in April 2002 the Chancellor bit this financial bullet and announced unprecedented increases in health care spending.[4] In so doing he appeared to tip the previous Treasury orthodoxy on its head, health care becoming an investment in improved health with its attendant economic and social benefits, rather than a public cost to be controlled. While many of the determinants of health undoubtedly lie outside health care systems, there is growing evidence that the contribution of health care to population health (both its quantity and quality) is greater than often acknowledged.[5]

The third key message from the Nuffield Trust Report is the need to prepare the people who work in the health services for the changes ahead. It is a sobering thought that the clinical leaders of health services in 2022 are currently students in our universities or young, newly qualified professionals embarking on their careers. What kind of health care world are we preparing them for? How will we update their skills and maintain their enthusiasm in a world of accelerating change? These are among the most complex problems of all. Already, the expanding health care system made possible by new financial resources is struggling to find sufficient people of the required calibre to fill the posts that are being created, the problem being the lag effect of workforce plans based on the assumptions of a previous age.

Demographic Change

In Scotland these workforce problems exist in the context of an ageing population now declining in absolute terms (Table 12.1). The Registrar General for Scotland reported that the number of births and deaths in 2001 were both the lowest ever-recorded in Scotland, with the number of deaths now exceeding the number of births by about 5000.[6]

TABLE 12.1 Key Demographic Data For Scotland

Population

1. Scotland's population reached a peak in 1974 and since then has been on a gradually declining trend, although with some fluctuations.

2. The gradual fall in population is projected to continue.

3. Scotland is the only country within the UK with recent and projected declines in population, and there are relatively few countries in the world which are currently declining in population.

4. Scotland has recorded a natural decrease (an excess of deaths over births), since 1997, while net migration loss has reduced.

5. The natural decrease is projected to continue to grow and is the main factor in the projected population decline.

6. Scotland's population is ageing (and is projected to continue ageing) with higher proportions in the older age groups and smaller proportions in the younger age groups.

7. The numbers of children have reached a new low and, despite the losses through death and migration for people born in earlier years, the population aged under 1 year is now lower than for any other single age up to 60 years.

8. The distribution of population within Scotland is changing. In general, the larger urban areas (except Edinburgh) are declining, and many areas around the bigger cities and some rural areas are increasing in population.

Births

9. Birth rates in Scotland are lower than in any other country in the UK, and this trend is projected to continue, but the rates are similar to the average for European countries, some of which (Spain, Italy, Germany, Austria and Greece) have lower birth rates than Scotland.

10. Falling birth rates reflect the fact that women are having fewer children and having them later and as a consequence average completed family size fell below two for women born after 1953.

11. The proportion of births to unmarried parents is continuing to increase, but most births are jointly registered by parents living at the same address.

Deaths

12. Death rates have fallen significantly in Scotland since 1981, but less rapidly than most other countries of the UK.

13. Stillbirths, perinatal and infant mortality rates continue to fall and are at historically low levels, but remain above the EU average.

14. Mortality rates are falling for both men and women, but male life expectancy at birth has remained 4–6 years less than that for women over the last 50 years.

15. The main causes of death in Scotland are cancers and heart disease; over the last decade there has been a big fall in the latter but not in the former.

Migration

16. Net emigration from Scotland is much lower than 40 years ago and even 15 years ago.

17. Recent 2001 Census results suggest that net emigration is more likely to be weighted towards males and the younger age groups than previously thought.

18. The pattern of net migration between Scotland and the rest of the UK varies markedly by age group for both males and females, with a net inflow peaking at age 19 years and a net outflow peaking at age 23 years.

19. Moves between Health Board areas within Scotland are highest for males and females in their 20s and 30s, with large peaks at student ages (18–22 years).

SOURCE: General Register Office for Scotland.[6]

Looking ahead the population projections for the country as a whole indicate that by 2020 the annual natural decrease 'will be 10 000 a year; the proportion of children under 16 years of age is projected to fall by 20 % by 2021, while the proportion of people aged 60 years and over is projected to increase by over 25 %.' Changes in the ratio of dependent to non-dependent Scots is masked by the increase to 65 years of the retirement age for women, but the dependency ratio increases rapidly after 2021. Scotland is the only country in the UK exhibiting some of these trends. They are unusual by comparison with other developed countries, indeed no other country in Europe apart from Germany has a declining population, and they will not be reversed nor changed quickly. Future planning for our health services as well its workforce must reflect these circumstances.

If there is a degree of predictability about the changes in the population of Scotland, the same cannot be said of its political governance. A former Secretary of State for Wales, Ron Davies, famously described political devolution as 'a process not an event'. It is impossible to say where we are in this process other than being close to its start. So much depends on who has political control of the UK Government and the devolved administrations and their respective policies on further constitutional change. The 'devolution' process also sits in the context of some broader changes in our political institutions. The expansion of the European Union, and the harmonisation of many policy areas are unlikely to leave health care untouched. Although the current EU treaties give its institutions competence in public health matters rather than health care, it is already obvious that competence in adjacent subjects – for example, employment, and the free movement of goods and services – is having a profound impact on Scottish health care policy.[7,8] The example of the Working Time Directive is perhaps the best example, as its strictures on doctors working hours is leading to both a fundamental reconsideration of how to staff Scottish hospitals, and questions about the organisation of hospital services throughout the country.[9]

How, then, might Scotland's health service prepare for the future? What are the steps it might take to increase its chances of navigating a course through the uncertain world ahead? In the paragraphs that follow we offer some suggestions in the hope that they may stimulate some debate among Scotland's health service community.

Improving health and reducing health inequalities

Firstly, we must continue to focus on improving Scotland's health status and attack the poverty, deprivation and inequality that blight the health of the Scottish population. A recent analysis of Scotland's health status compared with other European countries reminds us that Scotland was not always 'bottom of the health league table'; and that it is not bottom for every cause of death or age group. This demonstrates that there is nothing inevitable about Scotland's poor health status and that it is amenable to change through 'the organised efforts of society'. This analysis also showed that the most evident problems are seen in working aged adults where premature mortality is consistently the worst in Europe.[10] Achieving improvements will, however, require determined and sustained action. Action throughout the lifespan will be necessary for lasting change but improved prevention and treatment of the main causes of death in working aged adults must be an early priority.

We will not rehearse all the evidence and the statistics presented in chapter 2 which indicates the profound scale and complexity of the challenge posed by the relatively poor health status of Scotland's population, and the contribution which poverty and disadvantage make to that record. There is though one startling fact which highlights the intensity of the problem of ill health in Scotland – over half of the one million people who live in the 15 UK parliamentary constituencies with the highest rates of premature mortality (deaths under 65 years) are in nine Scottish constituencies and, in particular, in Glasgow.[11, 12] These Scottish constituencies are home to about 10% of Scotland's total population.

A recent authoritative analysis concluded that the 'research evidence clearly indicates that the major causes of health inequalities in Scotland are related to socioeconomic factors, such as income, education, and employment, and the subsequent impact that these factors will have on the material environment that a person experiences, such as their working environment, housing, transport, and nutrition.'[11] These are the factors that determine the life circumstances of individuals and the context for their health-related behaviours some of which – for example, smoking – have a serious long-term impact on morbidity and mortality. Since 1997 there has been a new determination in government health policy to address these issues, but it is evident that long-term, sustained action by different levels of government (local, Scottish, UK, and European) will be required if life circumstances are to be improved. The most recent paper from the Scottish Executive – *Improving Health in Scotland: the Challenge*[13] – published in March 2003 is an important statement of intent. The actions of the European political institutions in relation to agriculture and food (including tobacco), and employment, for instance, are important influences. In the post-devolution world of UK inter-government relations co-ordination may prove difficult if administrations are under different political control. The division of responsibilities between Westminster and Holyrood means that there are limits to the powers of any Scottish administration to challenge poverty and disadvantage since tax and social security policy remain in the competence of the UK Government. In the future these administrations may not share, as they do at present, a common policy perspective on social and health inequalities, with obvious implications for co-ordinated action. Similarly, closing the 'health divide' is not just a job for health ministers and the health service; co-ordinated action embracing the whole of government responsibilities is needed. Nor is it a job for government alone; individuals, communities, employers, voluntary organisations all have a part to play. Designing *effective* intervention policies to meet the challenge of health inequalities is perhaps the hardest problem of all though there is a growing body of evidence on successful interventions conveniently summarised in a recent publication from the Inter-Departmental Group on Health Inequalities, of the UK Government, led (significantly) by HM Treasury (see table 12.2).[14] Health and behavioural interventions can, in addition, be used to lessen the health impact of the uneven distribution of life circumstances in Scotland. Broad social justice measures go hand in hand with focused actions for prevention and treatment targeted at those who most in need.

In common with other parts of the UK the challenge in Scotland is to develop initiatives with the characteristics described in table 12.2, and because there remains so much uncertainty about the effectiveness of policy in this arena to explicitly embrace experimentation and evaluation of new approaches,[15] such as those currently underway concerned with early childhood (*Starting Well*); sexual health among young people (*Healthy Respect*); and the prevention of heart disease (*The Heart of Scotland*) – see chapter 3. Concern with health inequalities has not always been at the centre of the political agenda and so perhaps the biggest challenge of all is to sustain the current political commitment to reducing the adverse impact on health of poverty and disadvantage in Scotland.

TABLE 12.2 Key Findings on Successful Interventions to Tackle Health Inequalities

- Scotland's population reached a peak in 1974 and since then has been on a gradually declining trend, although with some fluctuations.

- Local assessment of needs, especially involving local people in the research process itself.

- Mechanisms that enable organisations to work together – ensuring dialogue, contact and commitment.

- Representation of local people within planning and management arrangements – the greater the level of involvement, the larger the impact.

- Design of specific initiatives with target groups to ensure that they are acceptable – that is, culturally and educationally appropriate – and that they work through settings that are accessible and appropriate.

- Training and support for volunteers, peer educators and local networks, thus ensuring maximum benefit from community-based initiatives

- Visibility of political support and commitment.

- Re-orientation of resource allocation to enable systematic investment in community based programmes

- Policy development and implementation that brings about wider changes in organisational priorities and policies, driven by community-based approaches.

- Increased flexibility of organisations, so supporting increased delegation and a more responsive approach.

SOURCE: *Tackling Health Inequalities*[14]

Crown copyright material is reproduced with the permission of the Controller of HMSO and the Queen's Printer for Scotland.

While we emphasise the importance of tackling poverty and health inequalities the analysis by Leon and colleagues [10] also reminds us that relatively poor health status of Scotland's population is not fully explained by the intensity of deprivation in the country. The implication of this important evidence is that attention to health improvement policies for the whole of the Scottish population as well as the disadvantaged is required. In practice this means focusing on identifying disease-specific risk factors at the individual level and helping people to modify them. The prime candidates in Scotland are smoking, alcohol, exercise and diet. There is ambivalence about alcohol in Scotland that needs to be acknowledged. It is a source of significant revenue, employment and pleasure, and an integral part of the way of life in many parts of the country. But it is also associated with increasing rates of liver cirrhosis, a trend in sharp contrast to other European countries.

Long-term planning

Secondly, we believe it would be desirable to establish a long-term scenario planning capacity – supported by but independent of government – which through its activities can be used to structure public and political discussion about priorities for investment and disinvestments in health care. The character of the issues discussed in this book does not lend itself to simple solutions, and, as the Wanless Review has illustrated, there is great uncertainty about the future. Is that review to be left on library shelves, referred to as a landmark study which informed the decisions of a UK Government at a particular point in its political life, or is it to be used as a starting point, a benchmark analysis, on which subsequent, and specifically Scottish analyses might be built? The scale and intensity of social deprivation in Scotland (notably Glasgow), the remote and rural character of much of the country, and its (uniquely) declining population, with the attendant social and economic implications, are three factors that suggest there is value in building on the Wanless analysis. There is another, and it is the need to build a better public understanding of the choices which must be made in health care. For understandable reasons politicians wish to be seen responding to every opportunity and every problem which the complexity that is health care creates. There is an inevitable clamour for additional resources but where are these resources to come from and at what opportunity cost? Scotland's health related public spending is already close to the European average as a share of its GDP, a target the Blair Government has adopted for the UK as a whole. Are the current plans to spend an increasing share of the national production on health as opposed to something else sustainable? Within the health services there are difficult choices to be made about the relative priority of competing needs whatever the level of spending, yet in recent years there has been a tendency for the Scottish Executive to announce new 'priorities' which now embrace mental health, cancer, heart disease and stroke, the elderly, children, the socially excluded, the learning disabled and so on. Each of these has important and legitimate claims on the health care cake, but there is a risk that if they are all priorities, none of them are. As we noted in chapter 1, The Scottish Office in the 1970s, through the work of its Health Service Planning Council, undertook a range of long-term analyses that attempted to construct an evidence-based context for political decision-making. A modern parallel in some respects has been the work undertaken on the geographical allocation of health care resources within Scotland under the Chairmanship of Professor Sir John Arbuthnott.[16] Perhaps the first task of a modern Scottish Health Services Planning Council could be to complement the work of the Arbuthnott Committee and take a long-term look at the relative needs for health care expenditure of different population or disease groups in Scotland. Significantly, the Planning Council of the 1970s, though a creation of government, had terms of reference that enabled it to undertake 'analyses at its own hand' so perhaps what is needed is a *health care* equivalent or arm of NHS Health Scotland, a well resourced body of recognised expertise, able through its own analyses to shape the policy agenda.

Structural change in the NHS

Thirdly, we suggest that further structural change in the health services should be minimised. Wholesale structural change is a characteristic of UK health care in the past three decades and is usually justified as an enabling measure to secure efficiency or quality improvements. A paper commissioned by the Scottish Executive in the context of its Review of Management and Decision Making (see chapter 1), concluded that there is, at best, only partial and incomplete evidence that structural change ever achieves the objectives claimed for it, and observed that, 'there are few 'right' answers to the problems of structuring health care systems, but there are many theories, ideas, prejudices, ideologies and experiences on which to draw. The search for new solutions to the recurring dilemmas of matching needs and resources has seen a growing sophistication in the systems used to control health care services [but] since there are no 'right' answers, a practical approach would be to experiment, to evaluate and to learn.'[17]

We suggest two areas that are ripe for experimentation, some of which is already happening. Both will depend on our ability to exploit the new opportunities of the information age – 'e-health'. Compared with many other service industries the NHS has invested less in its information systems, but in an age when electronic medical records and telemedicine are being developed we must think increasingly about virtual health care systems in which the delivery of clinical services are freed from traditional organisational boundaries. Experience suggests that technological challenges, great though they are, can be overcome; more subtle and complex are the behavioural changes required to exploit the new communications systems. That is why it is necessary now to blur the boundaries between hospital and primary care by developing service models that challenge their current institutionalised separation. The historical origins of this divide continue to cast a long shadow over the current health care system, and the difficulties encountered at the boundary are among the most intransigent of all – represented by breakdowns in communication, waiting lists, emergency admission pressures, and delayed discharges. The distinction between 'generalists' and 'specialists' is increasingly unhelpful; most medical graduates now undertake extensive postgraduate, 'specialist' training, before they take up their long-term careers. For many their clinical practice will involve the delivery of care in non-hospital settings for some or most of the time, and a few will need the specialist support facilities that only a hospital can provide. This 'community' of medical specialists should be organised to support the maxim that care should be delivered in or close to home if possible, and in hospital only if needs be.

A second and related candidate deserving encouragement is the development of care networks. Although Scotland is, in population terms, a small country, there are numerous distinctive communities with strong and understandable loyalties to local health services. At its best this is a very positive influence on health services, but at its worst it can foster community rivalries and parochialism (public and professional) that may not serve anyone's best interests. Managed Clinical Networks have emerged as a preferred model that attempts to square this particularly awkward circle and it is encouraging to see the progression of this idea. Evaluative studies currently underway may tell us more about the effectiveness of this model in the longer term. But we should not lose sight of the fact that there are a small number of services where it will make sense for Scotland to consolidate its clinical expertise into fewer centres that make best use of highly sophisticated technologies. Indeed, given the pressures on the health service workforce and NHS employers it may be inevitable, as part of both a fundamental reconsideration of how to staff Scottish hospitals and questions about the organisation of hospital services throughout the country.[9]

The Health Service workforce

Availability of trained healthcare staff will undoubtedly be the critical determinant of success for the NHS in Scotland and addressing this issue is our fourth concern. Despite devolution, Scotland cannot be considered in isolation and when it comes to recruitment we have to fish in the same pool as the rest of the UK. Taking doctors as an example, there are worrying signs about the ability of medical schools to meet increasing demand, this despite the fact that five new medical schools will open in England by 2005. Because each applicant for medicine applies to four schools it is easy to be lulled into a false sense of security about the supply of potential students; in reality the number of applicants for each place at medical school has fallen from 2.11 in 1995 to 1.55 in 2000. [18] Scotland has traditionally been a net exporter and seems destined to remain so even after 2005 (see chapter 11). In 2000, Scotland had a ratio of doctors per 1000 population (2.4) that was significantly higher than that of England (1.9). It is against this backdrop that the perceived need for workforce expansion must be viewed. *Our National Health* [19] set out the expectation that the total number of consultants in Scotland would rise by more than 600 over the following five years, with 'further increases' in the numbers of junior doctors. In England, however, *The NHS Plan* [20] talked of 7500 more consultants, 2000 extra GPs and 20 000 more nurses by 2004. It is already clear that these expectations cannot be fulfilled and that attempts to make up all of the shortfall (in doctors at least) by overseas recruitment are unlikely to succeed.

Other important variables in the workforce equation include job satisfaction, workforce retention, premature retirement, flexibility of working practices and contractual negotiations. Details of a proposed new contract between the NHS and GPs have been announced. The new contract is intended to offer a substantial increase in funding for primary care based on improvement in service quality. The contract applies throughout the UK, and if accepted, spending on general practice will increase from £6.1bn to £8bn this year.

While debate on the acceptance of the new GP contract continues, the die now appears to be cast as far as the consultant contract is concerned. Details of this contract were announced in 2002. In England and Wales, 70% of consultants and specialist registrars voted against accepting the contract, whereas in

Scotland the vote was 54% for and 46% against. Taking the vote of consultants alone the corresponding figures were 66% against in England and Wales, and 59% for in Scotland. The fact that the Scottish Executive is currently in discussion with Scottish consultants about implementing the new contract in Scotland signals a historic first break in the UK negotiation of terms and conditions of service since the NHS came into being in 1948. It remains to be seen whether agreement will result in divergence between Scotland and the rest of the UK and whether this will translate into significant influences on workforce recruitment and retention.

Scientific and Technological Advance

These future generations of health care providers will enter practice at a time when the successful Human Genome Project presents a major step forward in our ability to identify and then use knowledge about genetic risk factors in pre-symptomatic diagnosis, disease surveillance, optimisation of treatment, healthcare planning and drug discovery. NHS Scotland must prepare now to embrace the potential and understand the clinical, social, moral and ethical implications of the new genetics. As most major disorders have a significant genetic (hereditable) component, these recent and continuing advances have profound implications for population health and health service provision. Sequencing the human genome has been accompanied by the discovery of a multitude of single nucleotide DNA polymorphisms (that is, variations in DNA sequence). This has greatly enhanced the prospects for identifying complex disease genes, knowledge of which will allow individuals 'at risk' of those diseases to be identified. It also improves the prospects for preventive medicine and the tailoring of treatment to make it safer and more effective by taking account of specific genetic profiles and disease subtypes (pharmacogenetics). It is anticipated that single nucleotide polymorphism determinations will become part of the routine management of some common diseases within the next decade. [21] Realising the potential of these genetic advances will be far from straightforward. Genetic factors may be subtle, multifactorial and of low penetrance, and prove difficult to disentangle from environmental influences. Large databases and extensive collaboration will be needed, as exemplified by the Medical Research Council and Wellcome Trust initiative to establish a database of half a million individuals in the UK. Public confidence must be safeguarded, ethical issues given due consideration, and robust regulatory frameworks need to be in place (and are being put in place) to ensure that patient and public interests are appropriately balanced. Many of these issues will be addressed in a UK rather than purely Scottish context and a great deal of excellent work has already been undertaken.[22]

While there is a widely held perception that the UK is well positioned within Europe to retain a leading position in genome research,[23] there are also great concerns about the ability of the NHS to 'rise to the genomic challenge'. At present the NHS is focused almost exclusively and reactively on existing disease and it will need to change significantly if there is to be increasing emphasis on disease prevention.[24] Improved undergraduate and postgraduate education and training in genetics will be needed if advances in research and development are to be translated into better health and healthcare. All physicians and their teams, and not just clinical geneticists will be involved in this revolution in healthcare. Primary care professionals in particular will need to become genetically literate with development of skills in genetic risk assessment and communication, pharmacogenetics will become increasingly relevant in prescribing decisions.[25]

What of Scotland's position within the UK in respect of genome research and its translation into clinical and population benefit? 'Generation Scotland'[*] is a strategy that could capitalise on Scotland's biomedical expertise, stable population of 5.1 million, comprehensive medical records and linked disease registries and databases. The proposal would involve families where there is known to be forms of inherited disease and compare their DNA samples with those of healthy matched controls. It would shed important light on the cause of common diseases, such as cancer, coronary heart disease, mental illness, improve diagnosis, allow targeted intervention and treatment, and facilitate the development of new drugs and treatments. It would produce benefit for patients, their 'at-risk relatives' and future generations of Scots, as well as strengthening the Scottish science base and wealth creation.

The initiative will require a strong partnership between the public, the academic community, the NHS, Government and funding agencies, and commercial organisations. A multidisciplinary meeting hosted by the Royal Society of

---

[*] Developed by Professor David Porteous – Professor of Human Molecular Genetics and Medicine, University of Edinburgh

Edinburgh in 2002 gave broad endorsement to the concept while recognising several significant challenges, not least the need for effective public consultation, detailed consideration of ethical and security arrangements, and timely discussion with the Scottish Executive and potential funding partners. If the UK has a strong position within Europe in respect of genome research and its implications, arguably Scotland has a particularly strong position within the UK.

Research and Development

The challenges of the new genetics remind us how important it is to invest in health R&D so that Scotland's health system has the benefit of the best clinical and scientific brains working with it. Our final suggestion to prepare for the future is to ensure Scotland is competitive in the global market for these people, and as in the past, put Scotland at the forefront of clinical progress. Scotland has a strong tradition and an established reputation for excellence in medical training, clinical medicine and biomedical research. Its Universities with Medical Schools (St Andrews, Aberdeen, Glasgow, Edinburgh, Dundee) and Dental Faculties (Glasgow, Dundee) have been joined relatively recently by newer Universities with significant profiles in the training of nurses/allied health professionals.

Biomedical research in Scotland has continued to compete successfully for many years within a UK context, gaining funding from major national Research Councils, Government Agencies and Charities such as Cancer Research UK and the British Heart Foundation, that has been at least proportionate to the size of its population. It is imperative that Scotland continues to compete at both a national and international level if its biomedical research base is to remain strong and able to command top gradings in UK Research Assessment Exercises such as that carried out in 2001. The availability of Scottish response mode funding such as that provided by the Chief Scientist Office and the former Clinical Resource and Audit Group (now part of NHS Quality Improvement Scotland) offers useful additional flexibility but must never be allowed to overshadow the importance of competing within a UK context.

The fact that Scotland possesses four major clinical medical schools and one pre-clinical school offers exciting possibilities for further collaboration in biomedical research and the translation of discovery in basic science into the clinical arena. The company Cyclacel in Dundee, for example, is a direct extension of the excellence of oncological research in that centre. A £50M Research Institute for Medical Cell Biology will soon be built alongside the new Edinburgh Royal Infirmary and Medical School and may well form the nidus from which a major Biomedical Research Park can develop. A rebuilt Beatson Institute for Cancer Research will complement further the clinical strengths of the Glasgow Medical School and related NHS Oncology Services. Collaboration, always a feature of biomedical research in Scotland, seems destined to increase, while the combination of new fit-for-purpose buildings and co-location of related interests offers exciting prospects for translational research and real clinical benefit for Scottish patients.

As we said at the start of this chapter, predicting the future is hazardous. In the mid 1980s no one anticipated the introduction of the internal market in the NHS, HIV was perceived as a terrible threat to the whole community, no one had been identified as suffering from a new variant of CJD, and the personal computer was a novelty. Though people campaigned for a Scottish Parliament, it probably seemed a distant prospect. Events will also play their part, those unexpected turns that shape subsequent actions. As the chapters of this book have shown, there has been an extraordinary amount of change in the past 15 years. In view of this, perhaps the most important quality that Scotland's health care community may need in the years ahead is the capacity to embrace and welcome change even though its prospect may cause discomfort, not least because as CS Lewis[26] observed: 'the future is something which everyone reaches at the rate of 60 minutes an hour, whatever he does, whoever he is.'

REFERENCES

1.   Wanless D. *Securing our future health: taking a long term care view*: Final Report. London: HM Treasury, 2002.

2.   Nuffield Trust *Policy Futures for UK Health: 2000 Report*. London: Nuffield Trust, 2000.

3.   Stewart S (ed). *The possible Scot:making healthy public policy*. Edinburgh: The Scottish Council Foundation, 1998.

4.   HM Treasury. *Budget 2002*. House of Commons papers 2001–02, 592, 17 April. London: The Stationery Office, 2002.

5.   Bunker J. The role of medical care in contributing to health improvements within societies. *International Journal of Epidemiology* 2001, 30: 1260–1263.

6.   Registrar General for Scotland. *Scotland's Population 2001*. Annual Review of Demographic Trends. Edinburgh: The Stationery Office, 2002.

7.   McKee M, Mossialos E, Baeton R(eds). *The Impact of EU Law on Health Care Systems*.Brussels:PIE-Peter Lang, 2002.

8.   McKee M, Mossialos E. *EU Law and the Social Character of Health Care*. Brussels: PIE –Peter Lang, 2002.

9.   Scottish Executive. 2002. *Working for Health: The workforce development Action Plan* for *NHS Scotland*. www.scotland.gov.uk/library5/health/wfh-00.asp .

10.   Leon D, Morton S, Cannegeister S, McKee M. *Understanding the Health of Scotland's Population in an International Context*. London and Glasgow: London School of Hygiene and the Public Health Institute for Scotland, November 2002.

11.   *Health Inequalities in the New Scotland*. Glasgow: Health Promotion Policy Unit and the Public Health Institute for Scotland, April 2002.

12.   Shaw M, Dorling D, Gordon D, Davey Smith G. *The Widening Gap. Health Inequalities and Policy in Britain*. Bristol: The Policy Press,1999.

13.   Scottish Executive. *Improving Health in Scotland: the Challenge*. Edinburgh: The Stationery Office, 2003.

14.   *Tackling Health Inequalities: 2002 Cross-Cutting Review*. London:Department of Health, 2002.

15.   Macintyre S.Evidence-based policy making. *British Medical Journal* 2003,326:5–6.

16.   Scottish Executive. *Fair Shares for All*. (The Arbuthnott Report) Edinburgh: The Stationery Office, 2000.

17.   Woods KJ. *A Critical Appraisal of Accountability Systems in Integrated Health Care Systems*. Edinburgh:The Scottish Executive, September 2002. http://www.show.scot.nhs.uk/sehd/publications/DC20021001CritApprAccount.pdf

18.   Medical school applications – a critical situation. *British Medical Journal* 2002, 235:786–7.

19.   Scottish Executive Health Department. Our National Health – a plan for action, a plan for change. Edinburgh:The Stationery Office, 2000.

20.   Department of Health. *The NHS Plan. A Plan for Investment. A Plan for Reform*. London, The Stationery Office, 2000.

21.   Mathew C. Postgenomic technologies: hunting the genes for common disorders. *British Medical Journal* 2001,322:1031–1034.

22.   Zimmern R, Cook C. *Genetics and Health. Policy issues for genetic science and their implications for health and health services*. The Nuffield Genetics Scenario Project. London: The Nuffield Trust and the Public Health Genetics Trust, 2000.

23.   Richards T. The genomic challenge. *British Medical Journal* 1999,318:341–342.

24.   Fears R, Roberts D, Poste G. Rational or rationed medicine? The promise of genetics for improved clinical practice. *British Medical Journal* 2000,320:933–935.

25.   Emery J, Hayflick S. The challenge of integrating genetic medicine into primary care. *British Medical Journal* 2001,322:1027–30.

26.   Lewis CS. Of God. In *The Screwtape Letters*. Quoted in *A Dictionary of Modern Quotations*. Harmondsworth: The Penguin Press, 1971.

Secretary of State for Scotland

2003–	Mr Alistair Darling MP
2001–2003	Mrs Helen Liddell MP
1999–2001	Dr John Reid MP
1997–1999	Mr Donald Dewar MP
1995–1997	Mr Michael Forsyth MP
1990–1995	Mr Ian Lang MP
1986–1990	Mr Malcolm Rifkind MP
1979–1986	Mr George Younger MP

First Minister

2001–	Mr Jack McConnell MSP
2000–2001	Mr Henry McLeish MSP
1999-2000	Mr Donald Dewar MSP

Minister for Health in Scotland (post devolution)*

2001–	Mr Malcolm Chisholm MSP
1999–2001	Ms Susan Deacon MSP

Minister for Health in Scotland (pre devolution)

1997–1999	Mr Sam Galbraith MP
1995–1997	Lord James Douglas-Hamilton MP
1992–1995	Lord Fraser of Carmyllie
1987–1992	Mr Michael Forsyth MP
1986–1987	Lord Glenarthur
1982-1985	Mr John Mackay MP

---

* In May 1999 The Scottish Parliament came into being. There remained a Secretary of State for Scotland based in London but health was one of the responsibilities devolved to the Scottish Parliament under the ultimate authority of the First Minister.

Permanent Secretary

2003–	Mr John Elvidge
1998–2003	Sir Muir Russell
1988–1998	Sir Russell Hillhouse
1978–1988	Sir William Kerr Fraser

NHS Scotland Chief Executive

2000–	Mr Trevor Jones
1993–2000	Mr Geoff Scaife
1989–1993	Mr Don Cruickshank

Head of Scottish Home and Health Department

1992–1996	Mr Hamish Hamill
1990–1992	Sir Graham Hart
1984–1990	Sir William Reid

Chief Medical Officer (CMO)

2001–	Dr Mac Armstrong
1996–2000	Sir David Carter
1991–1996	Dr RE Kendell
1989–1991	Dr Kenneth Calman
1985–1988	Dr Ian S Macdonald

Chief Nursing Officer (CNO)

1992–	Miss Anne Jarvie
1998–1992	Mrs Yvonne Moores
1977–1988	Miss Margaret Gibson Auld

INDEX